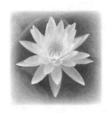

Servant Leadership in Nursing

SPIRITUALITY AND PRACTICE
IN CONTEMPORARY HEALTH CARE

D1411721

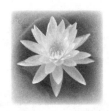

Servant Leadership
in Nursing

SPIRITUALITY AND PRACTICE
IN CONTEMPORARY HEALTH CARE

MARY ELIZABETH O'BRIEN
SFCC, PhD, MTS, RN, FAAN

Professor
School of Nursing
The Catholic University of America
Washington, DC

JONES AND BARTLETT PUBLISHERS
Sudbury, Massachusetts
BOSTON   TORONTO   LONDON   SINGAPORE

World Headquarters

Jones and Bartlett Publishers
40 Tall Pine Drive
Sudbury, MA 01776
978-443-5000
info@jbpub.com
www.jbpub.com

Jones and Bartlett Publishers
Canada
6339 Ormindale Way
Mississauga, Ontario L5V 1J2
Canada

Jones and Bartlett Publishers
International
Barb House, Barb Mews
London W6 7PA
United Kingdom

Jones and Bartlett's books and products are available through most bookstores and online booksellers. To contact Jones and Bartlett Publishers directly, call 800-832-0034, fax 978-443-8000, or visit our website, www.jbpub.com.

Production Credits
Publisher: Kevin Sullivan
Acquisitions Editor: Amy Sibley
Associate Editor: Patricia Donnelly
Editorial Assistant: Rachel Shuster
Senior Production Editor: Carolyn F. Rogers
Marketing Manager: Rebecca Wasley
V.P., Manufacturing and Inventory Control: Therese Connell
Composition: Graphic World
Cover Design: Scott Moden
Cover Image: © Atiketta Sangasaeng/ShutterStock, Inc.
Printing and Binding: Malloy, Inc.
Cover Printing: Malloy, Inc.

Library of Congress Cataloging-in-Publication Data
O'Brien, Mary Elizabeth.
  Servant leadership in nursing : spirituality and practice in contemporary health care / Mary Elizabeth O'Brien.
    p. ; cm.
  Includes bibliographical references and index.
  ISBN 978-0-7637-7485-1 (pbk.)
  1. Nursing services—Administration. 2. Nursing ethics—Religious aspects—Christianity. I. Title.
  [DNLM: 1. Nursing Care—organization & administration. 2. Christianity. 3. Leadership. 4. Religion and Medicine.
  5. Spirituality. WY 105 O13s 2010]
  RT89.O27 2010
  362.17'3068—dc22
                                      2009032445
6048

Printed in the United States of America
14 13 12 11 10   10 9 8 7 6 5 4 3 2 1

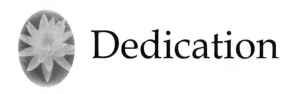 # Dedication

For all nurses who lovingly embrace the philosophy and practice of servant leadership in their ministry to the ill and infirm.

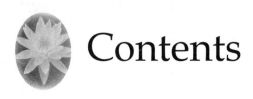

Contents

The greatest among you must become like the youngest and the leader like the one who serves.

           — *Luke 22:26–27*

Whoever wishes to become great among you must be your servant...for the Son of Man came not to be served but to serve.

           — *Mark 10:43, 45*

Here is my servant whom I uphold, my chosen in whom my soul delights.

           — *Isaiah 42:1*

Chapter 8 The Spirituality of Servant Leadership in Nursing 327

You are my servant whom I have chosen.

— Isaiah 43:10

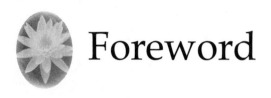

Foreword

This book is a treasure in so many ways. All nurses should send a resounding note of gratitude to Sister Mary Elizabeth.

She has collected in one volume an incredible amount of research on centuries-old nursing heroes and matched that with compelling research on contemporary nursing heroes. Her book manages to be both scholarly and inspiring at the same time.

I was struck by a quote from a 1914 article in the *American Journal of Nursing* by Dr. Charles Emerson, describing nursing as "a profession that does not yet know how great are the responsibilities that are to rest on its shoulders." In so many ways, I think that is still so true today. Nurses, in spite of more education and experience, still only partially glimpse the magnitude of their role, as Florence Nightingale so beautifully said, to "often hold God's precious gift of life in their hands." It may be that to realize this too clearly would overwhelm us.

As challenging as nursing can be in today's world, it is wonderful to have the resources in this book to inspire and encourage us as we read about the wonderful nurses who blazed the trail before us; however, it is even more inspiring and encouraging to couple this with actual quotes from today's nursing heroes. Most of us who have been in health care can think of other nurses in the various positions and specialties highlighted who also see their care of patients in exactly the same way.

The love of people that motivated the emergence of nursing is still so evident today. It is no wonder that in interview after interview nursing is the most trusted voice. Only this love keeps nurses practicing with the challenges that are so stressful today. We count on this love to continue to inspire nurses and to keep our healthcare system, in the face of increased technology, focused on the human being to be cared for.

This is a wonderful book to give to a nurse. It is also an excellent book for executives and board members. Reading it will help them appreciate the wonderful and saintly things being done each day and night in their facilities. It will help them make boardroom decisions that protect this great treasure for their communities.

We are indebted to the author for bringing together such an inspiring collection and relating it to contemporary nursing and leadership theory. It confirms the timeliness of this magnificent profession.

Sr. Carol Keehan, DC

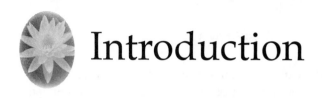 # Introduction

In 1977, Robert Greenleaf introduced a conceptualization of leadership that he labeled "servant leadership" with the publication of his seminal work *Servant Leadership: A Journey into the Nature of Legitimate Power and Greatness.* Greenleaf's philosophy purported that a true leader, in any venue, must be a servant of those he or she leads. Since that time the concept has been embraced by many business and educational communities for whom the practice of servant leadership has been found to be a highly successful leadership style. This is reflected in the plethora of books and articles on servant leadership published during the past three decades.

It is, however, only more recently that the practice of servant leadership has captured the attention of healthcare institutions and, more specifically, of nurses practicing in those facilities. Recent nursing servant leadership articles do, however, strongly support the adoption of servant leadership as the most appropriate leadership philosophy and practice for nursing and health care.

Ever since becoming acquainted with the philosophy of servant leadership, I have wanted to explore the concept as a potential leadership style for contemporary practicing nurses. In fact, my own clinical nursing practice, as well as my nursing education and nursing research experiences over the past 35 years, have suggested that the majority of nursing leaders are already practicing servant leadership although not using the label. To validate or contradict my perception I decided to conduct a phenomenological study of the philosophy and behavior of currently practicing nursing leaders entitled Called to Serve: The Lived Experience of a Nursing Vocation.

A unique characteristic of this book is the inclusion of the Called to Serve study data, which contain many powerful and poignant nursing servant leadership perceptions and anecdotes elicited in tape-recorded interviews with 75 nursing leaders. These data provided the foundation for an empirically based model of servant leadership for nursing that can be used to teach and guide the practice of servant leadership among nurses. The sample population of 75 nursing leaders interviewed for the study consisted of 4 administrators, 13 managers/supervisors, 10 head nurses, 18 charge nurses, 10 team leaders, 9 advanced practice nurses (clinical nurse specialists, nurse–midwives, nurse practitioners, parish nurses, and nurse anesthetists), 9 nurse educators, and 2 nurse researchers (pseudonyms are used in all cases where nurse leaders are named).

Chapter 1 broadly explores nursing as a vocation of caring, in terms of both history and current nursing practice. Servant leadership in general and servant leadership in nursing are also discussed. In Chapter 2, the spiritual heritage of servant leadership in nursing is explored from an historical perspective identifying nursing servant leader role models from the early Christian era, the Middle Ages, and the post-Reformation period. Chapter 3 examines the biblical roots of the nurse's call to serve, and Chapter 4 introduces the design of the study Called to Serve, and presents five nursing vocation attitudinal themes identified in initial data analysis. In Chapter 5, the newly developed model of servant leadership for nursing is presented including 9 nursing servant leadership themes and 16 subthemes upon which the model is based. Chapter 6 presents data describing nursing servant leadership themes embraced specifically by nurse administrators, nurse managers, nurse clinicians, advanced practice nurses, nurse educators, nurse researchers, and parish nurses. Chapter 7 includes data reflecting nursing servant leadership in a variety of healthcare venues such as the hospital, clinic, long-term care facility, community, and parish. Finally, in Chapter 8 the spirituality of servant leadership in nursing is explored and described.

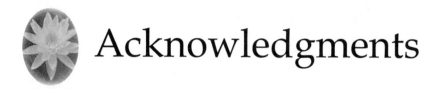# Acknowledgments

There are many people to be acknowledged in this work on servant leadership. First, deep gratitude is expressed to the nursing leaders who willingly participated in the research, and who shared poignant and inspiring perceptions and anecdotes reflecting the lived experience of servant leadership in their practice. I am also grateful to the many Catholic University School of Nursing students who assisted with the interviewing and to The Catholic University of America Office of the Vice Provost, which partially funded the servant leadership study with a University Grant-in-Aid.

I am especially indebted to Sister Carol Keehan, DC, President and Chief Executive Officer of the Catholic Health Association and consummate servant leader in nursing, who graciously gave of her time to review the manuscript and contribute a foreword for the book. And, as always, I am very thankful to the editorial and production staff of Jones and Bartlett Publishers: Kevin Sullivan, Amy Sibley, Rachel Shuster, and Carolyn Rogers, for caringly and carefully shepherding the manuscript to publication.

Finally, I must express my heartfelt gratitude for the true authorship of this work: to God the Father, who blesses me with the strength and energy to write; to his Divine Son, who provided the ultimate model of servant leadership for his followers; and to the Holy Spirit, without whose guidance and inspiration the thoughts in this book would never have come to light.

The Prayer of a Nurse Servant Leader

Gentle God,

Teach me to listen with my heart to
those who are anxious
and afraid.

Teach me to give generously of myself
to those seeking acceptance
and understanding.

Teach me to minister with mercy and
compassion to those who are
wounded in body or in
spirit.

Teach me to caringly assess the needs
of those who are suffering
and sorrowful.

Teach me to courageously advocate
for those who are marginalized
and underserved.

Teach me to wisely discern decisions
which will be healing and
comforting.

Teach me to lovingly strive to make
a difference for those seeking
solace and consolation.

Teach me to be unfailingly present to
the concerns of those
I serve.

And, teach me to joyfully embrace
my nursing vocation
of caring.

Teach me,
dear Lord,
to become a nursing servant leader
worthy of my
calling.

Amen.

1 Called to Serve: The Nurse's Vocation of Caring

The greatest among you must become like the youngest and the leader like the one who serves.

—Luke 22:26–27

Several of the nurses that I work with said that they saw servant leadership and nursing as synonymous.
—Caitlin, Nurse manager of a palliative care department

In a nursing vocation – a calling to serve – sometimes you have to extend yourself to do the right thing and be caring and compassionate in that calling. I think especially as a nursing supervisor in the hospital, empathy and compassion stand out. Once . . . we had a patient who was dying in the critical care unit, and one of the evening staff was hesitant to let the family members stay because it was past visiting hours. But, as the CCU (critical care unit) supervisor, I said they could stay because it was important; the patient was aware of what was happening. She knew that she was dying, and she knew that the family was there, and it meant a lot to the family also. I think you have to cross over and put yourself in the place of the patient and family to do the right thing and be compassionate and caring. . . . Sometimes we have to bend the rules a little bit so we make sure we are allowing that caring and compassion of our nursing vocation to be evident.
—Anne, supervisor of a critical care unit

The concept of servant leadership in nursing is both old and new, both ancient and modern. From the beginning of time individuals have been called forth from their societies to serve the needs of the ill and the injured. In Chapter 2 of this book, nursing's tradition of service is documented through exploring the lives of nursing leaders from the

1

advent of the pre-Christian and Christian communities through the Middle Ages and into the post-Reformation era.

In this chapter the 21st-century concept of servant leadership is examined in terms of its philosophy and behavioral characteristics both generally and in regard to servant leadership's specific relevance for nursing. First the seminal work of Robert Greenleaf, who popularized the term in 1977, is described. Also included are findings from an extensive examination of current servant leadership literature published by Greenleaf disciples and other students of the subject. Following this, the writings of contemporary nursing scholars of servant leadership are reviewed. In later chapters a nursing research study, identifying and describing the attitudes and behaviors of a cadre of contemporary nurse servant leaders, is described. From the narrative data obtained through open-ended interviews with the nursing leaders, a model of servant leadership for nursing has been created.

Since Greenleaf first purported the notion that a true leader, in any venue, must be a servant of those he or she leads, the concept has been embraced by a number of business and industrial organizations, as well as educational communities. It is only more recently, however, that the practice of servant leadership has captured the attention of healthcare institutions, and more specifically of nurses practicing in those facilities. Recent nursing servant leadership articles do, however, strongly support the adoption of servant leadership as the most appropriate leadership philosophy and practice for nursing and health care.

Both nursing history, reflecting the profession's tradition of service, and the attitudes and activities of today's nurses powerfully reveal the spirituality of servant leadership already existing in the nursing community. Poignant stories of caring and compassion, from the earliest understandings of the needs of the sick to the conceptualization of modern medicine, present an elegant mosaic of servant leadership in nursing. In the following pages, this mosaic is displayed in a rainbow of brilliant hues reflecting the myriad ministries carried out by servant leaders in nursing.

NURSING AS A VOCATION OF CARING

Before discussing the concept of servant leadership, with its characteristic attributes and activities, we need to first understand what philosophy of nursing—what philosophy of life—nursing servant leaders embrace in the practice of their caring ministries. What is it, in fact, that calls one to be a "servant" leader in nursing, rather than simply a leader or a follower? To answer that question one needs to look at the concept of the nurse's vocation—that is, the nurse's vocation of caring.

In beginning to explore the nursing literature examining and describing the meaning of the nurse's vocation, it is important to explain what is meant by the term *vocation*. In general dictionaries the term *vocation* is usually defined as relating to a job to which one might feel called or for which one is trained such as teaching or social work; definitions usually do not attach any spiritual dimension to the concept. In looking at the definition of vocation in a dictionary of theology, however, a spiritual underpinning is attributed to the concept, for example "In traditional Christian usage, *vocation* refers to a divine call to undertake a particular activity or embrace a particular 'state of life' on behalf of God or the community" (Holland, 1990, p. 1087).

When writing about nursing as a "vocation" most nursing authors appear to adopt an understanding of the latter spiritual or theological definition of the term; this is particularly true with literature whose purpose is to explore whether nursing is a "vocation" or a "job." One example is a 1999 debate published in *Nursing Times* entitled "Nursing is a vocation...Two nurses beg to differ." In the paper, written jointly by two currently practicing British nurses, one author states: "I am a nurse because it is my vocation.... This commitment is born of a mixture of personal needs, a sense of duty, and a spiritual belief.... All nurses are driven by vocation to some extent" (Barker & Wheeler, p. 33). A dissenting nurse comments "Nursing is just a job. It is a job that requires you to perform certain duties, for which you receive a financial reward.... If nursing were a vocation, financial reward would be immaterial (and) ... applicants would need only to demonstrate a calling to become a nurse" (p. 33). Thus, the nurse argues that perhaps only an "apprenticeship" might be appropriate as preparation for a nurse rather than academic training (p. 33). The paper does not resolve the vocation question but leaves the debate for the reader to ponder.

Interestingly, another British nurse author and researcher, Ann Bradshaw, in her book *The Nurse Apprentice 1860–1977*, supports the historical concept of nursing as a vocation and apprenticeship. While not denying the importance of contemporary nursing education, Bradshaw laments the fact that some nurses in the current professional community have lost the sense of vocation or the vocational call to serve that was common in earlier times. Her historical research explored British nursing practice prior to as well as following the advent of baccalaureate education. Bradshaw concludes that the concept of nurses perceiving nursing as a vocation was much more evident during the era of the 3-year diploma nursing programs, which consisted of an apprenticeship in a hospital with some formal classes provided to support practice. Nightingale's Christian faith underlying her philosophy of nursing, is also cited as central to the earlier perception of nursing as a vocation of service (Bradshaw, 2002).

Considering Bradshaw's understanding of Nightingale's Christian philosophy of nursing, Swedish theologian Mikael Lundmark has offered an interesting analysis of the nursing vocation by comparing the writings of Bradshaw and Katie Eriksson, who also finds in nursing central concepts of love and charity as identified by Saint Paul. Ultimately Lundmark concludes that both Bradshaw and Ericksson's models "prevent nursing practice from being reduced to a mechanistic application of techniques" and reinforce "a high ethical standard" (2007, p. 778). Their theories, Lundmark concludes "explicitly (Bradshaw) or implicitly (Eriksson) advocate a vocational understanding of nursing as being essential to nursing theory" (p. 778).

As the founder of professional nursing, and as a Christian, Florence Nightingale recognized nursing as a spiritual calling in her classic work *Notes On Nursing* published in 1859:

> And remember every nurse should be one who is to be depended upon … she must be a religious and devoted woman; she must have a respect for her own calling because God's precious gift of life is often literally placed in her hands. (pp. 70–71)

Nightingale scholar JoAnn Widerquist observed "Florence Nightingale did experience a call to service. Nightingale became a nurse in answer to her divine call … she influenced others entering nursing in its infancy to consider the work as a calling more than a profession" (1995, p. 4). Widerquist explained that Nightingale was probably influenced by the fact that a significant characteristic of Victorian religion was the "sense of vocation … this carried with it a powerful sense of the sacredness of time and the sin of wasting it. *Vocation* or *calling* was most often used to mean a spiritual or divine function or predisposition to undertake a certain work" (p. 4). Widerquist added that "Nightingale's concept of calling was that each person must do what he or she is best able to do in service to others within the will of God and His laws" (p. 5) and cited Florence Nightingale's 1893 comment: "A new art and science (nursing) has been created since and within the last 40 years and with it a new profession, so they say; we say *calling*" (p. 6).

In a qualitative study of 15 graduate nurses, the call to be of service was found to be "paramount" (Magnussen, 1998, p. 175). And Verna Carson notes that "service combines the nurse's professional preparation with the gift of his or her personhood. It calls for offering one's gifts and knowledge to others in such a way that the spiritual resources of the nurse are shared with others" (1989, p. 53). Carson adds:

> Viewing nursing as a service allows even the simplest nursing tasks to take on deeper meaning. For instance, providing a bath to a client too weak to bathe himself certainly meets needs of comfort and hygiene. But, if during the bath, the nurse is gentle in her approach, is aware of the client's feeling state and responds appropriately, then the bath becomes a way of serving the client and touching the very core of his spirit. (p. 53)

Christian nurses, it is suggested, are called to serve the ill and the infirm by the teaching and example of Jesus, as recorded in the gospels:

> The gospel message of Jesus is idealistic, yet it has survived escalating levels of knowledge and technology for almost two millennia. This is because the gospel of Jesus touches the heart. The message is simple but profound. We, as members of the human family, are called to care, called to love. Our greatest commandment is taught by Jesus: we must love God and love one another (Matthew 22:37–39). And, we, as nurses, are called to care, called to love, in a special way, those who are ill in their bodies, in their minds, or in their spirits. We, as Christian nurses, are called to love as Jesus loved, without discrimination, without reserve, and sometimes without reward. We are called to follow Him to the Cross, if need be, in order to live out this vocation of loving. (O'Brien, 2001, p. 2)

Jesus' words, as recorded in Matthew 25:35–36, 40, provide the impetus and the mandate for the call to nursing:

> For I was hungry and you gave me food, I was thirsty and you gave me something to drink, I was a stranger and you welcomed me, I was naked and you gave me clothing, I was sick and you took care of me, I was in prison and you visited me…. Truly I tell you, just as you did it to one of the least of these who are members of my family, you did it to me."

There are also a number of scripture passages in which Jesus' disciples are directly mandated to care for the health of those to whom they will minister; these include such passages as: "The Commissioning of the Twelve: 'Then Jesus summoned His twelve disciples and gave them authority over unclean spirits, to cast them out and to cure every disease and every sickness … (instructing them to) … cure the sick, raise the dead, cleanse lepers, cast out demons' (Mt. 10:1;5;8)" (O'Brien, 2003, pp. 9–10).

To truly explore the concept of nursing as a vocation of caring, however, one must begin by looking back, back to the words and thoughts of early nursing leaders, to those wise and prudent voices who sought early on to communicate the spirit and spirituality, as well as the scope and standards, of this young and immature profession of ministering to the sick.

THE HISTORY OF THE NURSING VOCATION OF SERVICE

Historically, nursing is described as being "a vocation of service, incorporating a clearly accepted element of ministry to those for whom the nurse cared. A nurse's mission was considered to be driven by altruism and empathy for the sick, especially the sick poor. The practicing nurse of the early and middle 1900s did not expect much in terms of worldly rewards for her efforts. She envisioned her caregiving as commissioned and supported by God; to Him alone were the thanks and the glory to be given. The vision of nursing as a spiritual ministry is reflected in Sr. Mary Berenice Beck's nurse's prayer:

> I am thine own, great Healer, help Thou me to serve Thy sick
> in humble charity; I ask not thanks nor praise, but only light to
> care for them in every way aright. My charges, sick and well,
> they all are Thine. (1945, p. xvii) (O'Brien, 2008, p. 2)

Other nursing authors of the era also described the vocational element of nursing. Nurse historian Minnie Goodnow (1916) wrote "Nursing is not merely an occupation, temporary and superficial in scope; it is a great vocation" (p. 17). She added: "It (nursing) is so well known to be difficult that it is seldom undertaken by a woman who has not, in the depths of her consciousness, an earnest purpose to serve humanity" (p. 17). Goodnow also advised that nursing is on a higher plane than that of an ordinary occupation, and thus "more is expected" of the nurse (Goodnow, 1913, p. 18).

Virtually all of the nurse authors of the late 1800s and early 1900s followed Florence Nightingale's lead in describing nursing as an elevated vocation or calling to serve the sick. Writing in 1885, Clara S. Weeks, who authored one of the first textbooks in nursing, described the confidential nature of the nurse–patient relationship with the admonition "No one (nurse) with any sense of delicacy can regard (the relationship) as otherwise than inviolably sacred what is thus tacitly left to her honor" (p. 22). In an 1898 text identifying "practical points in nursing," Emily Stoney commented that "The Profession of nursing is one in which there is no limit to the good that can be done; it is also one in which every woman [sic] embracing it must walk worthy of the vocation to which she is called" (pp. 17–18); and, in her 1921 book, *The Psychology of Nursing,* Aileen Cleveland Higgins, superintendent of the Stanford School for Nurses, wrote "The trained nurse, like cloisonné, is made up of many precious things. Virtue upon virtue, gift upon gift, power upon power, the ideal nurse possesses" (p. v).

Writing on "The Place of Religion in the Life of the Nurse," in a 1914 *American Journal of Nursing* article, physician Charles T. Emerson described nursing as "a profession that does not yet know how great are the responsibilities that are to rest on its shoulders" (p. 856). Emerson continued, "We need cultured nurses, educated nurses, and we need spiritual nurses … nurses who hear their call most clearly… (nurses who) have seen the highest spiritual vision of service to their fellow man" (pp. 863–864). He concluded: "Do this and society will call you blessed" (p. 864). In a 1922 address on the spiritual aspects of nursing, Rev. Wilson Stearly is quoted as speaking of the nurse as both professional and minister: "To the physician, the nurse … is a colleague in science and a coworker in the ministry and art of healing" (p. 336); and in a 1923 article in *The Public Health Nurse,* nurses were reminded that "all who embrace nursing as a life profession must have as the secret source of their ministering contacts the ability to do what (saints) did, namely, give their help in the name of God" (White, 1923, p. 283). In 1926, the journal entitled *The Trained Nurse and Hospital Review,* published a paper on the "Christ Spirit" in the hospital in which the author asserted: "Nurses go to the bedside from a season of prayer. They meet the waning hopes of the poor bedridden soul with the radiant beams of a morning glimpse of God" (Lumpkin, 1926, p. 628).

The spiritual vocation of the nurse was recognized in a 1939 *American Journal of Nursing* paper entitled "The Religious Function of the Nurse," which noted that the nurse "above any other professional worker" is called to "serve the religious needs of her patients" (Dicks, p. 1110); and a 1940 article in *The Trained Nurse and Hospital Review* pointed out the relationship between the nurse's profession and vocation stating: "The immense moral strength, the elevation of ideals, and the inspiration toward self-sacrifice and service that come from the teachings of Christ are of priceless aid to the nurse even from a professional standpoint" (Gill, p. 189).

As well as attention to professional duties, the inspiration of the New Testament makes nursing a "profession of kindness" asserted Mary Ranson in a 1952 article (p. 29). "There are only a few vocations that Christ explicitly promised to reward; yours is one of them," promised an author speaking to student nurses in 1954 (Hain, p. 57); and "Your role as a nurse is to take human suffering, lift it in hands that are tender, bless it with lives that are dedicated, enrich it with the incense of prayer, and offer it to God almighty," was a minister's message to nurses published in 1955 (Murphy, p. 58). Finally, in a 1956 nursing text dealing with moral issues, the authors asserted "Because the nurse's vocation is so singularly Christlike, it is imperative that she work through Him, and in Him, and with Him. The nurse will find the solution to most of her difficulties, will see her vocation in a new light, through personal contact with Christ" (Hayes, Hayes, & Kelly, p. 8).

In the early days of professional nursing, books and articles both by nurses and about nurses, such as those cited above, described nursing as a special calling, a vocation of service, characterized by the highest ideals of caring and commitment. This was partly to highlight the positive and elevated nature of this newly identified profession in order to counteract the preprofessional era of the unseemly women to whom nursing roles were often relegated. The spirituality of the nursing vocation was also applauded in order to remind those aspiring to the professional nursing role that much would be asked of them in their chosen work. This was especially true in earlier times when nurses were called upon to work long hours, in often less than comfortable conditions, for little pay. Even as working conditions and salaries improved, however, nurses themselves continued to envision their caregiving activities as constituting a service to humankind, chosen for altruistic rather than material reasons. Many Christian nurses perceived a direct link between their profession of caring for the ill and the Lord's teaching in Matthew 25:35–36; for other nurses, simply the humanitarian nature of the nurse's service provided satisfaction and fulfillment.

For the majority of nurses this ideal of service, whether religious or secular, has not changed even as both the art and science of the profession have evolved into a more sophisticated catalog of knowledge and skills. That fact is clearly and poignantly demonstrated in contemporary nurses attitudes and behaviors reported in later chapters of this book. While it must be admitted that a few of today's nurses have decried the service commitment of nursing, strong voices supporting and applauding the concept of the nursing vocation continue to be heard.

CONTEMPORARY NURSING AS A VOCATION TO SERVE THE SICK

During the past few decades, as society has witnessed a heightened emphasis on the professionalization of nursing, some opinions have surfaced in the literature decrying the "vocational" dimension of nursing the sick. One such perception was reflected in a commentary in the *American Journal of Nursing*, in which the author M. Belcher noted:

> When writers in nursing journals state that it takes compassion to be a nurse, that nursing is the sacrifice of oneself for others, and that nursing is a noble profession, I disagree.... Nursing pays us to place the needs of others before our own.... Self-sacrifice as the road to nobility has never been good for nurses. (Belcher, 2004, p. 13)

Belcher added "That so many nurses see nursing as a calling is a long-standing tradition that has nothing to do with the work we do" (p. 13).

Related to the observation cited above, a few other nursing authors during the last 50 years have raised the question of whether nursing can be both a profession and a vocation; some of these include "Nursing: Vocation or Profession" (Kluge, 1982); "Nursing Is a Vocation: Do Nurses Undermine Professionalism by Seeing Their Work as a Vocation? Two Nurses Beg to Differ" (Barker & Wheeler, 1999); and "Nursing is an Occupation Not a Vocation for Me" (Crowe, 2003). These articles, however, are based on the authors' personal opinions and not upon empirical research. In fact, far more current nursing literature argues for the concepts of professionalism and vocation coexisting in contemporary nursing practice.

In the 2002 book, *Nursing Apprentice 1860–1967* cited earlier, Bradshaw concluded, with some dismay, that perhaps it is the present emphasis on the professionalism of nursing that has led to some devaluing of the vocational ethic. In contrast to Bradshaw's perception, however, a study of nursing care as a calling conducted in Finland (Raatikainen, 1997) found that data elicited in interviews with 179 practicing hospital nurses revealed support for the perception of nursing as a vocation. Raatikainen reported:

> The nurses who were committed to their profession and experienced their job as a calling had good knowledge about their patients ... and were also good sources of support for their

patients ... they were aware of concern for spiritual questions (and also) worked closely within a team ... to possess proficient professional abilities.... They had a deep understanding of the whole process of patient care. (p. 1111)

The author concluded: "According to these results the calling experience is not in conflict with professional principles" (p. 1111).

During the latter half of the 1900s and the beginning of this millennium a number of other nurses wrote about the phenomenon of nursing as a vocation of service. Some articles were primarily reflections of the nurse author's clinical experiences of nursing as a personal calling, for example: "Nursing, A Calling" (Jones, 1984); "Answering God's Call" (Schmidt, 1997); "Hearing the Call to Nursing" (Jeffries, 1998); "Childhood Interest in Nursing Has Become Lifelong Vocation" (King, 2003); "Responding to God's Call" (McKoy, 2004); and "God's Call" (Folta, 2005). Other nurse authors examined the concept of a nursing vocation more broadly.

In a 1987 article Julia Lane, Dean of the School of Nursing at Loyola University of Chicago, described the nurse "who engages in the practice of nursing as a vocation or 'calling' and (described) how that sense of vocation may deepen and broaden care provided to patients" (p. 332). Lane asserted:

the person who feels "called" to nursing views the profession through a different lens. Nursing has a deep personal meaning in terms of religious or humanitarian values. The nurse makes the connection between what he or she is doing and the ultimate meaning and purpose of life. (p. 337)

"This," Lane adds "generally enables the nurse to reach out more sensitively, more hospitably, and more compassionately to other spirits in the world" (p. 337). Lane ends by describing nursing as a "noble vocation" (p. 337) as does Downe (1990) in her article entitled "A Noble Vocation" (1990). Downe asserted that if we are to support professional status for our nursing, "We should be linking that professionalism to better care for our clients ... if we are recognized for our skills, caring and dedication, in other words for our vocation," the professional status will be assured (p. 24). Downe concludes by suggesting:

perhaps the time has come to insist that caring for people and caring about the care we give is not a sign of weakness, but an essential part of humanity. Maybe our resurrection of the "vocational" element to our professionalism will ensure that our development leads not only to increased recognition and status as a group but more importantly, to the recognition that we are givers of essential care. (p. 24)

In a survey on vocation that asked "Why am I a nurse?", Eunice Siccardi interviewed 40 practicing nurses. Ninety-five percent of the group considered nursing a vocation, which many saw as a call from God and as directly related to the desire to help those who were ill and suffering (1995, p. 9). Jean Watson, in discussing transformative leadership, noted that a "fourfold path of leading, embedded in the hidden meaning of the word *vocation* (Latin for 'voice' as in giving voice to inner calling of caring–healing) may be the primary source of nursing's survival in this century" (2000, p. 1).

In a 2002 article in *Nursing Ethics*, Karolyn White, in her article "Nursing As Vocation," explored the topic from an ethical standpoint. White argued that "nursing is best understood as a vocational occupation" (p. 279). This conclusion is based on Blum's model of vocations, which suggests that "such occupations are socially expressed within practices embodying traditions, norms, and a range of meanings: industrial, social, personal, and moral. Vocational workers are those who identify in certain ways with these traditions, norms, and meanings" (p. 279). "Nursing care," White notes, "requires a duty to care for patients, which implies more than the mere legal notion of a duty to care" (p. 280). She adds:

To have a nursing vocation is to be dedicated and committed to assisting another who is disadvantaged in some way on the basis of need and because of what is genuinely best for them. To give succor in this way involves being a person who possesses the virtues of compassion, care, and concern. Vocations and those who enter them have different aspirations and a different focus from instrumental occupations.... This, it seems to me," the author concludes "is vital, particularly for nurses whose purpose is to care for the sick and needy. (p. 283)

An editorial in a 2004 issue of *Nursing Standard* entitled "Pride at Work," asserted that "Nurses are proud of what they do, and the reason that they carry on is simple—patients" (p. 13). This was one of the findings from a survey of 1338 nurses in the UK that showed that "94% ... are proud to be nurses" (p. 13). "Caring" was considered to be "the number one requirement it takes to be a nurse," and "Most (76%) nurses" responding to the survey believed that "nursing is a vocation" (p. 13). And in another 2004 *Nursing Standard* article, author Jane Salvage observed that although some nurses may "stay away from describing what they do as a vocation … it is time to rehabilitate the term" (p. 16). Salvage admits that in some quarters nursing's "vocational ideal has been undermined by social and cultural change: the triumph of scientific thought and the extinguishing of religion, mysticism, and metaphysics" (p. 16). "A consequence," she points out, "is the current focus on evidence-based practice, measurement, outcomes, and technical rationality. Coupled with growth of bureaucratic control over care delivery, this leaves little room for faith, devotion, or the apparently irrational" (p. 16). This, Salvage admits, "creates a paradox." Most nurses come into nursing "because they want to help people"; some have a religious motivation, others a humanitarian philosophy, but while not all call nursing a vocation, the majority of nurses "act out in their career choice their wish to be of service" (p. 16). In asking where that leaves nursing today, Salvage turns to our founder Florence Nightingale who "saw nursing as an 'act of charity,' a branch of the 'love of our kind' but … (was not) sentimental about it. The nurse had to acquire art, science, skill, and knowledge to turn her values into effective action" (p. 17). Salvage, thus concludes: "Even if they do not readily use the word *vocation*, nurses continue to heed their inner call to be of service. Our challenge now is to rehabilitate the idea of vocation … and forge a new collective ideal of service that can help transform health services and society" (p. 17).

In a recent survey of 131 student nurses, the question was asked: "Why do you want to be a nurse?" The two most significant categories of response were "to help or care for people" and "because they felt called or led." The authors reported:

> Almost one half of the student's statements indicated that the main reason they wanted to become a nurse was to help or care for people or "to serve." Typical responses were "to serve and help others," "I love people, and I love helping and giving to others," and "I want to help people when they are the most vulnerable." (Prater & McEwen, 2006, p. 66)

And, nursing as a Christian vocation is addressed by Doornbos, Groenhout, and Hotz in their book *Transforming Care: A Christian Vision of Nursing Practice* (2005). The authors explain:

> Christians are called to a life that embodies the sorts of concerns God portrays to us in Scripture. We are called to act in ways that model God's care for us to a world in dire need of

care and love…. This gives us a starting point for … how we should think about our lives in the context of nursing as a practice and as a vocation. (p. 106)

"To be a nurse," the authors assert:

is to choose to have, as a part of one's identity, a central focus on healing and the maintenance of health and appropriate care for those whose health is failing. This is a fundamentally moral goal and one to which Christians are called to contribute. So nursing is an honorable practice, one that can legitimately be the vocation to which a Christian is called. (p. 106)

Contemporary nursing leaders such as those quoted above repeatedly describe nursing as a vocation of service to others, the undergirding philosophy derived either from a religious or a humanitarian motive. Dean Julia Lane asserted that the nursing vocation prompts a nurse to "reach out more compassionately to other spirits in the world"; Karol White observed that having a nursing vocation means to be "dedicated and committed" to helping another in need; and Jane Salvage points out that even nurses who do not use the term *vocation* continue to respond to "their inner call to be of service." It thus seems most appropriate that nursing should embrace the practice of servant leadership currently being well received in a number of business and educational institutions.

SERVANT LEADERSHIP: A SACRED CALLING

The contemporary concept of servant leadership was first conceived by Robert K. Greenleaf; his classic book on servant leadership initially having been published in 1977. In posing the question "Who is the servant-leader?", Greenleaf answered: "The servant-leader is servant first…. It begins with the natural feeling that one wants to serve, to serve first…. That person is sharply different from one who is leader first…. The difference manifests itself in the care taken by the servant-first to make sure that other people's highest priority needs are being served" (1977, p. 27). The "best test" of this Greenleaf asserts is to pose the questions: "Do those served grow as persons? Do they, while being served, become healthier, wiser, freer, more autonomous, more likely themselves to become servants?" (p. 27). Greenleaf adds:

The natural servant, the person who is servant-first, is more likely to persevere and refine a particular hypothesis on what

serves another's highest priority needs than is the person who
is leader-first and who later serves out of promptings of con-
science or in conformity to normative expectations. (p. 28)

Ultimately Greenleaf's position was that a good leader in any
organization must, in fact, be a servant first; that is what it means, in
his conceptualization, to be a servant leader.

As noted earlier, over the past several decades, Greenleaf's servant
leadership concept has been embraced and operationalized by a number
of business and educational institutions and organizations, including
some healthcare facilities, in the conduct of their corporate management.
Numerous books and articles by Greenleaf disciples have been and
continue to be published addressing the various aspects of the servant
leadership spirit and spirituality (Agosto, 2005; Blanchard & Hodges,
2003, 2005; Hunter, 2004). Distinguished among these scholarly writings
are those of Larry C. Spears (2003, 2004a,b). Of significant importance
in understanding the concept of servant leadership is Spears' identification of the "Ten Characteristics of the Servant-Leader." In 2003, Spears
reported: "After some years of carefully considering Greenleaf's original
writings, I have identified a set of 10 characteristics of the servant-leader
that I view as being of critical importance to the development of servant-
leaders" (2003, p. 16). These characteristics include: "Listening, empathy,
healing, awareness, persuasion, conceptualization, foresight, stewardship, commitment to the growth of people, and building community"
(pp. 16–19).

In an article entitled "A Review of Servant Leadership Attributes: Developing a Practical Model" authors Robert F. Russell and
A. Gregory Stone (2002) presented an overview of the servant leadership
literature with the goal of developing a broad servant leadership model.
Larry Spears' 10 characteristics of the servant leader were noted;
however, Russell and Stone suggested, based on their literature
review, that a group of 20 servant leader attributes might be identified.
These included 9 functional attributes: "vision, honesty, integrity, trust,
service, modeling, pioneering, appreciation of others, and empowerment" (2002, p. 146). Also included were 11 "accompanying attributes of
servant leadership": "communication, credibility, competence, stewardship, visibility, influence, persuasion, listening, encouragement, teaching, and delegation" (pp. 146–147). Russell and Stone noted that three
of Spears' characteristics, listening, persuasion, and stewardship, are
included in their list and that others are "incorporated under broader
categories" (p. 146).

A number of research studies were conducted during the past decade that explored the following servant leadership topics:

- The examination of leadership practices and principals identified by servant leaders (Taylor, Martin, Hutchinson, & Jinks, 2007), which explored 12 categories of leadership: integrity, humility, servanthood, caring for others, empowering others, developing others, visioning, goal setting, leading, modeling, team building, and shared decision making (p. 408)
- A comparison of transformational leadership versus servant leadership (Stone, Russell, & Patterson, 2004)
- Two explorations of the role of values in servant leadership (Russell, 2001; Washington, Sutton, & Field, 2006)
- Construction of two instruments to measure servant leadership characteristics: a servant leadership assessment tool (Dennis & Bocarnea, 2005) and development of a servant leadership scale (Barbuto & Wheeler, 2006)
- A correlational study of servant leadership, leader trust, and organizational trust (Joseph & Winston, 2005)
- A case study of servant leadership at a religiously affiliated educational institution (Winston, 2004).

A research study exploring the role of nurse–midwives as servant leader care providers for Amish women was conducted by nurse–midwife Victoria L. Wickwire (2006). Employing the framework of servant leader characteristics identified by Spears, Wickwire developed a concept of care model that included the following concepts:

- Listening—Affirmation and engagement
- Empathy—Understanding and acceptance
- Healing—Wholeness and health
- Awareness—Encouragement and interaction
- Persuasion—Building consensus; trust
- Conceptualization—Helping others through change; commitment
- Foresight—Intuitiveness and incorporating lessons of the past
- Stewardship—Decreased misunderstanding; servant caring
- Commitment to the growth of people—Helping ministries and humility in caring
- Building community—Instill love; compassion (p. 145)

While the concept of servant leadership, as originally conceived by Greenleaf, is not inherently spiritual or religious in nature, one can indeed locate a human "sacredness" in its underlying philosophy: Servant leadership "begins with the natural feeling that one wants to serve, to serve first," and "The care taken by the servant leader [is] to make sure that other people's highest priority needs are being served" (Greenleaf, 1977, p. 27). Servant leaders are to place others' needs before their own and to serve those over whom they assume leadership. Surely these characteristics of the servant leader bring to mind the scripture model: "The Son of Man came not to be served but to serve and to give His life as a ransom for many" (Mark 10:45). This conceptualization is validated in writings such as those of servant leadership scholars Ken Blanchard and Phil Hodges (2003) who authored the book, *Lead Like Jesus: Lessons from the Greatest Leadership Role Model of All Time*. Blanchard and Hodges assert that "Jesus modeled the heart of a true servant leader by investing most of His ministry time training and equipping the disciples for leadership" (2003, p. 46). They point out that at the end of His ministry, Jesus told His disciples "I no longer call you servants ... I call you friends" because He wanted them to grow into greatness in their discipleship after He went to the Father (p. 46).

Echoing a similar theme is the 2008 book "*Black Belt Leader, Peaceful Leader: An Introduction to Catholic Servant Leadership*" by counselor and Aikido martial arts sensei Tim Warneka. In his book he presents a global image of servant leadership for the world community. Warneka observed poignantly, "Today's world cries out for people who can lead with a global perspective. We need leaders who lead from the heart as well as the mind ... leaders who can act ethically, intentionally, and with respect.... Most of all we need leaders who understand that the primary function of a leader is to *serve*, not to *be* served" (p. xi).

The 10 principles of servant leadership identified by Warneka are:

1. Love
2. Humanity
3. Right use of power
4. Leadership as spiritual practice
5. Leadership as a journey of faith
6. Building an embodied peaceful presence
7. Valuing community
8. Seeking personal transformation
9. Understanding the universal
10. Lifelong learning (2008, p. 32).

When looking at the description of servant leadership as described by Greenleaf, Spears, Russell and Stone, Blanchard and Hodges, Warneka and others, one is struck by the relevance that the theory has for professional nursing. The identified characteristics, attributes, and principles of servant leadership seem to read like a list of ideal behavioral characteristics of the contemporary nursing leader. And indeed they are representative of many nursing servant leaders' practice as is clearly demonstrated in the research findings discussed in later chapters.

SERVANT LEADERSHIP IN NURSING

During the past few decades nurses have written extensively about the various understandings of leadership and leadership theory; nurse authors have written significantly little, however, about the concept of servant leadership. Leadership is defined in a 2008 edition of the book *Nursing in Today's World* as "the ability to guide, motivate, and inspire, and to instill vision and purpose" (Ellis & Hartley, p. 471). To provide leadership, the authors add, one must "be able to influence the beliefs, opinions, and behaviors of others and to persuade others to follow [one's] direction" (p. 471). Leadership is also defined as a "process of influence"; a leader "influences others to move in the direction of achieving goals" (Carroll, 2006, p. 3). Leadership, it is pointed out, is "not limited to people in traditional positions of authority" (p. 3).

In a chapter entitled "Leadership and Followership," nurses Theresa Valiga and Sheila Grossman identify six leadership competencies that they note are derived from a presentation given by Warren Bennis, an influential scholar of leadership. The competencies, which are not incompatible with the theory of servant leadership, include:

1. Leaders must foster a clear vision with an endowed purpose that is owned by the people involved with the leader.
2. Leaders must keep reminding people of what is important.
3. Leaders must be optimistic and see possibilities.
4. Leaders must create a culture of candor.
5. Leaders must mentor others and acknowledge their ideas and accomplishments.
6. Good leaders must be in tune to getting results. (2007, p. 9)

In describing leadership as a "peak and perk of professional development" for nurses, Mary Schira observed that "although a leader may be seen as someone who takes charge during a time of crisis or difficulty, most leaders are individuals who work every day among a group of people to encourage high levels of performance and quality" (2007, p. 290). Schira lists as the "characteristics and attributes we value in leaders: communication, openness, motivation, vision, passion, risk taking, environment control, and shares rewards" (pp. 291–293).

Nursing authors suggest that there is "more than one way" of leading (King & Cunningham, 1995, p. 3); that "leadership behavior impacts staff nurse empowerment, job tension, and work effectiveness" (Laschinger, Wong, McMahon, & Kaufmann, 1999, p. 28); and that leadership is the "key to quality outcomes" in nursing (Perra, 2001, p. 68).

A type of leadership style, somewhat akin to that of servant leadership, that is generally included in the nursing leadership literature is that of transformational leadership. Transformational leadership theory describes leadership behavior in which "both leaders and followers act on one another to raise their motivation and performance to higher levels" (Carroll, 2006, p. 9). It is pointed out that transformational leadership "depends on the concept of empowerment, in which all parties are allowed to work together, to the best of their ability, to achieve a collective goal. The process transforms both the leader and the follower … [and allows for] innovation and change" (Carroll, 2006, p. 9). Some attributes of transformation are identified as "self-knowledge, authenticity, expertise, vision, flexibility, shared leadership, charisma, and the ability to inspire others" (Dossey, 2005, pp. 6–14). In a study of transformational leadership in two different kinds of nursing units, it was found that leaders in "nursing developmental units" demonstrated more transformational leadership behaviors than those in "conventional clinical settings" (Bowles & Bowles, 2000, p. 76). It was concluded that the leaders in nursing developmental units may have been more skilled and have more environmental support for transformational behaviors than those in conventional settings (p. 76).

In discussing the "evolution of leadership in nursing," British nurse manager Nadeem Moiden observed that as new nursing leadership theories emerge, they are compared with older theories and a "more achieved style of nursing leadership may emerge" (2002, p. 25). Staff nurse Claire Welford points out that nursing leadership needs to assure that the workplace will become a place where all participants are positively motivated and "led through change" (2002, p. 11). For change to occur, however, nursing leaders need to "move away from traditional leadership practices and behaviors" (Fedoruk & Pincombe, 2000, p. 20). A theory that could undergird the establishment of supportive and growth producing nursing environments is that of servant leadership.

Although the concept of servant leadership described earlier seems most appropriate to explain the desired spirit and practice of leaders in the professional nursing community, there is, as noted, a paucity of nursing literature exploring or identifying this concept within professional nursing. In a recent computer search of the extant nursing and allied health literature only 22 articles were found addressing the practice of servant leadership in nursing; several of these were brief and did not demonstrate how servant leadership might be practiced in the nursing community.

In a 1-page commentary on servant leadership in *Professional Nurse,* Stephen Prosser described the concept of servant leadership generally and identified Spears' 10 characteristics of servant leadership but did not discuss the relevance of the concept to nursing (2002, p. 238). In another commentary found in *Reflections,* the journal of Sigma Theta Tau, president Fay L. Bower also described Greenleaf's conceptualization of servant leadership and related his leadership style to her understanding of leadership in the honor society of nursing (1994, pp. 4–5). In an article in a 2004 issue of *Patient Care Staffing Report,* entitled "Shared Governance and Servant Leadership are Drawing Nurses to New Hospital," the chief nursing officer at a newly opened facility is described as expressing her vision of leadership, mentioning that "servant leadership" would be a "watchword" at the hospital. How the concept would be incorporated was not elaborated (Weber, 2004, p. 3).

Related to the report of employing servant leadership in a hospital setting four other articles were found that also supported the initiation of servant leadership in healthcare facilities. In the journal *Health Progress,* it was noted that two hospitals belonging to the Catholic Health Association "have developed programs to better integrate servant leadership into their culture" (Yanofchick, 2007, p. 7). A newsletter of a rural medical center highlighted the positive value of implementing a "culture of servant leadership" (Englert, 2007, p. 1). The importance of servant leadership in the long-term care setting has been described as "an alternative to the traditional power-based approach" as "it encourages collaboration and valuation of all workers" (Downs, 2007, p. 39). Sarah Mullally, chief nursing officer for England, challenged British nurses to adopt patient-focused leadership styles, one of which was servant leadership. Mullally observed:

> Servant leaders … inspire, create collaboration, coach, are consistent, are confirming, and promote continuous development and improvement. Servant leaders create matrix organizations and promote reconciliation and have a genuine concern for others. They recognize the possibility of human failure and see discipline as part of the developmental process. (2007, p. 7)

The servant leadership concept applied to organizational health in general was described by Spears in an article in *Reflections on*

Nursing Leadership, including explanations of his 10 characteristics of the servant leader. Spears noted "Servant leadership truly offers hope and guidance for a new era in human development and a prescription for creating healthy organizations" (2004b, p. 26). *Nursing Management,* a British journal, published a paper entitled "The Servant Leader" that provided some examples from the National Health Service (Howatson-Jones, 2004).

Two nurse-authored articles found in the *Nurse Leader* and the *Health Care Manager,* respectively, addressed selected characteristics of servant leadership as applied to nursing. In the *Nurse Leader,* Patricia Campbell and Pamela Rudisill identified and described how 6 of Spears' 10 characteristics of servant leadership might be applied in the role of the nursing leader:

1. Listening was described as important for nursing leaders who may not consider all variables "within and outside of our control"
2. Awareness, it was suggested, "permits the nurse leader to plan and implement strategies to address needs in a proactive manner"
3. Persuasion, the authors noted reflected a leader perceived by staff as "a consistent, fair and reasonable individual … who can exhibit a strong and persuasive influence"
4. Foresight was viewed as essential for nurse leaders "who must be visionary leaders with a road map in place for followers"
5. Stewardship was described as "the responsibility and accountability for managing resources in an appropriate manner"
6. Commitment to the growth of individuals, the authors assert, permits "the involvement of nursing staff in the decision-making process" and "results in positive outcomes." (2005, pp. 27–28)

In the article published in the *Nurse Manager,* entitled "Servant Leadership: Serving Those Who Serve Others," authors Sandra Swearingen and Aaron Liberman describe the history, philosophy, and application of the servant leadership concept, the latter discussion focusing on the meaning of Spears' 10 characteristics of servant leadership for the nursing community (2004):

1. In discussing listening, the authors not only suggest that the nurse leader must listen to his or her "own inner voice" but add "truly listening to what nurses are saying about their profession is the first step of solving many of its problems."
2. Empathy was noted as important to the "distinct generations working in the profession."

3. Healing was seen as "desperately needed to heal relationships among those that heal others."

4. Awareness was related to the current need for nurse leaders to be "aware of the influences on their industry and the resulting problems that stem from the state of health care today."

5. Persuasion was related to "avoidance of top-down leadership," which is "oppressing the nursing profession" and the fact that "consensus building in nursing leadership is an area that needs development."

6. Conceptualization included the "vision to create healthy, healing, work cultures."

7. Foresight was associated with the fact that "leadership must take lessons from the past, incorporate them with the present, and foresee the consequences of the decisions on the future."

8. Stewardship was viewed as "first and foremost a commitment to serving the needs of others."

9. Commitment to the growth of people was related to the idea that "nurses … need and want mentorship. There is always something new to learn."

10. Describing the importance of building community, the authors point out "most healthcare workers spend more waking hours at work than they do in their own homes … there is a need to build communities to meet the needs of all stakeholders in the organization." (pp. 102–105)

A 2004 fundamentals of nursing text contains a chapter on leadership, delegation, and collaboration that includes a subsection entitled "Servant Leadership." In the discussion it is pointed out that "a number of authors believe that the servant leadership approach is valuable in healthcare applications" (Friedman & Mullens, p. 485). In a 2006 nursing text on leadership and management, the author applauds servant leadership as a new and innovative kind of leadership strategy for nurses: "When applied to health care, servant leadership is an attractive alternative to the traditional bureaucratic environment experienced by nurses" (Huber, 2006, p. 22). Huber further describes servant leadership as a model that "enhances the personal growth of nurses, improves the quality of care, values teamwork, and promotes personal involvement and caring behavior" (p. 22).

The understanding of servant leadership for nursing articulated by Huber is also supported by Mark Neill and Nena Saunders in their paper: "Servant Leadership: Enhancing Quality of Care and Staff Satisfaction" (2008). Neill and Saunders observed that "servant leadership encompasses a powerful skill set that is particularly effective in implementing a team approach to the delivery of nursing practice" (p. 395). They add that the "model not only encourages the professional growth of nurses" but also "simultaneously promotes the improved delivery of healthcare services through a combination of interdisciplinary teamwork, shared decision making, and ethical behavior" (Neill & Saunders, 2008, p. 395).

The philosophy and practice of servant leadership has been identified as doing the following:

- Supporting nursing research (Jackson, 2007)
- Supporting nursing education (Robinson, 2009; Neill, Hayward, & Peterson, 2007)
- Facilitating healing (Ramer, 2008)
- Supporting and transforming healthcare organizations (Schwartz & Tumblin, 2002; Deckard, 2009).

A 2005 commentary published in *Clinical Systems Management* observed that while the concept of servant leadership has received attention in the press, "little empirical research exists to support the theory or the anecdotal evidence used in the popular press material" (Farling, Stone, & Winston, p. 19). The authors add: "The concept of servant leadership lacks support by well designed and published empirical research" (p. 19). Both the paucity of literature exploring the concept of servant leadership in the professional nursing community and the commentary in *Clinical Systems Management*, asserting the need for empirical research on servant leadership, provided impetus, support, and encouragement for the nursing study discussed in the later chapters of this book.

To date the literature on servant leadership in general, as well as servant leadership in nursing, has focused primarily on the leadership of an individual whose role is that of work supervisor—one whose position places him or her in charge of other employees in an organization. This is certainly relevant for many nursing leaders. Nurses in the hospital setting are administrators, supervisors, head nurses, charge nurses, team leaders, or individuals who may hold a variety of other positions that place them in charge of other staff members. The same is true in the educational setting where nursing faculty members may be deans, associate deans, area chairs, program managers, research team leaders, and so forth.

It is important to remember, however, that essentially all nurses are leaders related to their roles in caring for patients, family members, study participants, and students. Thus, nurses ministering at the bedside, or in such settings as a clinic, the operating room, or the emergency department, are also servant leaders for those patients and, in some cases family members, committed to their care. Research nurses are servant leaders for their study participants during a patient's participation in a protocol. And in the educational setting, individual faculty members are charged with the responsibility of being servant leaders for their students. Nurses' lived experiences of carrying out the servant leadership role in these various nursing settings are presented in Chapters 5, 6, and 7 of this book.

The present chapter has demonstrated, through extensive review of the literature, that nursing has been and is perceived by nurses as a vocation of caring, both historically and in contemporary professional practice. The literature also demonstrates the relevance of the theory of servant leadership to nursing practice. The relationship between the concept of understanding nursing as a vocation and the concept of practicing servant leadership among nursing leaders is evident. There is a marriage of attitudes, behaviors, practices, and goals between the centuries-old profession of nursing the sick and the decades old theory of servant leadership. Nurses are sometimes described as "born" to be nurses; servant leaders, it would seem, might also be so described as being "born" to be servant leaders. Nursing leaders combine a deeply felt desire to care for the sick with a clear and unambiguous goal of serving all those to whom they minister. Professional nurses are indeed called to be servant leaders in their ministry of caring for the ill and the infirm.

REFERENCES

Agosto, E. (2005). *Servant leadership: Jesus and Paul*. St. Louis, MO: Chalice Press.

Barbuto, J. E., & Wheeler, D. W. (2006). Scale development and construct clarification of servant leadership. *Group & Organizational Management, 31*(3), 300–326.

Barker, S., & Wheeler, J. (1999). Nursing is a vocation: Do nurses undermine professionalism by seeing their work as a vocation? Two nurses beg to differ. *Nursing Times, 95*(25), 33.

Beck, M. B. (1945). *The nurse: Handmaid of the divine physician*. Philadelphia: J. B. Lippincott.

Belcher, M. C. (2004). I'm no angel: I am a nurse and that's enough. *American Journal of Nursing, 104*(7), 13. (Appended article and investigator's letter (s) of response — original and as edited by AJN and published in the *American Journal of Nursing, 104*(10), 93.)

Blanchard, K., & Hodges, P. (2003). *The servant leader: Transforming your heart, head, hands and habits*. Nashville, TN: Countryman.

Blanchard, K., & Hodges, P. (2005). *Lead like Jesus: Lessons from the greatest leader of all time.* Nashville, TN: Thomas Nelson.

Bower, F. L. (1994). Servant leadership...President's message. *Reflections, 20*(4), 4–5.

Bowles, A., & Bowles, N. B. (2000). A comparative study of transformational leadership in nursing development units and conventional clinical settings. *Journal of Nursing Management, 8*(2), 69–76.

Bradshaw, A. (2002). *The nurse apprentice 1860–1977.* Aldershot Hampshire, UK: Ashgate.

Campbell, P. T., & Rudisill, P. T. (2005). Servant leadership: A critical component for nurse leaders. *Nurse Leader, 3*(3), 27–29.

Carroll, P. (2006). *Nursing leadership and management: A practical guide.* Clifton Park, NY: Thomson Delmar Learning.

Carson, V. B. (1989). Nursing-science and service: A historical perspective. In V. B. Carson (Ed.), *Spiritual dimensions of nursing practice* (pp. 52–73). Philadelphia: W. B. Saunders.

Crowe, P. (2003). Nursing is an occupation not a vocation for me. *Nursing Times, 99*(35), 18.

Deckard, G. J. (2009). Contemporary leadership theories. In N. Borkowski (Ed.), *Organizational behavior, theory and design in health care* (pp. 203–222). Sudbury, MA: Jones and Bartlett.

Dennis, R. S., & Bocarnea, M. (2005). Development of the servant leadership assessment instrument. *Leadership and Organization Development Journal, 26*(8), 600–615.

Dicks, R. L. (1939). The religious function of the nurse. *American Journal of Nursing, 39*(10), 1109–1112.

Doornbos, M. M., Groenhout, R. E., & Hotz, K. G. (2005). *Transforming care: A Christian vision of nursing practice.* Grand Rapids, MI: William B. Eerdmans.

Dossey, B. M. (2005). Florence Nightingale's tenets: Healing, leadership, global action. In B. M. Dossey, L. C. Selanders, D. Beck, & A. Attewell (Eds.), *Florence Nightingale Today: Healing Leadership, Global Action* (pp. 9–15). Silver Spring, MD: American Nurses Association.

Downe, S. (1990). A noble vocation. *Nursing Times, 86*(40), 24.

Downs, F. C. (2007). The servant leadership worldview in long-term care nursing. *Annals of Long-Term Care, 15*(8), 36–39.

Ellis, J. R., & Hartley, C. L. (2008). *Nursing in today's world: Trends, issues and management.* Philadelphia: Lippincott Williams & Wilkins.

Emerson, C. T. (1914). The place of religion in the life of the nurse. *American Journal of Nursing, 14*(10), 856–864.

Englert, J. (2007, February). Rural facility received Baldrige for 2006: Culture of servant leadership at core of success. *HealthCare Benchmarks and Quality Improvement* [Newsletter]. Tupelo, MS: North Mississippi Medical Center, 1–2.

Farling, M. L., Stone, A. G., & Winston, B. E. (2005). Servant leadership: Setting the stage for empirical research [Abstract]. *Clinical Systems Management, 7*(5–6), 19.

Fedoruk, M., & Pincombe, J. (2000). The nurse executive: Challenges for the 21st century. *Journal of Nursing Management, 8*(1), 13–20.

Folta, R. (2005). God's call. *Christian Nurse International, 11*(1), 7.

Friedman, L. H., & Mullens, L. A. (2004). Leadership, delegation and collaboration. In R. Daniels (Ed.), *Nursing fundamentals: Caring and clinical decision making* (pp. 477–489). Clifton Park, NY: Delmar Learning.

Gill, M. K. (1940). Religion in the life of the student nurse. *The Trained Nurse and Hospital Review, CV*(3), 189–192.

Goodnow, M. (1913). *First year nursing: A textbook for pupils during their first year of hospital work.* Philadelphia: W. B. Saunders.

Goodnow, M. (1916). *Outlines of nursing history.* Philadelphia: W. B. Saunders.

Greenleaf, R. K. (1977). *Servant leadership: A journey into the nature of legitimate power and greatness.* New York: Paulist Press.

Hain, R. (1954). Capping exercises. *The Catholic Nurse, 3*(1), 53–57.

Hayes, E. J., Hayes, P. J., & Kelly, D. E. (1956). *Moral handbook of nursing.* New York: Macmillan.

Higgins, A. C. (1921). *The psychology of nursing.* New York: G.P. Putnam's Sons.

Holland, P. D. (1990). Vocation. In J. A. Komonchak, M. Collins, & D. A. Lane (Eds.), *The New Dictionary of Theology* (pp. 1087–1092). Collegeville, MN: Liturgical Press.

Howatson-Jones, I. (2004). The servant leader. *Nursing Management, 11*(3), 2–24.

Huber, D. L. (2006). Leadership principles. In D. L. Huber (Ed.), *Leadership and nursing care management* (pp. 1–32). Philadelphia: Saunders Elsevier.

Hunter, J. C. (2004). *The world's most powerful leadership principle: How to become a servant leader.* New York: Waterbook Press.

Jackson, D. (2007). Servant leadership in nursing: A framework for developing sustainable research capacity in nursing. *Collegian: Journal of the Royal College of Nursing Australia, 15*(1), 27–33.

Jeffries, E. (1998). Hearing the call to nursing. *Nursing, 3*(2), 71–72.

Jones, I. H. (1984). Nursing a calling. *Nursing Times, 80*(7), 49.

Joseph, E. E., & Winston, B. E. (2005). A correlation of servant leadership, leader trust and organizational trust. *Leadership and Organization Development Journal, 26*(1), 6–22.

King, J. (2003). Childhood interest in nursing has become lifelong vocation. *The Catholic Herald,* January 16, 6.

King, K., & Cunningham, G. (1995). Leadership in nursing: More than one way. *Nursing Standard, 10*(12–14), 3–14.

Kluge, E. W. (1982). Nursing: Vocation or profession. *The Canadian Nurse, 78*(1), 34–35.

Laschinger, H. K. S., Wong, C., McMahon, L., & Kaufmann, C. (1999). Leader behavior impact on staff nurse empowerment, job tension and work effectiveness. *Journal of Nursing Administration, 29*(5), 28–39.

Lane, J. A. (1987). The care of the human spirit. *Journal of Professional Nursing, 3*(6), 332–337.

Lumpkin, G. T. (1926). The Christ spirit which makes the hospital great. *The Trained Nurse and Hospital Review, 77*(6), 628–630.

Lundmark, M. (2007). Vocation in theology-based nursing theories. *Nursing Ethics, 14*(6), 767–780.

Magnussen, L. (1998). Women's choices: An historical perspective of nursing as a career choice. *Journal of Professional Nursing, 14*(3), 175–183.

McKoy, Y. D. (2004). Responding to God's call. *Journal of Christian Nursing, 21*(2), 35–37.

Moiden, N. (2002). Evolution of leadership in nursing. *Nursing Management, 9*(7), 20–25.

Mullally, S. (2001). Leadership and politics. *Nursing Management, 8*(4), 21–27.

Murphy, J. F. (1955). How is your fervor for Christ? *The Catholic Nurse, 3*(4), 57–59.

Neill, M. W., Hayward, K. S., & Peterson, T. (2007). Students perceptions of the interprofessional team in practice through application of servant leadership principles. *Journal of Interprofessional Care, 21*(4), 425–432.

Neill, M. W., & Saunders, N. S. (2008). Servant leadership: Enhancing quality of care and staff satisfaction. *Journal of Nursing Administration, 38*(9), 395–400.

Nightingale, F. (1859). *Notes on nursing.* London: Harrison.

O'Brien, M. E. (2001). *The nurse's calling: A Christian spirituality of caring for the sick.* Mahwah, NJ: Paulist Press.

O'Brien, M. E. (2003). *Parish nursing: Healthcare ministry within the church.* Sudbury, MA: Jones and Bartlett.

O'Brien, M. E. (2008). *Spirituality in nursing: Standing on holy ground* (3rd ed.). Sudbury, MA: Jones and Bartlett.

Perra, B. M. (2001). Leadership: The key to quality outcomes. *Journal of Nursing Care Quality, 15*(2), 68–73.

Prater, L., & McEwen, M. (2006). Called to nursing: Perceptions of student nurses. *Journal of Holistic Nursing, 24*(1), 63–69.

Pride at Work. (2004). *Nursing Standard, 18*(28), 13–16.

Prosser, S. (2002). Servant leadership. *Professional Nurse, 18*(4), 238.

Raatikainen, R. (1997). Nursing care as a calling. *Journal of Advanced Nursing, 25*(1), 1111–1115.

Ramer, L. M. (2008). Using servant leadership to facilitate healing after a drug diversion experience. *AORN Journal, 88*(2), 253–258.

Ranson, M. (1952). The roots and branches of nursing. *The Catholic Nurse, 1*(1), 29–30.

Robinson, F. P. (2009). Servant teaching: The power and promise for nursing education. *International Journal of Nursing Education Scholarship, 6*(1), 1–15.

Russell, R. F. (2001). The role of values in servant leadership. *Leadership and Organization Development Journal, 22*(2), 76–83.

Russell, R. F., & Stone, A. G. (2002). A review of servant leadership attributes: Developing a practical model. *Leadership and Organization Development Journal, 23*(3), 145–157.

Salvage, J. (2004). The call to nurture. *Nursing Standard, 19*(10), 16–17.

Schira, M. (2007). Leadership: A peak and perk of professional development. *Nephrology Nursing Journal, 34*(3), 289–284.

Schmidt, K. (1997). Answering God's call. *Journal of Christian Nursing, 14*(1), 11.

Schwartz, R. W., & Tumblin, T. F. (2002). The power of servant leadership to transform health care organizations for the 21st century economy. *Archives of Surgery, 137*(12), 1419–1427.

Siccardi, E. (1995). Why am I a nurse: A 'mini' survey on vocation. *Christian Nurse International, 11*(1), 9–10.

Spears, L. C. (2003). Introduction: Understanding the growing impact of servant-leadership. In R. K. Greenleaf, *The Servant-Leader Within: A Transformative Path* (pp. 13–27). New York: Paulist Press.

Spears, L. C. (2004a). Practicing servant-leadership. *Leader to Leader, 34*(Fall), 7–11.

Spears, L. C. (2004b). Prescription for organizational health. *Reflections on Nursing Leadership, 30*(4), 24–26.

Stearly, W. R. (1922). The abiding and spiritual aspects of nursing. *The Public Health Nurse, XIV*(7), 333–338.

Stone, A. G., Russell, R. F., & Patterson, K. (2004). Transformational versus servant leadership: A difference in leader focus. *Leadership and Organization Development Journal, 25*(4), 349–361.

Stoney, E. A. M. (1898). *Practical points in nursing: For nurses in private practice.* Philadelphia: W. B. Saunders.

Swearingen, S., & Liberman, A. (2004). Nursing leadership: Serving those who serve others. *Health Care Manager, 23*(2), 100–109.

Taylor, T., Martin, B. N., Hutchinson, S., & Jinks, M. (2007). Examination of leadership practices of principals identified as servant leaders. *International Journal of Leadership in Education, 10*(4), 401–419.

Valiga, T. M., & Grossman, S. (2007). Leadership and followership. In R. A. Patronis Jones (Ed.), *Nursing leadership and management* (pp. 3-12). Philadelphia: F. A. Davis.

Warneka, T. H. (2008). *Black belt leader, peaceful leader: An introduction to Catholic servant leadership.* Cleveland, OH: Asogomi.

Washington, R. R., Sutton, C. D., & Field, H. S. (2006). Individual differences in servant leadership: The roles of values and personality. *Leadership and Organization Development Journal, 27*(8), 700–716.

Watson, J. (2000). Leading via caring-healing: The fourfold way toward transformative leadership. *Nursing Administration, 25*(1), 1–6.

Weber, D. (2004). Shared governance and servant leadership are drawing nurses to new hospital. *Patient Care Staffing Report, 4*(7), 1–3.

Weeks, C. S. (1885). *A textbook of nursing: For the use of training schools, families and private students.* New York: D. Appleton and Company.

Welford, C. (2002). Matching theory to practice. *Nursing Management, 9*(4), 7–11.

White, F. S. (1923). At the gate of the temple. *The Public Health Nurse, XV*(6), 279–283.

White, K. (2002). Nursing as vocation. *Nursing Ethics, 9*(3), 279–290.

Wickwire, V. L. (2006). *Amish childbearing beliefs and practices and the implications for nurse–midwives as servant-leader care providers.* Unpublished doctoral dissertation, Andrews University.

Widerquist, J. (1995). Called to serve. *Christian Nurse International, 11*(1), 4–6.

Winston, B. E. (2004). Servant leadership at Heritage Bible College: A single-case study. *Leadership and Organization Development Journal, 25*(7), 600–617.

Yanofchick, B. (2007). Servant leadership: Bring it home. *Health Progress, 88*(5), 6–7.

2 The Spiritual Heritage of Servant Leadership in Nursing: A Tradition of Service

Whoever wishes to become great among you must be your servant . . . for the Son of Man came not to be served but to serve.

—Mark 10:43, 45

There is a sacredness in the work we do as nurses, as servants, in our ministry of caring. There is a sacred trust that we hold in the relationship between the nurse and the patients and families. There's also that sacred trust in our relationships between those of us who are leaders and our staff members, our patients, or our students. In a way, it's like no other professional relationship. Because we need to provide the physical care, the very best care or teaching that we can, but we also need to protect and advocate for those we care for whether it's in direct nursing care, or supervising, or teaching about the nursing role. We have the responsibility to care holistically for others, not just physical but emotional and spiritual needs as well. It makes me think of the Florence Nightingale quote, from nursing history, that the nurse often holds in her hands "God's precious gift of life." What a truly sacred trust has been given to us in doing our ministry of nursing; what a sacred heritage has been left to us in caring for the sick.

—Martha, nurse educator specializing in adult health

It is often said that we stand on the shoulders of those who have gone before us. How true this is for contemporary servant leaders in nursing. In later chapters the attitudes and behaviors of contemporary nursing servant leaders are identified and described. First, however, it is important to reexamine and remind ourselves of the magnificent caring, and often heroic characteristics, of nursing servant leaders of the past. A select group of servant leaders who cared for the sick is highlighted in the following pages; many more could be added to their number, some of whose names may never have been recorded. The legacies of servant leadership left by this small cadre of nursing leaders, have, nevertheless, provided and continue to provide inspiration, support, and encouragement for their nurse followers.

Perhaps no other profession has as rich a heritage of servant leadership as nursing. Even prior to the Christian era, when nursing of the sick began to become a formalized calling, ancient civilizations included individual leaders whose unique vocation was attending to the needs of the ill. While these first servant leaders, both before and following the advent of Christianity, were generally not referred to as *nurses*, the vocational role they embraced was that of "nursing" the sick, in whatever way was needed and appropriate, within their respective societies.

Nursing in the pre-Christian era was carried out extensively, but not exclusively, in such cultures as ancient Egypt, Greece, Rome, and Israel (O'Brien, 2008). Identified healers, whose primary calling was the care of the sick, included such practitioners as Buddhist herbalists, Hindu male nurses, and Irish druidic priests and priestesses. "Archeological study of the pre-Christian cultures has also revealed two related yet distinct types of nurses. One group consisted of skilled women who 'nursed for hire'; more commonly identified, however, were 'nurses' whose positions were those of slaves in wealthy households" (Dolan, Fitzpatrick, & Herrmann, 1983, p. 81). These nurses practiced their art and science "according to the established medical models of their respective societies" (O'Brien, 2008, p. 22).

It is suggested that the attitudes and behaviors of nurses in these pre-Christian cultures significantly influenced the attributes of service and charity later adopted by caregivers of the early Christian era such as the deacons and deaconesses, widows, virgins, and Roman matrons; those individuals who chose to dedicate their lives to providing care for the ill members of their church communities (Bullough & Bullough, 1987).

JESUS AS SERVANT LEADER: THE ADVENT
OF CHRISTIAN CARE OF THE SICK

Then Jesus went about all the cities and villages ... proclaiming the good news of the Kingdom, and curing every disease and every sickness.

—Matthew 9:35

Jesus, although the recognized leader of a new religious community, later to be labeled Christianity, placed service, especially service to the sick, as central to His mission and ministry. Jesus is described as the "enduring model of servanthood. . . . The form of Christ's servanthood included self-emptying, identification with the needy and self-giving" (Johnson, 1988, p. 133). Thus, for Jesus' early disciples nursing of the sick was not only considered a vocation but was "accorded a place of honor and respect, associated as it was with one of the primary messages of Jesus: to love one's neighbor" (O'Brien, 2008, p. 25). Jesus empirically validated the importance of caring for the sick as manifested through His many healings recorded in the Gospels: the cure of the royal official's son (John 4:46–54), the raising of Jairus' daughter (Luke 8:40–42), the healing of Peter's mother-in-law (Luke 4:38–39), the cure of the bent-over woman (Luke 13:10–17), the cleansing of a leper (Luke 5:12–16), and many others (O'Brien, 2006, pp. 30–31). It has been estimated that the healing narratives comprise over a third of all the Gospel stories (Wilkenson, 1998).

Jesus' teaching also significantly influenced the care of the sick by emphasizing the "brotherhood of man, thus giving a new dignity to humanity and making all men responsible for the care of the needy" (Walsh, 1929, p. 1). The Christian philosophy was for all persons to "help each other and to give special consideration to the poor, seeing Christ in them. The early Christians exemplified a consciousness that they belonged to one great family and were truly 'members of one another'" (Sellew & Nuesse, 1946, p. 68). And the "practical test of the new faith was not to be ministered unto but to minister" (Stewart & Austin, 1962, p. 38)

It is important to note that Jesus admonished His followers to go out and *cure the sick* (Matthew 10:5–10) and to *care for the ill* (Matthew 25:36). Christian nurses receive their "professional commission directly from the Lord" (O'Brien, 2006, p. 30). Nurse historian Josephine Dolan asserted that Jesus provided the example for Christian nurses as to how to care for those who are ill: "Instead of saying the word and healing the sick, Christ gave individual attention to the needs of all by touching, anointing, and taking the hand" (1973, p. 47). Dolan added "the least gesture of human kindness" was important to Jesus and "even a cup of cold water given in His name did not pass unrewarded" (p. 47). "Thus, Christ in His own ministry of healing and teaching prepared the way for His followers to serve, with care and tenderness, the needs of their ill brothers and sisters" (O'Brien, 2008, p. 25).

Jesus taught His disciples to place "great emphasis, not only on tending the sick in their own households but also on the duty to ... seek out sick strangers and minister unto them" (Pavey, 1952, p. 94). Several nurse historians have pointed out that Jesus' parable of the "Good Samaritan" (Luke 10:25–37) demonstrated the importance He placed on service to the sick and injured stranger as a virtue to be embraced by His followers (Walsh, 1929; Jamieson & Sewall, 1954; Seymer, 1949). The ideal of Christian charity "inspired many hundreds and even thousands of men and women ... to devote their entire lives to the single object of assisting others. Nursing with such an ideal as motivation would carry greater prestige and become more important than it had been earlier" (Bullough & Bullough, 1997, p. 11).

In Christianity, Sister Charles Marie Frank asserts, "Nursing as an organized service to society had its inception and development" (1959, p. 60). This thought is echoed by M. Patricia Donahue in the comment: "Christ's teachings of love and brotherhood transformed not only society at large but also the development of nursing. 'Organized nursing' was a direct response to these teachings and epitomized the concept of pure altruism initiated by the early Christians" (1996, p. 74).

It is asserted that "there is little evidence that any organized group of women nurses existed before the Christian era; ideals such as service, charity, and self-sacrifice, derived from Christian teaching, now supported "groups of workers whose main function was to care for the sick and the needy" (Deloughery, 1977, p. 5).

In their book *Lead Like Jesus,* current scholars of servant leadership Ken Blanchard and Phil Hodges advise that Christians who seek to be servant leaders must be "willing to follow Jesus as (their) leadership role model" (2005, p. 11). "The call by Jesus to servant leadership" they assert, "is clear and unequivocal. His words leave no room for plan B.... For followers of Jesus, servant leadership isn't an option; it's a mandate. Servant leadership is to be a living statement of who we are in Christ, how we treat one another, and how we demonstrate the love of Christ to the whole world" (p. 12).

NURSE SERVANT LEADERS OF THE EARLY CHRISTIAN ERA

During the early years following the advent of Christianity, many follow-ers of Jesus took on the mantle of servant leadership in terms of caring for those who were sick and suffering. Notable among these servant leaders were the deacons and deaconesses appointed to serve the community of the young Christian church, Roman matrons who had converted to Christianity following the death of a spouse, and a variety of other altru-istic men and women who chose to give their lives in service of the sick.

Veronica of Jerusalem (First Century AD): Parish Nursing

The heroism and courage of these early nursing servant leaders is, I believe, initially reflected in the actions of the holy woman Veronica of Jerusalem, who according to legend was present during Christ's painful journey to Calvary and who cleansed His bleeding face with her veil. As described by Franciscan Matthew Miller "Veronica, a woman, risking the physical punishment of the guards, bravely broke through their ranks and with tender, womanly sympathy wiped the bleeding countenance of the Master" (1954, p. 19).

In my heart I have always thought of Veronica as a nurse. I believe that only one deeply imbued with the calling to provide care for the sick and suffering would have had the courage and the compassion to step out of an anonymous crowd, risking the wrath of spear-wielding Roman soldiers, to comfort her injured rabbi. I view Veronica as a servant leader among parish nurses, for she might well be considered a member of Jesus' first congregation of followers in Jerusalem. Her nursing activity of wiping the Lord's face was a comfort measure carried out to support and console the leader of her newly created parish community.

In looking at the older nursing literature, one finds that Veronica is frequently cited as a model for nurses, including a 1939 editorial in *The Trained Nurse and Hospital Review* in which Veronica is extolled as a nurs-ing example (Heyward, p. 346) and a 1953 article that encourages nurses to care for patients even as Veronica cared for her Lord (The Nurse's Mass, p. 54). Two 1954 articles both describe Veronica as the nurse's role model (Miller, p. 20; Hawley, p. 17). A 1958 article, describing the nurse as a "modern Veronica," suggests that nurses should show their patients the "compassion which Veronica showed to Christ on the *Via Dolorosa*" (Meyer, p. 47). Several articles published in the 1960s demonstrated simi-lar themes. One author pointed out that on the journey to Calvary "no one offered Jesus physical comfort except Veronica.... Could it be that she was experienced in giving care to those who suffered?" (Ridgway, 1960, p. 67). Another paper asserted that Veronica was the model for "our public health nurses" (George, 1964, p. 57).

In her 1978 nursing history, Josephine Dolan asserted that nursing practice was indeed fostered by the examples of early caregivers such as Veronica who wiped the face of Jesus and who "will be recorded for all time for (her) example in comforting the afflicted" (p. 49). Finally, British spiritual writer Caryll Houselander pointed out that it was Veronica's compassion that inspires the "Veronicas of today." Nurses were identified as such contemporary "Veronicas" by Houselander: "Nurses who comfort the dying in hospitals ... who go into the homes of the sick and the poor to serve" (1955, p. 69).

Several years ago I searched the literature attempting to find documentation of the legend of Veronica of Jerusalem. While she is not identified in any of the four gospels formally accepted into the canon of scripture, there is a woman named Veronica (*vera icon,* meaning true image) noted in an apocryphal (hidden) text entitled *The Gospel of Nicodemus* (Schneemelcher, 1963, p. 457). And, in a 1984 text on the apocryphal works, a passage from a 14th-century French Bible is cited that describes Jesus as passing a holy woman named Veronica, who, upon seeing His suffering, used her veil to wipe His bleeding face (Ford, p. 6).

In seeking to determine if Veronica's simple action of wiping the Lord's bleeding and perspiring face had relevance for today's nurses, I asked a group of newly practicing nurses whether their experiences of wiping or washing a patient's face contained a spiritual dimension reflective of Veronica's act. A few examples of the young nurses' powerful and poignant responses reflect the spiritual meaning of the caregiving activity:

> Washing a patient's face makes me think of Jesus telling His disciples "Whatever you do for the least of my people, you do for me." This is just one way, through one small gesture, that I may do as I would for Jesus. When I wash someone's face all of the normal boundaries are dissolved. Their need for my care creates a spiritual relationship. To do this out of love and respect is a very beautiful connection between two human beings; "For whoever does this for the least of these does so for me." (O'Brien, 2003, p. 106)

> To wash a patient's face may seem like a little thing, but it is the little things done with great love, that make a difference with God. (p. 107)

Washing a patient's face shows the patient how much you
care about their comfort and brings you closer to the true
personality.... That's when the spiritual part comes in ... the
reverence for their life. (p. 107)

Whether the legend of the holy woman Veronica is accurate in
all of its details or not, the image of a caring, compassionate woman,
brave enough to step out of a group of curious onlookers to comfort
her wounded spiritual leader, whom some considered a criminal, is a
magnificent guide for nurses, especially those engaged in contemporary
parish or congregational nursing.

Phoebe (58 AD): District Nursing

Phoebe, a deaconess of the early Church, has been described by nurse
historians as the first "visiting nurse" and also as "the first district nurse."
Describing Phoebe's deaconess role, historian Minnie Goodnow observed
that "From her time, visiting nursing has been done in one form or
another in all civilized countries" (1916, p. 22). Phoebe's diaconate was
first identified in scripture by St. Paul who wrote to the Roman Christian
community: "I commend to you our sister Phoebe, a deacon of the church
at Cenchreae, so that you may welcome her in the Lord as is fitting for
the saints, and help her in whatever way she may require from you, for
she has been a benefactor of many and myself as well" (Romans 16:1–2).
While Paul does not specify Phoebe's activities, historians argue that her
work as an early woman deacon of the church must have included visiting and nursing the sick in their homes, "suggestive of the role played
by our visiting nurses today" (Dietz & Lehozky, 1967, p. 23), as this was
a key activity for female deacons of the time. It is believed that Phoebe
spent a significant amount of time in nursing the sick poor who were
unable to leave their homes (Grippando, 1986, p. 4).

In their comprehensive four-volume history of nursing, M. Adelaide
Nutting and Lavinia Dock reinforced the concept of Phoebe's early servant leadership in nursing:

She was the first parish worker, friendly visitor and district
nurse and from her day the work of visiting nursing has never
been unknown. Converts to the primitive church ... regarded
it as a sacred duty to comfort the afflicted; it was the special
duty of the deaconess to attend the sick in their own homes.
(1935, p. 102)

It should be noted that the title of deacon or deaconess (*diakonos* in Greek) is translated as servant. The deacons and deaconesses of the early church were "considered to be the 'servants' of the poor and needy in the best sense of that word" (Walsh, 1929, p. 3). Thus, Deaconess Phoebe can indeed be considered the first servant leader among visiting nurses.

Helena (AD 250–330): Gerontological Nursing

Helena, a Roman matron, and mother of the Emperor Constantine, under whose influence she was converted to Christianity, is described as having devoted her life to the care of the sick poor after her husband's death. Helena established a number of shelters for individuals who sought to visit the holy land. She is described as being possessed of both "unusual ability as well as sanctity" (Frank, 1959, p. 65), and is believed to have found "relics of the True Cross" (Dolan, 1963, p. 72).

Helena supported the sick poor both financially and through her nursing care. Her special concern, however, was related to the needs of the aged and infirm sick poor, and she is reported to have started the first Roman "nursing home" for elders, described at the time as a *gerokomion* (Dolan, 1973). She "encouraged nurses to become specially skilled in what we would now identify as gerontological nursing" (Dolan, Fitzpatrick, & Herrmann, 1983, pp. 46–47). Thus, Helena became a servant leader in gerontological nursing well before the term was familiar to the professional nursing community.

Paula (AD 347–404): Hospice Nursing

Frank identifies another Roman matron, Paula, as having founded the first hospice for pilgrims (1959). As one of a "renowned group of Roman matrons," Paula was also one of the "most learned women of her time" (Frank, p. 73). According to history, Paula, during her lifetime, built numerous hospices along major roads of the time for those who became ill and/or close to death while traveling. Saint Jerome is reported to have written of her:

> She was piteous to them that were sick and comforted and served them humbly…. She was oft by them that were sick, and she laid their pillows aright; and … she rubbed their feet and boiled water to wash them. And it seemed to her that the less she did to the sick in service, so much the less service did she to God. (Nutting & Dock, 1935, p. 141)

Paula worked as a nurse and as a servant in her hospices (Nutting & Dock, p. 141). In the hospices "she served personally the sick. Some have regarded her as the first to teach nursing as a distinct art rather than as a generalized service to the poor" (Sellew & Nuesse, 1946, p. 75). Jerome outlived "famous Roman Patrician nurses" such as Paula; after her death, he wrote an "inspiring tribute to Paula's benignity and goodness" (Nutting & Dock, p. 142).

While the 4th-century concept of "hospice" was somewhat different from what the contemporary healthcare system understands in using the term *hospice*, the underlying philosophy remains. The hospice of the early Christian era was a place of rest, comfort, care, and security for traveling pilgrims, especially those who were seriously ill or dying. Today's hospices are also places of rest, comfort, care, and security for those traveling on a final journey from this world to eternal life. Paula's servant leadership in hospice nursing remains a sterling witness for current hospice nurses.

Radegonde (AD 519–587): Monastic Nursing

Radegonde, who was both daughter of a Thuringian king and had been married to a king who was massacred, ultimately devoted her life to the care of the sick and needy. She founded Holy Cross Monastery within whose walls she took the sick poor, especially lepers, to care for them (Goodnow, 1916). Radegonde's monastic community grew to over 200 sisters, who she inspired and trained to follow her in the care of the ill and the infirm. In Radegonde's monastery "the care of the sick was the chief activity. . . . Radegonde bathed the patients herself, giving special care to the lepers" (Dolan, Fitzpatrick, & Herrmann, 1983, p. 47). Her example led many other women "of noble birth to care for the sick" (Dolan, Fitzpatrick, & Herrmann, p. 48).

Today's monasteries generally include an infirmary, where only their own ill or aged members are cared for. Abbess Radegonde's 6th-century servant leadership in admitting noncommunity members to be cared for within the monastery setting set a precedent for the establishment of early hospitals such as the great *Hôtels-Dieu* of Lyon (AD 542) and Paris (AD 650), many of which were completely staffed by monastic nurses. Nurse historian Minnie Goodnow also pointed out that since "there appeared to have been no physicians in Thuringia, Radegonde prescribed as well as tended the sick" (1916, p. 22). Thus, Radegonde of Thuringia was a servant leader nurse practitioner of her era as well as a monastic nurse.

Dymphna of Belgium (AD 605–620): Psychiatric and Mental Health Nursing

Although she died at the age of only 15, Dymphna of Belgium might indeed be considered the first identified servant leader in the area of psychiatric and mental health nursing. While accounts of Dymphna's life and emigration to Belgium vary somewhat in details, certain points emerge repeatedly in the literature.

Dymphna is described as a beautiful only daughter of a pagan Irish king and a Christian mother. The king, grief stricken at the loss of his wife to illness, became mentally unstable. It was reported that the king desired to take Dymphna as a replacement for his lost wife, and in seeking to escape the possibility of incest, she fled to Gheel, Belgium, seeking refuge. Dymphna was followed by her enraged father and ultimately beheaded by him when she refused to return to Ireland.

In his 1929 *History of Nursing*, physician James Walsh, observed that, on arriving in Belgium, Dymphna immediately undertook the work of assisting Irish missionaries in working with the "Teutonic barbarians" who had moved to the country from the north. "She took a great deal of interest in their children (especially) those that were half-witted or feeble minded" (p. 98). Dymphna has also been described as having a deep concern for adults who were mentally ill, and she had a special gift for caring for them in their illnesses. It is suggested that this may have been related to her experiences with her own father's grief-imposed madness.

Walsh noted that although Dymphna did not live long enough to formally establish medical and nursing care for the mentally ill in Belgium, "the blood of the martyr proved to be the seed of Christians." The Belgian women were certain that even after her death "Dymphna would be interested in their children," so they brought the disturbed children to a shrine erected to honor her (Walsh, p. 98). Walsh added that the Belgian people "did not expect a cure to take place all at once so they left the children near the shrine to be cared for by neighboring families." "This," he concluded "represented the beginning of an important movement for the care of the insane (sic) in families, which has continued ever since" (pp. 98–99).

Historians Dolan, Fitzpatrick, and Herrmann reported that, soon after Dymphna's death in Gheel, accounts of "miraculous cures, especially of those who were mentally ill and emotionally disturbed" abounded, and relatives began to bring ill family members to Dymphna's tomb in hopes of healing (1983, p. 59). A shrine and church were built in Dymphna's honor and also a building to house the mentally ill pilgrims.

As the number of pilgrims grew, however, the *Chambre des malades* could not accommodate all of the ill, and "the housewives of Gheel accepted these patients as boarders and as foster members of their families" (Dolan, Fitzpatrick, & Herrmann, 1983, p. 59).

This practice of hospitality for the mentally ill, the forerunner of deinstitutionalization for psychiatric patients, continued for centuries, and the Gheel community ultimately was granted it's own mental health facility to oversee the community's family foster care. This facility, the State Psychiatric Hospital Center for Family Care, was placed under supervision of the Belgian government (Matheussen, Morren, & Seyers, 1975, p. 1). Gheel's foster family care has become a model for home health care of the mentally ill, grounded in the fact that "the people of Gheel have learned from childhood to live with the patients; their reception and care have been passed on from generation to generation" (Foster family care in Gheel, 1991, p. 15). In Gheel, it is said, the mentally ill have never been shunned or stigmatized. They are accepted as full members of the community.

It seems both appropriate and acceptable to label the young Dymphna a servant leader in the arena of psychiatric nursing for her witness of caring for the mentally ill, which led to the foster family care system in Gheel; the system remains functional today. This is reflected in two recent articles on the Gheel system of deinstitutionalization published in scholarly journals. In 2003, the *Community Health Journal* published a paper entitled "The Legend and Lessons of Gheel, Belgium: A 1500 Year Old Legend, a 21st Century Model," which explains how the Gheel foster family care system for mental patients provides a model case study that can help other communities "identify significant factors that contribute to successful community mental health programs" (Goldstein & Godemont, 2003, p. 1). In a 2007 article on deinstitutionalization for the mentally ill, the author points out that "the oldest example of community care for mental patients, the historic colony for mental patients in Gheel, Belgium" contains important lessons for contemporary mental health care (Tuntiya, 2007, p. 1).

NURSE SERVANT LEADERS OF THE MIDDLE AGES

Peter Gerard (1050–1120): Military Nursing

Peter Gerard, sometimes labeled Blessed Gerard, has been described alternately as a monk and/or an "intensely devout" layman (Jensen, Spaulding, & Cady, 1959, p. 73). His canonical status notwithstanding, Peter Gerard is identified as the founder of the most significant military order of the 11th century, the Knights Hospitallers of St. John of Jerusalem.

The hospitaller military orders were those nursing communities of men called forth by the needs of the injured crusaders of the era. The crusaders were considered to be in the service of God "ready to fight the infidel wherever he was to be found so that the holy ground on which Christ trod might again belong to His followers" (Deloughery, 1977, p. 11). It was recognized at the time that large numbers of crusaders wounded in battle would need care not only on the battlefields and in the military camps but also in hospitals on their return from combat.

There were three different ranks of hospitaller order members, all of whom took vows of poverty, chastity, and obedience, and wore a distinctive habit consisting of a black robe with a white linen cross having 8 points "symbolic of the eight beatitudes" that the knights were to live by (Nutting & Dock, 1935, p. 181). These beatitudes were spiritual joy, to live without malice, to weep over thy sins, to humble thyself to those who injure thee, to love justice, to be merciful, to be sincere and pure of heart, and to suffer persecution" (Donahue, 1996, p. 126). The hospitallers were considered a "religious fraternity formally abjuring the world, and dedicated themselves at the altar as servants of the poor and of Christ" (Nutting & Dock, 1935, p. 181). Nurse historian Anne Austin cites from the Rule of the Order written by the first Master General Raymond du Puy:

> I ordain that all the brethren engaging in the service of the sick shall keep with God's help the three promises that they have made to God … poverty, chastity, obedience … and to live without any property of their own because God will require of them at the last judgment the fulfillment of these three promises. (1957, p. 73)

The three groups of hospitallers were the "knights" who went into the battlefield to care for seriously wounded crusaders, the "priests" who were ordained to provide for the spiritual needs of the ill crusaders, and the "serving brothers" (*freres sergents*) whose primary responsibility was nursing in hospitals founded to serve recovering crusaders (Pavey, 1952, pp. 163–164; Seymer, 1949, p. 40).

Peter Gerard is reported by historians as having founded the Knights Hospitallers of St. John around 1070 AD. A particular role for the early community members was care of the crusaders in a hospital in Jerusalem (Seymer, 1949). The hospital, guided by the patronage of St. John, was placed under the directorship of Blessed Peter Gerard (Dolan, Fitzpatrick, & Herrmann, 1983, p. 63).

Blessed Peter Gerard may not have been formally trained as a nurse, but his life commitment as director of one of the first and most important hospitaller communities well equips him to be described as a distinguished servant leader in military nursing. What a superb legacy Blessed Gerard left for military nurses of this century.

Hildegard of Bingen (1098–1179): Infirmary Nursing

Hildegard of Bingen, an important nurse leader of the 12th century, was as a young child given over to the care and mentorship of an anchoress, Jutta, living within a large Benedictine monastery (Dolan, 1978). As Hildegard grew into young adulthood she undertook the nursing of the sick in the monastery infirmary. Within a short time Hildegard's reputation as a nurse and healer grew notably, and the ill began flocking to the monastery to experience Hildegard's ministrations. Ultimately Hildegard took religious vows as a Benedictine nun and founded her own monastery where her nursing and her writing about nursing-related topics flourished.

Hildegard wrote two works based on all that she had learned during her work with the sick in the monastery infirmaries. These were entitled *Liber Simplicis Medicinae* and *Liber Compositae Medicinae,* which included "the general diseases of the human body and their causes, symptoms and treatment" as well as general physiology and psychology (Dolan, Fitzpatrick, & Herrmann, 1983, p. 77). Another medical book by Hildegard was *Liber Operum Simplicis Hominis,* "which was concerned with anatomical and physiological subjects" (Donahue, 1996, p. 147).

Hildegard's works lay ignored for many centuries until some German Benedictine sisters translated her writings in the 1960s. Currently Hildegard's wisdom and contributions to nursing are widely recognized, especially her awareness of the body-mind-spirit connection. "This concept is most timely in light of our present-day emphasis on holistic health care, uniting rather than isolating the needs and problems of body, mind, and spirit" (O'Brien, 2008, p. 33).

Catherine of Siena (1347–1380): Community Health Nursing

Catherine of Siena, a 14th-century Dominican tertiary, is identified by many contemporary nurses as the "Patroness of Nursing." While Catherine is sometimes extolled as a scholar and advisor to theologians, it was her care for the sick poor, especially lepers and those who became ill during the period of the European Black Plague, that superbly equips her to be a servant leader role model for contemporary community health nurses.

During the plague years, Catherine "organized groups of young men as stretcher bearers to transport the stricken from all over the city to the wards of the hospital, which she supervised" (Donahue, 1996, p. 136). Throughout the epidemic it was reported that Catherine "could be seen going about the streets of Siena at night. With a lighted lantern she would look for forsaken victims so that she might comfort them" (Dolan, Fitzpatrick, & Herrmann, 1983, p. 72). Catherine is also described by historians Nutting and Dock as having "walked night and day in the (hospital) wards, only resting a few hours now and then in an adjacent house" (1935, p. 230).

Physician and nursing historian James Walsh wrote of the spiritual nature of Catherine's ministry to the sick:

> According to ... legend, her devotion to the ailing poor was so pleasing to the Master, who had gone about healing the ailing, that she had a number of visits (from) ... Christ ... (who) put a ring on her finger as an indication that she was to be His heavenly spouse (1929, pp. 121–122).

And, an appreciation of Catherine, written in 1853, by Blessed Raymond of Capua asserted, "Catherine was wonderfully compassionate to the wants of the poor, but her heart was even more sensitive to the sufferings of the sick" (Austin, 1957, p. 94).

Catherine of Siena might well be identified as a servant leader in the area of community health nursing for her commitment and care of those suffering from contagious diseases of the time such as leprosy, and especially for her leadership role in organizing workers to carry plague sufferers from their homes and the streets to the hospital for care. Catherine never feared for her own health but only for that of her brothers and sisters in the Siena community.

NURSE SERVANT LEADERS OF THE POST-REFORMATION ERA

Following the religious reformation of the early 16th century, a number of nursing communities and movements emerged to meet the needs of the sick, especially the sick poor, in both cities and urban areas. Within these groups, there were significant nursing leaders who may well be described as servant leaders of their respective communities. While the choice of individuals is significantly limited by time and space, nine key servant leaders are here identified as ministering in hospital nursing, missionary nursing, professional nursing, Red Cross nursing, academic nursing, trauma nursing, public health nursing, frontier nursing, and combat nursing. It is recognized that many other nursing servant leaders can be identified during the time period from the 1500s to the 1900s. Some are well known to the nursing community; others' names were recorded only in the hearts of those they served. The latter were servant leaders, nonetheless, and while not individually identified by the professional nursing community, they are indeed remembered by the One who alone calls each person by name.

Camillus De Lellis (1550–1614): Hospital Nursing

Camillus De Lellis is especially known as a servant leader for his founding of a religious community of men, the Nursing Order of Ministers of the Sick. They are sometimes called the "Camillans" who cared for the sick in hospitals. As with Catherine of Siena, Camillus and his community cared for plague victims in Italy. Camillus' community is notably identified with hospital nursing at the renowned Santo Spirito hospital in Italy.

Camillus De Lellis had been a soldier whose leg was seriously injured in battle. After the injury Camillus went to the San Giacomo Hospital in Rome to seek treatment for his leg; being poor at the time, he offered to work at the institution in return for his care. It is reported that he remained at the hospital for four years "finally receiving an appointment as superintendent of the servants, which in that period included nurses — all male" (Dolan, 1963, p. 150). As Camillus recognized the value of loving service to the sick, he encouraged others to join him in forming a religious community of men to serve the ill and injured. Camillus was ordained a priest prior to founding the community.

One of Camillus' first goals was "directed toward preparing and providing hospital nurses" (Dolan, Fitzpatrick, & Herrmann, 1983, p. 96). While Camillus also sent his nurses to minister to the sick poor in the streets and to military troops, he was always committed to those who were hospitalized because of his early experiences in hospital nursing at San Giacomo. When living in Rome he and his community served as nurses at Santo Spirito each day. It was reported that "A visitor (to Santo Spirito) one day asked Camillus if he did not find the noises and the odors of the hospital trying. 'Trying!,' he exclaimed. 'There is no music sweeter to me than the voices of the sick, all clamoring at once to be assisted; no perfume more delicious than the odor of drugs and ointments that bring relief to the sick" (A Sister of Mercy, 1917, p. 97).

Surely Camillus De Lellis, with his love and concern for those hospitalized for their illnesses and injuries, which led to the founding of a nursing community dedicated to hospital nursing, may be identified as a servant leader for today's hospital nurses. Most nurses, regardless of our current roles, have had some experience in hospital nursing. Thus, we are deeply aware of the care and commitment it took for Camillus to embrace with love the "noises and odors of the hospital," especially the hospital of the Middle Ages.

Vincent de Paul (1580–1660): Home Care Nursing

While Vincent de Paul was not himself engaged in full-time care of the sick, he was founder of a community of religious sisters, the Daughters of Charity, one of whose primary ministries was nursing of the sick in their homes. Nurse historians Nutting and Dock devote an entire chapter in their classic four-volume history of nursing to "Saint Vincent de Paul and the Daughters of Charity" (1935). Nutting and Dock point out that although not himself a nurse, early on in his ministry, Vincent settled near a charity hospital in France run by the nursing Brothers of St. John of God, asking to assist as a volunteer. Nutting and Dock add: "Hither came Vincent every morning to dress wounds and to wait upon the patients" (1935, p. 406).

It was during this period of volunteer nursing that Vincent became acutely aware of the many sick poor confined to their homes with no one to care for them. And it was thus that Vincent gathered a small band of women, initially calling them the Ladies of Charity, whose mission was to visit and care for the sick poor in their homes. As observed by Vincentian Father Robert Maloney, Vincent's vision of ministry was focused on following the "liberation which Christ brings to the poor" (1992, p. 25); thus, he admonished his followers that they should "cherish the poor as their masters, since Our Lord is in them and they in Our Lord" (pp. 26–27). Vincent continually reflected the servant leadership characteristic of giving of yourself in his philosophy of "living and dying in the service of the poor" (Maloney, 1995, p. 52).

In 1633, the Ladies of Charity were formally established as a religious community, labeled the Daughters of Charity, with one of the women, Mlle. Le Gras, later known as Louise de Marillac, as the superior. Saint Louise became the guide and teacher of the new Daughters of Charity. As described by nurse historian Josephine Dolan "She would give the Dames de Charite instructions. She accompanied them on their rounds, helping them, advising them, assisting them in their duties, and making suggestions about other ways of giving care to patients" (1973, p. 100).

Vincent de Paul's institution of the Daughters of Charity was a revolutionary concept in terms of women's religious communities of the era. Previously, women religious remained cloistered in their convents. Vincent, however, asked his sisters to leave their convents to go wherever they were needed in the care of the sick and the poor. Citing a conference of Saint Vincent de Paul to the Filles de la Charite, Nutting and Dock report that the founder commented: "You are not religious in the strict sense, and can never be because of the service to the poor.... You have no grating to set you off from the dangers of the world; you must erect one in your own inner self, which will be far better" (1935, p. 423). The importance of Vincent's teaching in this regard is evidenced in a now famous quote from the Daughters of Charity rule: "Your convent will be the house of the sick; your cell, a hired room; your chapel, the parish church; your cloister, the streets of the city, or the wards of the hospital" (Daughters of Charity, 1993). Nutting and Dock noted that when it was suggested to Vincent that the Daughters of Charity, who dressed in the garb of the day, wear a veil as other sisters, he replied: "Modesty is their veil" (1935, p. 423). In her book, *Nursing, the Finest Art*, historian M. Patricia Donahue asserts that the Daughters of Charity "became widely known as visiting nurses, since they ... cared for the poor and the sick in their homes" (Donahue, 1996, p. 186).

Jeanne Mance (1606–1673): Missionary Nursing

Jeanne Mance, although born into an aristocratic French family, became early in life concerned about those who were poor and sick. She was initially taught nursing of the sick in 1638 when she became a member of a ladies organization formed to care for the ill during a severe epidemic near her home in France (Dolan, 1978, p. 99). Jeanne had for some years been touched by the stories she had heard of the needs of settlers in the New World or New France, as Canada was sometimes referred to. Thus, in 1641 she accepted, with the support of a wealthy French woman, the mission to travel to Montreal, Canada, to teach nursing and to build a hospital. This facility was to provide care for both new world colonists and also for the Iroquois Indians (Dolan, 1978).

During her missionary work, Jeanne returned several times to France to recruit nursing sisters to help care for the sick in Canada. The sisters' mission was to "staff the Hotel Dieu in Montreal with Jeanne Mance as administrator" (Dolan, Fitzpatrick, & Herrmann, 1983, p. 98).

The establishment of this hospital is described by Patricia Donahue as "the story of Jeanne Mance, a romantic figure in Canadian nursing" (1996, pp. 221–222). On first arriving in the New World, Donahue notes that missionary Jeanne Mance began her nursing in a "tiny cottage hospital inside the (settlers') fort (where) she tended to men wounded by (Iroquois Indians') arrows' (p. 222). Donahue adds: "She compounded her own medicines, treated chilblains and frostbite, practiced bloodletting, and cared for the Iroquois Indians as well as the colonists" (p. 222).

In this small hospital Jeanne Mance nursed the sick for close to 15 years. "She earned the reputation of being the 'first lay nurse of Canada' and of North America as well" (Donahue, 1996, p. 225). Following this period of her nursing, Jeanne moved to the more spacious Hotel Dieu where she also faithfully served the sick of the area until her death in 1673. Although she was not a vowed religious, as a missionary nurse, Jeanne Mance is reported to have sought to spread the Christian faith among the Indians. She cared not only for their bodies but also for their souls.

History has not left us a record of the many fears, anxieties, and general difficulties Jeanne must have experienced in the ministry, but one can indeed guess that her mission to the New World must not have been easy for one born into wealth and comfort. Yet, Jeanne returned home to France on only a few occasions, and those trips were made only to recruit others to help with her nursing ministry. The life of servant leader and missionary nurse Jeanne Mance provides inspiration, support, and guidance for today's missionary nurses throughout the world.

Florence Nightingale (1820–1910): Professional Nursing

It is difficult to describe the servant leadership of Florence Nightingale, the founder of professional nursing, in a few paragraphs. From the time she was young Florence felt called to serve others; her vocational call to care for the sick was said to have occurred even before her 17th birthday (Selanders, 1993, p. 8). Florence was a deeply spiritual and prayerful woman and was inspired by the nursing ministries of both the Daughters of Charity and the Kaiserswerth Deaconesses whom she wished to imitate (Dolan, 1973, p. 167) and with whom she studied nursing.

Florence's desire for service, in the form of nursing the sick, was not viewed favorably by her family, yet she never wavered in moving toward that goal. This desire was supported not by human encouragement but by Florence's trust in the greatness of God as her source of strength and "Spirit of Truth" (Widerquist, 1992, p. 49). She "pursued a mission of service to humanity throughout her lifetime" (Donahue, 1996, p. 198).

Florence Nightingale is, of course, especially remembered as a servant leader who not only cared for the wounded soldiers in the Crimea but who also taught and modeled for a cadre of nurses who accompanied

her in both the art and the science of skilled nursing. Many were the acco-
lades awarded by the British government for her leadership and selfless
commitment in coping with the dreadful conditions she and her nurses
faced in the Crimean mission.

Florence's servant leadership in establishing professional nursing,
however, was her greatest gift to those who would follow her. In the
words of nurse historians "Miss Nightingale was the originator of the
concept of the nursing process. She insisted that prepared and educated
persons were necessary to function properly in the nurse's role" (Dolan,
Fitzpatrick, & Herrmann, 1983, p. 165). To that end she established the
first training school for nurses at St. Thomas Hospital in London and
authored a book entitled *Notes on Nursing* that laid out the basic principles of good physical and psychological nursing care for the ill person.
Such an educational thrust for nursing the sick provided a radical depar-
ture from the earlier concept of nursing being carried out by less than
desirable women who were not trained to do anything else. Florence
Nightingale single-handedly elevated nursing to a profession, consisting
of its own unique art and science.

Perhaps one of the greatest legacies that Florence Nightingale's
servant leadership left to the professional nursing community was a deep
and abiding faith in God and in the human person as a temple of God's
spirit. These beliefs are evidenced in her oft-quoted mandate:

> Nursing is an art; and if it is to be made an art, it requires as
> exclusive a devotion, as hard a preparation, as any painter's or
> sculptor's work. For what is the having to do with dead can-
> vas or cold marble compared with having to do with the living
> body—the temple of God's spirit? (Baly, 1991, p. 68)

Clara Barton (1821–1912): Red Cross Nursing

Although not herself a professional nurse with the training of Florence
Nightingale, Clara Barton was surely a nursing servant leader in her
founding of the important ministry of Red Cross nursing. Barton did, however, have an interest in caring for the sick from childhood, and as an adult
she worked to organize supplies to be provided for soldiers wounded in
the Civil War. It is reported that "when the Sixth Massachusetts Regiment
arrived in Washington on April 19, 1961, she was there to feed them and
dress their wounds" (Dolan, Fitzpatrick, & Herrmann, 1983, p. 173). Barton
also "personally nursed in federal hospitals and with armies on the battle-
field and cared for the wounded of the Confederate Army. Her impartiality

was expressed in the nursing care she extended (to all)" (Donahue, 1996, p. 255). Donahue asserts that Clara Barton's work "embodies the ideals now characteristic of the Red Cross" (p. 255), which she founded in United States in 1882. Clara "became (the Red Cross's) first president and held this office until 1904" (Donahue, 1996, p. 257).

Ultimately because of her "heroism in caring for the wounded under fire during the Civil War, and her later founding of the American National Red Cross," Clara Barton was labeled the "Angel of the Battle-field" (Deming, 1969, p. 23). In the early days of the war there were few physicians available to care for the wounded soldiers, and Barton is described as having stepped into that gap:

> Solely, as an individual, with no organization behind her, she raised volunteer nurses and supplies and drove her wagon trains to wherever the battle was raging. She and her fellow workers bandaged and nursed thousands of fallen soldiers in the midst of battle, often with shells bursting around them. (Deming, 1969, p. 25)

Barton was a servant leader of the highest order in serving those who were most in need of nursing care, compassion, and comfort. Her legacy is truly that of service in leadership, which has been, and will continue to be, modeled for centuries by Red Cross nurses who follow in her footsteps.

Isabel Hampton Robb (1859–1910): Nursing Education

Isabel Hampton Robb, perhaps the foremost servant leader of her era in nursing education, began her career as a teacher. After a brief time, however, she decided to undertake a nursing ministry and enrolled in the Bellevue Hospital Nurses' Training School in New York City. After graduating and working in several hospital-related positions, Hampton Robb was asked to become principal of the newly created Johns Hopkins School of Nursing.

In her role as principal at Johns Hopkins, Hampton Robb intro-duced a number of innovations into the education and practice of nurs-ing, including more time for the students to rest, study, recreate, and eat. "Her aim," which Dolan asserts "she had the ability and the persistence to achieve, was quality nursing care that combined a happy balance of intellectual and manual skills" (1978, p. 211). Hampton Robb's most important goal was to increase the quality of care for patients through the ministrations of well-educated and well-rounded graduate nurses.

Related to her desire to improve the quality of professional nursing care, she authored the important textbook for students, *Nursing: Its Principles and Practice for Hospital and Private Use* (1884). Hampton Robb later wrote two additional books for nurses: *Nursing Ethics* (1900) and *Educational Standards for Nurses* (1907).

Hampton Robb's penchant for leadership was also reflected in her instrumental involvement in founding several important nursing associations. She became "the first president of the newly formed "Nurses' Associated Alumnae of the United States and Canada, which was a nationwide union of nurse training school alumnae associations" (Dolan, Fitzpatrick, & Herrmann, 1983, p. 211). This organization's name "was changed in 1911 to the American's Nurses' Association" (Dietz & Lehozky, 1967, p. 118). Hampton Robb helped found two organizations to support the development of a graduate nursing program at Teacher's College and "was one of the original members of a committee to found the *American Journal of Nursing*" (Donahue, 1996, p. 321). The journal's success was greatly aided by the "authority and prestige" of Hampton Robb (Deloughery, 1997, p. 97).

Hampton Robb's lifelong commitment to service and excellence in both nursing practice and nursing education support her identity as a caring and innovative servant leader in the early days of nursing's professional and academic development.

Edith Cavell (1865–1915): Trauma Nursing

One of the greatest nursing heroines and servant leaders in trauma nursing during WWI was British nurse Edith Cavell, who trained at the Royal London Hospital. Her father was an Episcopal vicar. In 1907 Edith traveled to Brussels, Belgium, in order to become director of a new school of nursing, *L'Ecole d'Infirmière Dimplonier* (Bullough & Bullough, 1978, p. 124).

When "World War I began in Europe in July, 1914, Miss Cavell was offered a safe conduct to England, but she chose to remain in Brussels, which after 12 years was her home" (Dietz & Lehozky, 1967, p. 147). Nurse historians Dietz and Lehozky report that Cavell "at once made plans to oppose the enemy" (p. 147) after Brussels was captured and occupied by the Germans. However from the beginning of the war her training school-affiliated hospital cared for both allied and German soldiers without discrimination (Dolan, Fitzpatrick, & Herrmann, 1983, p. 293). Many of these soldiers required skilled trauma nursing to survive the wounds of war; Cavell provided this to all brought to her care.

Cavell also, however, began early on to cooperate with underground efforts to try and save the lives of wounded allied soldiers whom the occupation forces planned to either kill or to imprison in forced labor camps when they were well enough to leave the hospital. Edith is reported to have "treated the men alone in the back of the hospital to hide them from the Germans and to protect her nurses … (and) in the evening she went into the village to care for the sick and the injured, becoming known as 'The Poor Man's Nightingale'" (Arthur, 2006, p. 33). Edith also assisted British and French soldiers ready for hospital discharge to escape to England or Holland. "Miss Cavell helped to organize an underground system whereby, when it was time for the soldiers to leave, guides would take them away in the late afternoon or at night in groups of four or five, disguised as laborers and carrying forged identification papers. Since the German guards at the border could not speak French, those crossing the border were seldom questioned" (Dietz & Lehozky, 1967, pp. 147–148).

As more wounded soldiers began to escape, Edith became aware that she was under suspicion of aiding their flight from Belgium by the German commandant of the occupying forces; nevertheless, she did not stop her ministries of both trauma nursing and safe discharge planning. Supporters warned Edith to stop, but she responded "We must go on, for if these men are caught and shot, it would be our fault" (Judson, 1941, p. 232).

Ultimately, Cavell was arrested by the Germans and held in solitary confinement for 10 weeks at the Prison de St. Gilles in Belgium. Despite repeated attempts at intervention from governmental officials of both Britain and the United States, Cavell was sentenced to death for treason, according to the German Military Code: she was "sentenced on the charge that she had given the soldiers shelter and had aided them with money, food and clothing and had further given them medical care when they were ill" (Judson, 1941, p. 263). Cavell did not defend herself; she admitted that she had, in fact, done as accused.

During her last hours in prison, Cavell wrote a letter to her nurses advising "Cultivate among yourselves loyalty and *esprit de corps.*" She also asked forgiveness if anyone had a grievance against her and ended "I loved you much more than you thought" (Judson, 1941, p. 279). Cavell's last recorded words before her death were contained in the assertion: "I have nothing to regret. If I had to do it over again, I would do just as I did…. I know now that patriotism is not enough; I must have no hatred and no bitterness toward anyone" (Judson, p. 276).

Finally, biographer Helen Judson writes, on October 12, 1915, Cavell "was carried away (by the German guards) in the gray dawn … to be shot secretly at the *Tir National* as though she were too dangerous to live" (1941, p. 281). Judson added, "She gave her life that no nurse leaves the school (she directed) untouched by the spirit of service in which Edith Cavell laid the foundation.... They killed her body, but her soul dwells in the school" (pp. 282–283).

Cavell's magnificent servant leadership soul also dwells in the hearts of all nurses today, especially in the hearts of trauma nurses caring for those wounded in battle or other traumatic occurrences.

Lillian Wald (1867–1940): Public Health Nursing

Lillian Wald—nurse, social worker, and advocate for the poor—must be considered the first and most distinguished servant leaders in public health nursing in this country. Lillian, a native New Yorker, graduated from the New York Hospital Nurses Training School in 1891. She had sought nursing education because of her awareness of the myriad health needs of poor immigrants living in the Lower East Side of New York. Wald began to work in the community initially by conducting classes in home nursing for the disenfranchised immigrants (Dolan, 1978, p. 346).

Wald was particularly touched by witnessing the condition of one particular woman living in a run-down tenement on the Lower East Side. While teaching a class one day, she was asked by a child to come with her and help because her mother was very sick. "Lillian followed the girl ... into a rickety tenement at the rear of a narrow alley.... On a crumpled bed, stained with blood and grime, lay the girl's mother. Her face was chalk white and tense with pain. Next to her sat her husband, a lame beggar whose face was lined with sorrow" (Rogow, 1966, p. 28).

After providing basic care, food, and other necessities for the mother and her family, Wald knew that this was where she wanted to both live and serve her neighbors suffering in poverty. She "conceived the idea of establishing a neighborhood nursing service for the sick poor of the Lower East Side.... Her concept was that the nurse's visit should be like that of a very interested friend rather than that of an impersonal paid visitor" (Dolan, Fitzpatrick, & Herrmann, 1983, p. 227). Dolan, Fitzpatrick, and Herrmann add, "The experiment was a success, and the world famous Henry Street Settlement was opened in 1893" (p. 228). This would provide the foundation for the Henry Street Visiting Nurse Service (Dolan, 1978, p. 346). The group ultimately was formalized under the New York City government, and the nurses were given badges to wear that read: "Visiting Nurse, Under the Auspices of the Board of Health" (Rogow, 1966, p. 34).

In envisioning the idea of the visiting nursing service, and public health nursing in general, Wald said to a nurse friend who sought to accompany her, "Let us, two nurses, move into that neighborhood; let us give our service as nurses, and let us contribute our sense of citizenship to what seems an alien group in a so called democratic community" (Duffus, 1939, p. 35). Wald's nurse friend Mary Brewster moved into the community with her, and their public health nursing ministry was born. In the end the activities of the Henry Street Visiting Nurse Service went beyond nursing to include social work and education: "The scope of the settlement went far beyond the care of the sick and the prevention of disease. It aimed at rectifying those causes that were responsible for the poverty and misery itself" (Donahue, 1996, p. 305).

Lillian Wald not only served as nurse, social worker, educator, and researcher but also as author of two books describing her servant leadership: *The House on Henry Street* written in 1911 and *Windows on Henry Street* published in 1934. She left a legacy of care and commitment for the underserved that continues to inspire public health nurses worldwide.

Mary Breckinridge (1881–1965): Frontier Nursing

Surely one of the most important and beloved nursing servant leaders of the early 1900s was Mary Breckinridge, founder of the Frontier Nursing Service in Hayden, Kentucky, in 1928. Mary Breckinridge completed her basic nursing education at St. Luke's Hospital in New York, graduating in 1910. After graduation Mary married and had two children: a daughter who died shortly after birth and a son who died at the age of only four. Following these tragedies Breckinridge decided to dedicate her life to the care of children.

At the close of WWI, Mary volunteered to travel to France with an American nursing committee seeking to assist those devastated by the occupation. During her stay she became acquainted with a number of British-trained nurse–midwives; at that time there was no such education for nurses in the United States. After some consideration, Breckinridge decided to introduce nurse–midwifery to rural areas of America where there was no medical care available for poor mothers and babies. To accomplish this goal, Breckinridge moved to London and trained to become a certified midwife.

At the end of her training Breckinridge returned to the United States and to Leslie County, Kentucky, a poverty-stricken rural area of the state where at the time "medical care was virtually nonexistent, with no hospitals and only one licensed physician to serve the entire area" (Raines

& Wilson, 1996, p. 124). It was here in 1925 that Breckinridge created the "Kentucky Committee for Mothers and Babies ... three years later its name would be changed to the 'Frontier Nursing Service'" (McKown, 1966, p. 175).

Breckinridge and her first frontier nurses traveled on horseback to the mountain hollows as there was no other way to reach the mothers and babies in need. McKown reported that "The first nurse–midwives who came to assist her were recruited from England, since there were none in America" (and many did not know how to ride); thus "every new nurse was advised to take five riding lessons before reporting for duty, so she would know at least how to sit quietly on a horse and hold the reins" (p. 176). Mary and her first frontier nurses visited "hundreds of cabins, delivering babies, providing prenatal care as well as other types of preventive care such as typhoid vaccines, and instructing families in methods to improve the sanitary conditions of their homes" (Raines & Wilson, 1996, p. 125).

In a chapter entitled "Nurses on Horseback," a story is told of a mountaineer husband who made his way to one of the early frontier nursing stations, late on a snowy winter night, to seek help for his wife who was in prolonged labor; he admitted that "they didn't aim to ask the nurse "ride out" in such bad weather. The frontier nurse immediately responded that she would come. She is described as dressed in a "heavy sheepskin coat, boots and breeches" and carrying "forty pound saddle-bags over her shoulder and a layette under one arm" (Poole, 1960, p. 119). The frontier nurse is said to have followed the man on horseback for almost 3 hours along a snow-covered mountain trail to arrive at the log cabin where the laboring mother awaited. But, the author adds, "(The Nurse) took it all as a matter of course. She was used to it. It was part of her job. She'd been out on scores of nights like that. For hers' was one of the nine stations of the Frontier Nursing Service, and that is the kind of service they aimed to give to the mountaineers" (p. 119).

Donahue points out that "Each of the 'nurses on horseback' had certification as a nurse midwife, and the nurses gave antepartal, intrapartal, and postpartal care to the woman of their districts" (1996, p. 311). Breckinridge's goal was to "provide a program of good health care for all persons in an area of severe social and economic deprivation" (Dolan, 1978, p. 358).

Ultimately Breckinridge built a center for frontier nursing in an area near Hayden, Kentucky, and established the first graduate nursing school of midwifery in the country. She had also started a small clinic where seriously ill patients could be cared for. Several years later this was replaced by the Hayden Hospital and Health Center. In the hospital Breckinridge commissioned the construction of Saint Christopher's Chapel containing a stained glass window displaying an image of St. Christopher carrying the Christ child across a stream. The stream, Breckinridge observed was "like ours" (Breckinridge, 1981, p. 362). Breckinridge explained: "If the Frontier Nursing Service had a patron saint, it could be none other than Saint Christopher, on whose help we counted when we carried children on the pommels of our saddles through treacherous fords" (p. 362).

Today Mary Breckinridge's legacy of servant leadership in frontier nursing lives on in the hearts and spirits of the many nurses who have embraced, and continue to embrace her vision. While horses have now been replaced by jeeps, and the Hayden Hospital by the more modern Mary Breckinridge Hospital, today's frontier nurses continue to serve disenfranchised families in the rural mountains of Kentucky.

Geneviève de Galard (1925): Combat Nursing

One of the greatest heroines and servant leaders in the history of combat nursing is the French Air Force nurse lieutenant Geneviève de Galard who volunteered to serve as a flight nurse during the French campaign with the Viet Minh in 1953. She was stationed in Hanoi and assigned to fly casualty evacuation flights for French soldiers wounded in the battle of Dien Bien Phu. Her primary task was "to fly to Dien Bien Phu twice a day to care for the wounded as they were taken out for specialist care to Hanoi or Saigon" (Nurse heroes of the century, 1999, p. 34).

On one of the later evacuation flights, on March 27, 1953, as the war seemed to be all but lost, de Galard's plane was hit by artillery and seriously damaged although able to land. The plane, and thus its flight nurse, were stranded at Dien Bien Phu as repairs to the equipment were impossible. De Galard immediately reported to the closest field hospital and volunteered her services. At first it has been reported that the commanding officer was hesitant to allow her to stay as she would be the only woman at the front; however, he finally relented.

"Although her superior officers attempted to protect her, de Galard refused to stay in the safety of the fortress; she frequently risked her life, amid mortar shelling, to care for wounded soldiers on the battlefield. She refused numerous opportunities to be liberated, choosing instead to stay with her patients" (O'Brien, 2003, p. 95). In the field hospital Lieutenant de Galard "was in charge of the most seriously injured. Corridors were filled with men on stretchers. In the recovery room and surrounding areas they lay on the floor between already full beds…. Lt. de Galard wrote: 'It was like the catacombs'" (Nurse heroes of the century, 1999, p. 35).

de Galard was the "only woman in the underground hospital at Dien Bien Phu. She endured heavy bombardment, lived through the last hours of the siege, and was captured by the Viet Minh" (p. 34).

De Galard was imprisoned with a group of 50 soldiers and spent her time in captivity caring for the wounded and writing letters for the men. They were finally liberated after close to 3 weeks imprisonment and allowed to return to France. Air Force Nurse Geneviève de Galard's courage and compassion in combat nursing was highly praised by both her superior officers and the men for whom she cared.

De Galard received numerous honors following the war including France's Knight's Cross of the *Légion d'honneur* and the *Croix de guerre*. She was also honored by being made an honorary member of the French Foreign Legion, a "*Legionnaire de 1ère classe*, and was given, in all the news media, the complimentary title the 'Angel of Dien Bien Phu.'" In 1954, de Galard was invited by the U.S. Congress to come to America to be awarded the Medal of Freedom by President Dwight D. Eisenhower (France's heroine, 1954, p. 47).

When speaking to U.S. reporters de Galard said: "I do not deserve this honor . . . I come as a symbol of all those out there" (France's heroine, 1954, p. 47). She "insisted that she had only done 'what any nurse would do'" (O'Brien, 2003, p. 95). Geneviève de Galard is a nursing servant leader and role model extraordinaire for all nurses past and present who minister to those serving their country in combat nursing.

This chapter began with the admission that there were many servant leaders throughout the history of our profession whose names have never been recorded. They were servant leaders whose service, care, and commitment were known only to God and to those to whom they ministered in nursing. A mentality of humble, anonymous service, prevalent in the early nursing community, is reflected in the comments of the final servant leader highlighted above, Geneviève de Galard. As Galard herself asserted: "I do not deserve this honor . . . I have only done what any nurse would do."

This posture of hidden servant leadership is demonstrated also in the writings of some early nursing authors who published inspiring materials without attaching their names. Two classic examples from the early literature are "Mary's Nurse," an epic poem written by an anonymous author from the early 1900s, about a nurse caring for a mother-to-be on Christmas Eve, which was allocated two full pages, as a centerfold, in the fledgling *American Journal of Nursing* in 1929 (p. 1445). The other was "The Nurse's Mass," a poignant and moving 1953 article in which the unnamed nurse author likens the nurse's activities to those of a priest. The nurse author servant leader's humility is displayed not only in her anonymity but also in the content of the piece in which she marvels at God's "gift" of being allowed to be a nurse and comments, "I have nothing to give for what have I, that He did not first give me?" At the close of the article the author adds: "Here are my hands, for which there will be no task too lowly" (p. 59).

How blest we are, as today's nurses, to have the strong shoulders of such servant leaders as these on which to stand.

REFERENCES

Arthur, T. (2006). The life and death of Edith Cavell, English emergency nurse known as "The other Nightingale." *Journal of Emergency Nursing, 32*(1), 30–35.

A Sister of Mercy. (1917). *Camillus De Lellis: The hospital saint.* New York: Benziger Brothers.

Austin, A. L. (1957). *History of nursing sourcebook.* New York: C.P. Putnam's Sons.

Baly, M. (Ed.) (1991). *As Miss Nightingale said...Florence Nightingale through her sayings: A Victorian perspective.* London: Scutari Press.

Blanchard, K., & Hodges, P. (2005). *Lead like Jesus: Lessons from the greatest leadership role model of all time.* Nashville, TN: Thomas Nelson.

Breckinridge, M. (1981). *Wide neighborhoods: A story of the Frontier Nursing Service.* Lexington, KY: University of Kentucky Press.

Bullough, V. L., & Bullough, B. (1987). Our roots: What we should know about nursing's Christian pioneers. *Journal of Christian Nursing, 4*(1), 10–14.

Daughters of Charity. (1993). *Daughters of charity vocation Program* [Video]. Emmitsburg, MD: Author.

Deloughery, G. L. (1977). *History and trends of professional nursing.* St. Louis, MO: C.V. Mosby.

Deming, R. (1969). *Heroes of the International Red Cross.* New York: Meredith Press.

Dietz, L. D., & Lehozky, A. R. (1967). *History and modern nursing* (2nd ed.). Philadelphia: F.A. Davis.

Dolan, J. A. (1963). *Goodnow's history of nursing.* Philadelphia: W.B. Saunders.

Dolan, J. A. (1973). *Nursing in society: A historical perspective.* Philadelphia: W.B. Saunders.

Dolan, J. A. (1978). *Nursing in society: A historical perspective* (2nd ed.). Philadelphia: W.B. Saunders.

Dolan, J. A., Fitzpatrick, H. L., & Herrmann, E. K. (1983). *Nursing in society: A historical perspective.* Philadelphia: W.B. Saunders.

Donahue, M. P. (1996). *Nursing: The finest art, an illustrated history.* St. Louis, MO: C.V. Mosby.

Duffus, R. L. (1939). *Lillian Wald: Neighbor and crusader.* New York: Macmillan.

Ford, A. E. (1984). *La Vengeance de Nostre Seigneu.* Toronto, Ontario: Pontifical Institute of Mediaeval Studies.

Foster family care in Gheel. (1991). *Flanders: The Magazine of the Flemish Community, 9,* 15–17.

France's heroine. (1954). *Catholic Nurse, 3*(1), 46–47.

Frank, C. M. (1959). *Foundations of nursing.* Philadelphia: W.B. Saunders.

George, M. (1964). A way of the Cross for nurses. *Catholic Nurse, 12*(3), 56–58.

Goldstein, J. L., & Godemont, M. L. (2003). The legend and lessons of Gheel, Belgium: A 1500 year old legend, a 21st century model. *Community Mental Health Journal, 39*(5), 441–447.

Goodnow, M. (1916). *Outlines of nursing history.* Philadelphia: W.B. Saunders.

Grippando, G. (1986). *Nursing perspectives and issues* (3rd ed.). Albany, NY: Delmar.

Hawley, W. L. (1954). The lay apostolate in nursing. *Catholic Nurse, 2*(3), 17–20.

Heyward, M. E. (1939). The golden jubilee at the Catholic University School of Nursing. *Trained Nurse and Hospital Review, 11*(4), 346–347.

Houselander, C. (1955). *The way of the Cross.* New York: Sheed & Ward.

Jamieson, E. M., & Sewall, M. F. (1954). *Trends in nursing history: Their relationships to world events.* Philadelphia: W.B. Saunders.

Jensen, D. M., Spaulding, J. F., & Cady, E. L. (1959). *History and trends of professional nursing.* St. Louis, MO: C.V. Mosby.

Johnson, B. C. (1988). *Pastoral spirituality: A focus for ministry.* Philadelphia: Westminster Press.

Judson, H. (1941). *Edith Cavell.* New York: Macmillan.

Maloney, R. P. (1992). *The way of Vincent De Paul: A contemporary spirituality in the service of the poor.* Hyde Park, NY: New City Press.

Maloney, R. P. (1995). *He hears the cry of the poor: On the spirituality of Vincent de Paul.* New York: New City Press.

Mary's nurse. (1929). *American Journal of Nursing, 29*(12), 1444–1445.

McKown, R. (1966). *Heroic nurses.* New York: G.P. Putnam's Sons.

Matheussen, H., Morren, P., & Seyers, J. (1975, January). *The state psychiatric hospital: A center for family care in Gheel.* Gheel, Belgium (paper supplied by the Belgian Embassy, Washington, DC).

Meyer, A. G. (1958). The Catholic nurse: A modern Veronica. *Catholic Nurse, 7*(1), 45–47.

Miller, M. (1954). Modern Veronicas. *Catholic Nurse, 2*(3), 20–22.

Nurse heroes of the century. (1999). *Nursing Times, 95*(44), 34–35.

Nutting, M. A., & Dock, L. L. (1935). *A history of nursing* (Vol. 1). New York: G.P. Putnam's Sons.

O'Brien, M. E. (2003). *Prayer in nursing: The spirituality of compassionate caregiving.* Sudbury, MA: Jones and Bartlett.

O'Brien, M. E. (2006). *The nurse with an alabaster jar: A biblical approach to nursing.* Madison, WI: NCF Press.

O'Brien, M. E. (2008). *Spirituality in nursing: Standing on holy ground* (3rd ed.). Sudbury, MA: Jones and Bartlett.

Pavey, A. E. (1952). *The story of the growth of nursing.* Philadelphia: J.B. Lippincott.

Poole, E. (1960). Nurses on horseback. In H. Wright & S. Rapport (Eds.), *Great adventures in nursing* (pp. 118–139). New York: Harper & Brothers.

Raines, K. H., & Wilson, A. (1996). Frontier Nursing Service: A historical perspective on nurse-managed care. *Journal of Community Health Nursing, 13*(2), 123–127.

Ridgway, E. (1960). Veronica. *Catholic Nurse, 12*(3), 67.

Rogow, S. (1966). *Lillian Wald: The nurse in blue.* Philadelphia: Jewish Publishing Society of America.

Schneemelcher, W. (1963). Edgar Hennecke: New Testament apocrypha (Vol. 1). Philadelphia: Westminster Press.

Selanders, L. C. (1993). *Florence Nightingale: An environmental adaptation theory.* Newburg Park, NY: Sage.

Sellew, G., & Nuesse, C. J. (1946). *A history of nursing.* St. Louis, MO: C.V. Mosby.

Seymer, L. R. (1949). *A general history of nursing.* New York: Macmillan.

Stewart, I. M., and Austin, A. L. (1962). *A history of nursing: From ancient to modern times.* New York: G.P. Putnam's Sons.

The nurse's Mass. (1953). *Catholic Nurse, 2*(2), 53–54.

Tuntiya, N. (2007). Free-air treatment for mental patients: The deinstitutionalization debate of the nineteenth century. *Sociological Perspectives, 50*(3), 469–488.

Walsh, J. J. (1929). *The history of nursing.* New York: P.J. Kenedy & Sons.

Widerquist, J. G. (1992). The spirit of Florence Nightingale. *Nursing Research, 41*(1), 49–55.

Wilkenson, J. (1998). *The Bible and healing: A medical and theological commentary.* Grand Rapids, MI: William B. Eerdmans.

3 The Biblical Roots of the Nurse's Call to Serve

Whoever serves me must follow me, and where I am, there will my servant be also.

—John 11:56

Nurses have special gifts ... gifts of compassion, empathy, and service. All those fit together in being a nurse. I think I was called by God to serve as a nurse. There is nothing greater, and I say this with all humility, than to wash someone's feet. To be able to do that and think about the bible story of Our Lord doing that to the disciples brings tears to my eyes, that we are in the humble capacity to wash someone else's feet. What a privilege it is to give someone a bath or rub a back or give a hug when they are lonesome. I think that is what makes nursing a blessed vocation, and what makes it so important. It is a privilege that we are asked to enter people's lives when they are most vulnerable.

—Margaret, supervisor of a chemotherapy treatment area

Nurses, perhaps more than members of any other professional occupation, with the exclusion of religious ministry, are called to serve—called to serve those who are fragile and vulnerable in body, mind, or spirit, and, at times, in all three dimensions of human functioning. In the following chapter both historical and contemporary nursing literature cited reflect that call. The spirituality of the nurse's call to serve is a thread that runs throughout this book; the theme is especially vibrant when presented in the poignant words of practicing nurses as documented in the later chapters containing interview data. To grasp the underlying spirituality of a nurse's call to serve, however, it is important to look at the biblical roots of the concepts of service and servanthood as included in both Old and New Testament translations of the Bible.

59

The word *service* is derived from the Greek *diakoneo* meaning to serve; it was usually considered as referring to "personal service such as ... caring for another" (Doohan, 1993, p. 875). Biblical service may refer to "all sorts of work from the most inferior and menial to the most honored and exalted" (Leviticus 23:7; Numbers 3:6) (Service, 1993, p. 538).

Comments related to the concepts of service, serving, and the servant role are frequently found in both Old and New Testament Bible passages. In a concise concordance to the New Revised Standard Version of the Bible, the term *servant* is cited 33 times as included in Old Testament works, such as the books of Exodus, Numbers, 1 Samuel, Job, the Psalms, Isaiah, and Jeremiah. *Servant* is identified as occurring in 16 New Testament passages, including Luke, John, Acts, Romans, Galatians, Collossians, Timothy, Hebrews, and Revelation (Kohlenberger, 1993, p. 250). The term *servants* appears in 9 Old Testament works and 12 New Testament books. The word *serve* occurs 23 times in the Old Testament and 9 times in the New Testament (p. 250). A number of other service-related citations include such labels as "servant of God," "servant of the Lord," "all servants," "king's servants," and "temple servants."

Some examples of biblical servant figures identified in the Old Testament include: "the patriarchs Abraham, Isaac, and Jacob (Exodus 32:13) ... (and) Moses (Deuteronomy 34:5), Joshua (Judges 2:8), Samuel (1 Samuel 3:9), David (2 Samuel 7:5), Solomon (1 Kings 3:7), and Job (Job 1:8)" (Matera, 1995, p. 929). In New Testament passages, Jesus presents the concept of servanthood as "expressing humankind's relationship to God. God is the Lord to whom the believer owes unreserved service" (Matera, 1985, p. 929). Examples of Jesus' teachings noted by theologian Frank Matera are "No one can serve two masters" (Matthew 6:24) and "Nor is a servant above the master" (Matthew 10:24). Matera adds "the faithful servant does the master's will (Matthew 24:45–46) and realizes that in the presence of God even the best disciple is only an unprofitable servant (Luke 17:10)" (1985, p. 929).

As the citations above demonstrate, the concepts of service and servanthood are incorporated throughout the Old and New Testaments of the Bible. The meaningfulness of many of these service-related passages for the nursing community has been and continues to be reflected in the published body of nursing literature from the 1800s to the contemporary era.

THE THEOLOGY OF THE NURSE'S CALL TO SERVE

In reviewing the writings of our early nursing authors, one finds the concepts of service and servanthood identified frequently as central to the nurse's role of caring for the sick. Often these references have an explicit biblical association; at times, the linkage is implicit. Generally the service-associated concepts have a religious sentiment as their undergirding philosophy.

In two nursing textbooks from the late 1800s, the concept of service is implied in passages discussing the nurse's calling:

> In training for this difficult calling one of the first requisites is a very strong inclination practically to help the sick. In herself the nurse must realize an ever present impulse to benefit the suffering and must feel assured that her (sic) highest happiness consists in thus actively doing good. (Billroth, 1895, p. 20)

> The calling of the nurse is a noble one....the essentials of a good nurse are love of God and of fellow creatures....if you are not willing to minister to any and every one of your fellow creatures in distress, you are not fulfilling your highest mission as a nurse. (Pope, 1898, pp. 11, 13)

In a 1914 text *Modern Methods in Nursing*, Georgiana Sanders wrote:

> In few callings has the character of the individual so much to do with her success or failure as in the profession of nursing.... It is a career that ... frequently exacts the sacrifice of every other sentiment to the fulfillment of duty. (pp. 32, 36)

In a 1919 *Manual of Nursing*, it was pointed out that "The well-informed nurse will see at a glance the enormous field of usefulness that is open to her; surely such a work is akin to Divine service" (Humphry, p. v); and writing in 1921 on the topic of the "Spirit of Service," supervising nurse Bertha Mascot asserted that any nursing experience can provide "a clarion call to all nurses, regardless of what field they may be in, to make the most of their opportunity to put across the gospel of service to all mankind" (p. 20).

In 1922, articles in the *Trained Nurse and Hospital Review* and the *American Journal of Nursing* spoke to the "spirit" of service:

> I am knowledge and skill, honor and constancy, the first requisites of the woman you wish to become; but more than all of these, nay because I am all of these, I am the Spirit of Service for I am the trained nurse. (American Red Cross Bulletin, 1922, p. 33)

> The self-effacing woman engaged in the private duty field is doing one of the noblest of God's works....(the nurse) shall each but do service for spirit and heart (A Private Duty Nurse, 1922, pp. 901–902).

The poetic meditations of three nurses published in the *Trained Nurse and Hospital Review* during the 1920s also reflected the spirit and vision of service. In the first, the nurse author asks the Lord for "just one little star" to wear with her "uniform new" when she has finally "crossed the bar," noting: "Morning and evening, noontime and night, working to give a service just right" (Satyer, 1922, p. 235). In an anonymously authored poem, a nurse author meditates on the stress of her work in the hospital, a "mansion of woe," but adds "Compassion and Tenderness aid me, I know there is a God" (1922, p. 213). And in musing on the spirituality of the nurse's lamp, registered nurse Addie McQuhae asks of the Lord: "O seal thy motto on our hearts and send us forth again, with mercy and with charity, to help our fellow men" (1927, p. 386).

In both 1922 and 1925 December (Christmas) issues of the *Trained Nurse and Hospital Review* the concept of religiously affiliated service is highlighted, perhaps related to the blessings of the season: "We have before us the vision of service (as) the 'Great Commission'" (Woods, 1922, p. 494). Another stated:

You have found your purpose, a purpose which the Son of God
Himself has blest and shared. Among the multitudes who live
for themselves alone yours is the opportunity to spend and be
spent in the service of your fellow men. (Perry, 1925, p. 581)

In nurse educator Bertha Harmer's 1925 *Textbook of the Principles and Practice of Nursing*, the author's preface begins with the assertion that the aim of the book is to present the student with the basic principles of nursing "founded upon the ideals of service" (p. v). In a 1926 article on "What makes a hospital great," it is observed that the institution of the hospital must create in the nurse "a higher and holier conception of humanity. Every man (sic) she is called upon to serve must be her brother ... it must be God's call to serve her fellow man for the love of humanity and the glory of the Master" (Lumpkin, p. 629).

In four other 1926 nursing journal issues poetry penned by the practicing nurses of the era included the concept of religiously affiliated service as implicit to their musings: "For in your life of consecrated service, it is the Master's image that you see" (Imeldine, 1926, p. 192); "In the city hospital's hot ward, a gentle worker for the gentle Lord" (Window in English cathedral, 1926, p. 280); "Giving herself, not counting the cost.... for God established His universe, naming His co-creator nurse" (Gunn, 1926, p. 300); "In silence and in darkness where no eye may see or know, then her footsteps shod with mercy, and swift kindness come and go" (Wead, 1926, p. 933).

In 1927, nursing journal articles continued to reflect nurses' respect and care for the importance of service. In a graduation address, cited in the *American Journal of Nursing*, the speaker blessed the new nurses with the words: "May God illuminate you with the courage to work for the benefit of all mankind, without regard for earthly reward; and may quiet faith, like the lamp of the sanctuary, never be extinguished in your worship of this most noble purpose. Serve it always with all your soul" (Fraga, p. 354). In a Christmas story told of a young British student nurse who was forced to spend the holiday serving at a hospital, the author quotes the student as saying, at the end of her shift, "I am thankful for … the opportunity to serve those less fortunate than myself, and I know that in such service I will find happiness." The nurse author adds of the student nurse: "She had seen the vision of service; she had accepted it and claimed it as her own. She had interpreted it in the spirit of Christ, her Master" (Wead, 1927, p. 643).

Nurses' poems reflecting the meaning of service were also included in four 1929 issues of the *American Journal of Nursing*. One nurse, who wrote that all of her life revolved around a "call," mused: "To care for the sick … to give, is there any other incentive to live?" (*Johns Hopkins Nurses' Alumnae Magazine*, 1929, p. 786). A second nurse poet began her piece by dedicating herself and her work to the Lord, praying: "Take, then, mine eyes and teach them how to see, the clearest way to nurse the sick for thee" (Homans, 1929, p. 1028). In the third poem, Dorothy Hayward (1929) wrote about a nurse's hands, noting that they were temples molded by the "Sculptor's" tool and were thus used in "guarding flickering fires where life's flame lies trampled much" (p. 536). In a fourth poetic work, entitled "The Faithful Nurse," it was observed that nursing is "a gift of God," and nurses tread where "Jesus trod," in their ministry of healing. The poem concludes: "Long may the schools produce this type of nurse, who lives to serve, not for a heavy purse" (Booth, 1929, p. 380).

Finally, nursing journal articles into the 1930s and following decades of the 1900s continued to applaud the concept of religiously or biblically derived service as central to the ministry of the practicing nurse. In a 1930 issue of the *American Journal of Nursing*, a brief poem entitled "The Dedication of the Nurse" is included. It begins with the thought that "Recognizing the sacredness of the healing" art and the devotion required, the nurse will seek "alleviation of suffering, cure of disease and useful prolongation of human life" (Modern Hospital, p. 1234). A 1937 textbook, *The Art and Science of Nursing*, asserted that the nurse must be "entirely unselfish; willing to give up nearly everything for those to be served;

willing to expend most of one's time, all of one's strength, in the service of others" (Rothweiler, p. 27). The author of a 1938 text for hospital nurses advised: "We are the echo of Our Lord's words: 'Come to me all you that labor and are burdened'... We have to say to ourselves: 'I have someone to tend, someone to whom I can be of help, someone I can serve.' What a grand thing it is to be able to serve" (Mother Catherine De Jesus-Christ, p. 2). Writing in 1939 for the home care nurse, Mary Louise Habel and Hazel Doris Milton, pointed out that the nurse's "professional duties" should include the fact that "every effort should be made to maintain the highest ideals of service to mankind ... (the nurse's) obligation is to serve those who are sick" (p. xi).

THE BIBLICAL MEANING OF SERVANTHOOD IN NURSING

Kathy Schoonover-Shoffner, editor of the *Journal of Christian Nursing*, described the meaning of biblical servanthood for nurses in a 1997 article "A Call to Servanthood." Schoonover-Shoffner admits that for some the idea of servanthood may present a negative image, such as that of a person of lower rank or abilities. "Servanthood in scripture," she points out, "is not associated with weakness and inferiority but with power, greatness, and nobility—not because of who the servant is but because of the one served" (p. 14). The point is made, nevertheless, that servants of the Lord, as described in the Bible, often had to pay a high price for their servanthood: "Abraham was called to leave his home," "Moses (lived in the desert) for forty years," and "David suffered as a hunted fugitive for fourteen years" (Schoonover-Shoffner, 1997, p. 14). Schoonover-Shoffner concludes that nurses can learn three things from such biblical examples: "First, biblical servanthood means obedience to God"; "Second, servanthood points to times of hardship"; and "Third, servanthood requires humility" (1997, p. 15). The anecdotes and case study examples of practicing nurse servant leaders, presented in later chapters, contain perceptions and experiences reflective of all three of Schoonover-Shoffner's identified characteristics of servanthood: obedience to God, times of hardship, and humility.

Florence Nightingale, in her calling to serve the sick, also reflected the concepts of obedience, hardship, and humility: obedience to "what she believed to be a call from God" (Widerquist, 1995, p. 4); hardship in both going against the will of her family to serve the sick and in undertaking the dangerous mission to the Crimea; and humility, in committing her life to a ministry that had previously been considered by many as work befitting only women of unseemly or questionable character. As Nightingale scholar JoAnn Widerquist graphically put it:

> It took (Florence Nightingale) many years of constant struggle to find the particular vocation her call to service would take. Trying to answer God defined her life, and opened the door for modern nursing. (1995, p. 4)

In their book *Called to Care*, Judy Shelly and Arlene Miller assert that the ministry of nursing is indeed "servant work," adding that sometimes it is not easy work (2006, p. 245). They offer examples such as the "critical care nurse who works double shifts to care for a sick colleague" or "the nurse practitioner who gives up a lucrative position to work in an inner-city clinic" (p. 245). Shelly and Miller also support Schoonover-Shoffner's thought that the important point about servanthood is the identity of the person being served; they admit that while many

> servant-nurses remain unheralded and invisible ... the key to servanthood comes in whom we are serving. Jesus said, "Truly, I tell you, just as you did it to one of the least of these who are members of my family, you did it for me" (Matthew 25:40) (2006, p. 245).

The nurse's servanthood is embedded within the concept of his or her nursing ministry—a ministry of caring, of healing, and of compassion for those who are ill or injured. This chapter began by suggesting that perhaps the only vocation other than nurse that has service as a major component is formal religious ministry. Widerquist and Davidhizar, in discussing the ministry of nursing, liken much of a nurse's intervention to that of the pastoral care worker; both groups are concerned about the biopsychosocial and spiritual dimension of the person (1994, p. 648). Both nurses and pastoral caregivers, Widerquist and Davidhizar suggest, may use similar approaches, which "(a) provide concern and comfort, (b) assist the patient and family to find meaning in the illness, (c) provide hope, (d) facilitate expression of feelings, (e) respond to spiritual distress, and (f) promote actions aimed at seeking forgiveness" (1994, p. 649). While the latter concept of assisting one to seek forgiveness may seem to fall more within the domain of work of the religious minister, a nursing study of the spiritual needs of older adults revealed "forgiveness" as the "most frequently identified spiritual need" (O'Brien, 2008, p. 263). In some cases elders felt the need to receive forgiveness from a person whom they felt they may have offended during their lives; for other older individuals there was a felt need to express forgiveness to someone by whom they had been hurt. A difficulty with this need for an older adult was that frequently the person to whom or from whom they sought to give or receive forgiveness had predeceased the elder. Thus, it often fell to the geriatric nurse to assist the elder patient in giving over that particular need to God or in being a bridge to bring an elder together with a pastoral caregiver who might help ease their forgiveness-related concern.

The nurse, both historically and in contemporary society, must accept the role of servanthood if he or she is to function fully in a compassionate and caring ministry of nursing. Servanthood is not always easy, but it is truly the grace — the blessing and the gift of the practicing nurse.

BIBLICAL ROOTS OF NURSING SERVICE IN THE OLD TESTAMENT

The Old Testament scriptures contain important lessons for nursing servant leaders. These lessons are found especially in Deuteronomy, Joshua, and 1 Samuel. In the book of Deuteronomy a clear and unambiguous message about serving the Lord is conveyed: we should fear God, serve God alone, and that we should serve Him with our whole heart and soul. In Deuteronomy 6:13, the admonition is given "The Lord your God you shall fear; Him you shall serve, and by His name alone you shall swear." Deuteronomy 10:12 reinforces the teaching: "So now, O Israel, what does the Lord require of you? Only to fear the Lord your God, to walk in all His ways, to love Him, to serve the Lord your God with all your heart and with all your soul." And the passage in Deuteronomy 13:4 follows suit: "The Lord your God you shall follow, Him alone you shall fear, His commandments you shall keep, His voice you shall obey, Him you shall serve and to Him you shall hold fast."

The key concepts in the Deuteronomy passages — fear and love of God, obedience to His will and commandments, service to God alone, and service carried out with one's whole heart and soul — are also reflected in other Old Testament books as noted earlier. In the book of Joshua we are taught that we must "Love the Lord," "keep His commandments," "hold fast to Him," and "serve Him with all (our) heart and with all (our) soul" (22:5). The first book of Samuel also includes verses that support the concept of loving faithful service: "Direct your heart to the Lord and serve Him only" (7:3); "Do not turn aside from following the Lord, but serve the Lord with all your heart" (12:20); and "Only fear the Lord and serve Him faithfully with all your heart" (12:24).

Fear

Those of us who are followers of the Judeo-Christian tradition hold fast to the truth that our God is a loving and merciful and compassionate God. Thus, the concept of fear, which appears in all three passages of the book of Deuteronomy, as well as in the first book of Samuel, may seem somewhat disconcerting. A common understanding of fear is that it is an unpleasant emotion reserved for situations of great anxiety or uncertainty for ourselves or for those we love. How is it then that the Old Testament texts continually admonished God's chosen people, the Israelites, to fear Him? What does this mandate to fear mean for us as nurses?

First, we must acknowledge that the concept of fear can have both positive and negative consequences. If a person is fearful of undertaking new tasks or activities out of an undue anxiety related to the unknown, that individual might miss many satisfying and rewarding life experiences. On the other hand, if one declines to participate in some dangerous behavior, such as driving while intoxicated, because of a healthy fear of an accident, the outcome may be life-saving for both the intoxicated individual and other drivers.

Fear, as understood by biblical scholars has its own unique meaning vis-à-vis our relationship with our Creator. While fear is sometimes understood in the Bible as bringing about "emotional distress … with intense concern for impending danger or evil," such as in Joshua 9:24 (Louw, 1993a, p. 225), an "other area of meaning relates to allegiance to and regard for deity" (p. 225). Essentially the Old Testament references to fear of the Lord reflected a posture of "profound respect with implications of awe" before God (Louw, 1993a, p. 225). Fear of the Lord, identified as one of the seven gifts of the Holy Spirit, is described as "related to the virtues of hope, love, and temperance (and) brings proper use of pleasures and the senses, on the basis of a sensitivity to the activity of God and reverence for God's majesty" (Evans, 1993b, p. 438). The point is emphasized that "Born of poverty of spirit, this special kind of fear does not block intimate union with God but inhibits offense of God" (Evans, 1993, p. 438). Thus, such fear is "an element and not a contradiction of love" (p. 438). Fear is "the awe that a person ought to have before God" (Achtemeier, 1985, p. 305).

Nurse servant leaders rarely suffer from fear related to emotional distress associated with their role in the healthcare system. Nurse leaders do, however, frequently relate experiences and perceptions that reflect "sensitivity" to the presence of God and "awe" before His majesty. Any nurse who has served in a leadership role for a significant period of time has encountered situations that lead to the "awe that a person ought to have before God."

One example of this awe was revealed in a poignant story related by Anne Marie, the head nurse of an experimental Alzheimer's unit in a large urban medical center. Anne Marie told of caring for an early Alzheimer's patient, a man beginning the "slippery slope" into dementia while still in his midforties. Anne Marie described the courage and brave heart of the patient who, as a scientist, was very aware of the tragedy of his diagnosis. She spoke of the patient's spirituality, his amazing trust in the goodness of God in the midst of his illness. Anne Marie expressed a sense of awe, not only in the attitude of her patient, but in the goodness of God who provided her patient with the strength and spirit to be able to celebrate his life and give thanks for it in the midst of such great suffering.

Loving Obedience

Two other biblical concepts, both explicit and implicit in the service-related passages in the books of Deuteronomy and Joshua, are those of love (Deuteronomy 6:13, 10:12) and obedience (Deuteronomy 13:4 and Joshua 22:5). There are many kinds of love, and it is noted that human loves "in all their rich variety fill the passages of biblical narrative" (Fredriksen, 1993, p. 467). The kind of love expected of the Israelites in the Old Testament is considered a response to God's covenantal commitment to His people: "Chosen by God's love (Deuteronomy 7:7–8;10:15) Israel is to respond in kind; loving God who redeemed them and revealed His will to them, teaching His ways to all future generations" (Deuteronomy 6:4–7) (Fredriksen, 1993, p. 468).

Flowing directly from the concept of love of the Lord is that of obedience to His will and commandments; that is, to a commandment as "verbal or written requirement or order" (Unterman, 1985, p. 176). It is suggested by theologian Robin Maas that "the common-sense under-standing of obedience simply as compliance with the bidding of another" is not adequate for understanding the meaning of obedience in the spiritual life (1993, p. 709). "Obedience in the spiritual life," she asserts "is a matter of receiving and responding appropriately to a message or a word from God" (p. 709). Maas adds that since the word of God in Scripture always requires a "decisive response, the requirement of obedience serves as a kind of spiritual test" … for an individual and is "thus closely associated with faith" (1993, p. 709).

A spirit of loving obedience to the will of God is a virtue that nurse servant leaders are called upon to practice frequently. Daily, and sometimes hourly, nursing leaders are forced to face and to accept painful suffering, life-threatening diagnoses, and sometimes death among the patients with whose care they are charged.

Maggie, a pediatric nurse practitioner and charge nurse of a large pediatric oncology unit, spoke of the continual need to accept God's will in witnessing the suffering and death of her small patients. Maggie commented: "It's so hard sometimes. It just hurts so much to see them suffer. You can't help but think 'Why?' And the parents ask 'Why?' But then you know that somehow God, in His love, will take care of these little ones and bring them to His kingdom where they will never hurt again. Even when you don't always understand, you have to trust and you have to be obedient and you have to accept God's will."

Serving with the Heart and Soul

Passages in Deuteronomy 6:13, 13:4, and 1 Samuel 7:3 contain the admonition that the one hearing the word must serve God alone. This mandate seems again to flow from both love and obedience, for one who truly loves and is truly obedient can only be truly the servant of one alone who is the Lord. All three concepts, that of love, obedience, and faithful service to one Master, are also congruent with and supported by the teaching in Deuteronomy 10:12 and Joshua 22:5, which advise that we must love and serve the Lord our God with all our heart and all our soul; service with all our heart is also taught in the first book of Samuel (12:20 and 12:24).

These are important descriptors of biblical love, and service for the heart and the soul are key elements in controlling and supporting human behavior. The heart is identified spiritually as symbolizing "the center or core of the human person. It is the locus not only of our affectivity but also of our freedom and consciousness, the place where we accept or reject the mystery of ourselves, human existence, and God" (Callahan, 1993, p. 469). The heart is also described as the center for "decisions, obedience, devotion, and intentionality … within the heart, human beings meet God's word and thus it is the location where conversion takes place" (Edwards, 1985, p. 377).

The soul, in distinction to the heart, is a specifically spiritual concept which has been described as "the human individual's inherent capacity for selfhood, self-awareness, and subjectivity, the principle of human knowing and responsible freedom" (Noffke, 1993, p. 908). Noffke observed that "the human person as presented by the Old Testament is an undivided unity of flesh and spirit" (p. 909). For an Old Testament writer "soul indicated the unity of a human person" (Neyrey, 1985, p. 983).

Nursing's call to serve, while certainly a vocation incorporating activities of the mind and the body, is also very much an affair of the heart and the soul. It is the love and the tenderness of the nurse's heart and the selflessness and self-sacrifice of the nurse's soul that are the catalysts for so many caring behaviors that go far beyond what one might consider the accepted "line of duty" in nursing. Nurses, especially nursing leaders, serve patients, families, and other staff members with their intelligence, their technical skill, and their gifts for organization and management. But it is the caring of the nurses' hearts, and the faith and trust and hope in their souls, that provide for the truly touching and tender moments of healing for those they serve.

An example of a nurse serving with his heart and soul is that of Patrick, a mental health nurse, who worked with chemotherapy patients at a large city healthcare facility. Patrick explained that he became deeply involved with and attached to his chemo patients who were suffering from a variety of cancer diagnoses. Patrick's role was to counsel and support the patients throughout the chemo treatment and potential recovery. In this role he often became the patient's surrogate family member, friend, colleague, and chaplain, as well as their nurse. Deep and caring relationships developed during Patrick's caregiving. When the chemotherapy treatments were successful, Patrick would rejoice with his patients; when they failed he would grieve with them and their loved ones as well. In Patrick's own words, this nursing touched his "very heart and soul," sometimes with joy, sometimes with sadness, but always with an "intimacy" that was precious and treasured to his nurse's heart.

Finally, the most important word, which the above descriptors support and clarify is that of service — to be a servant of the Lord. In the Old Testament, service was understood as consisting of "tasks performed by lesser persons for those who controlled their existence" (Malina, 1985b, p. 930). For followers of the Lord, service consisted of a variety of activities mandated by God's commandments and by the communication of His will through the priests and the prophets. A badge of honor for one of God's chosen people was to be called a servant of the Lord. The title was self-selected by many individuals as reflected in such biblical passages as 1 Samuel 3:9: "Speak, Lord, for your servant is listening."

The desirability of being the Lord's servant is validated in passages from both the Psalms and the Book of the Prophet Isaiah: "Let your face shine upon your servant; save me in your steadfast love" (Psalms 31:16); "The Lord redeems the life of His servants; none of those who take refuge in Him will be condemned" (Psalms 34:22); "Make your face shine upon your servant, and teach me your statutes" (Psalms 119:135); "You are my witnesses, says the Lord, and my servant whom I have chosen" (Isaiah, 43:10); "See my servant shall prosper, he shall be exalted and lifted up, and shall be very high" (Isaiah 52:13); and "My servants shall sing for gladness of heart" (Isaiah 65:14).

To be called the "servant of the Lord" is perhaps the greatest title that any nurse servant leader can attain. It is the blessing and the grace of the nurse's call to care and to serve the ill and the infirm, the sick and the suffering, the hopeless and the despairing. Blessed are the nursing servant leaders for they "shall be exalted and lifted up."

BIBLICAL ROOTS OF NURSING SERVICE IN THE NEW TESTAMENT

In the New Testament scripture Jesus is quoted as even admonishing Satan who tempted Him in the wilderness to "Worship the Lord your God, and serve Him only" (Matthew 4:10). Much of the Lord's teaching on service of God, however, employs Jesus' own ministry as a model for those who would serve Him and His Father in heaven. When brothers James and John requested special seating near the Lord in glory, the other disciples became angry. "So Jesus called them and said to them, 'you know that among the Gentiles, those whom they recognize as their rulers lord it over them, and their great ones are tyrants over them. But it is not so among you; but whoever wishes to be great among you must be your servant, and whoever wishes to be first among you must be slave of all. For the Son of Man came not to be served but to serve, and to give His life as a ransom for many" (Mark 10:42–45).

When a dispute about greatness began among His disciples, Jesus taught them again using His own mission as a model: "The greatest among you must become like the youngest, and the leader like one who serves. For who is greater, the one who is at the table or the one who serves? Is it not the one at the table? But I am among you as one who serves" (Luke 22:26–27).

What a blessed example Jesus left for His nurse servant leaders in reminding us that His entire life, His reason for embracing a human persona, was to serve and not to be served. Caring service is the heart and soul and raison d'etre of the nursing profession. Nurses are called "not to be served but to serve." That is the gift and the joy and the treasure of the nurse's calling.

In sharing His own life and ministry with His disciples, Jesus not only taught and modeled the importance of the concept of being a servant, He also presented graphically the difficulties that could go along with adoption of such a mission and role. This was clearly evident in the oft-cited "grain of wheat" Scripture passage when Jesus admitted:

> Unless a grain of wheat falls into the earth and dies, it remains just a single grain; but if it dies it bears much fruit. Those who love their life lose it, and those who hate their life in this world will keep it for eternal life. Whoever serves me must follow me, and where I am there will my servant be also. (John 12:24–26)

In these words, it appears that Jesus was already preparing His followers for the fact that He would physically suffer and die in this world, and they, as His disciples, must be prepared to experience suffering and death as well.

The disciples' preparation for difficulties is also reflected in the Lord's description of the "world's hatred":

> If the world hates you, be aware that it hated me before it hated you. If you belonged to the world, the world would love you as its own. Because you do not belong to the world, but I have chosen you out of the world, therefore the world hates you. Remember the word that I said to you, servants are not greater than their master. If they persecuted me, they will persecute you. (John 15:18–20)

Nurse servant leaders may suffer the kind of difficulties that Jesus and His disciples experienced, the "hatred" and "persecution of the world." Nurses are, however, able to identify with the "grain of wheat" analogy; the scripture passage in which the Lord taught that it is only when something precious to us "falls to the ground and dies" that it "bears fruit." I wrote about a "grain of wheat" experience in my own nursing career in which I admitted how difficult the "death" of a hope could be (O'Brien, 2008, pp. 68–70). I believe that these "grain of wheat" experiences may happen to us in nursing a number of times, when for example, a patient for whom we have cared for weeks or even months, and for whom we anticipated a successful recovery, dies unexpectedly. It is on occasions such as this that our faith is tested, but it is also supported by the teaching of a Lord who Himself "fell to the ground and died" in order to provide salvation for all of humankind.

After many hours of preaching to His disciples, and sharing with them the potential difficulties of being His follower and servant, however, Jesus offered a precious gift to those who would choose to follow

Him in His analogy of the vine: "I am the true vine, and my Father is the vinegrower.... If you abide in me and my words abide in you, ask for whatever you wish and it will be done for you. My Father is glorified by this, that you bear much fruit and become my disciples. As the Father has loved me, so I have loved you; abide in my love.... I have said these things to you so that my joy may be in you, and that your joy may be complete" (John 15:1, 7–9, 11).

Jesus concluded His message by imparting a new dimension to the concept of faithful servanthood: "You are my friends if you do what I command you. I do not call you servants any longer because the servant does not know what the master is doing; but I have called you friends, because I have made known to you everything that I have heard from my Father" (John 15:14–15). This change in the servants' status seems also reflected in Peter's first letter in which he encouraged the early Christian community: "As servants of God, live as free people" (1 Peter 2:16). In this freedom, however, Peter warned: "Whoever Speaks must do so as one speaking the very words of God; whoever serves must do so with the strength that God supplies so that God may be glorified in all things through Jesus Christ. To Him belong the glory and the power forever" (1 Peter 4:11). The "word of God" is biblically understood as meaning the "law as communication from God," and also "the gospel and the person of Jesus Christ" (Muddiman, 1993, p. 818); the word of God in scripture generally denotes "God's revelation of His will and purpose" (Smith, 1985, p. 1141).

It is a blessed thought to know that we, as nurses, may speak with the "words of God" to our suffering patients and serve them and our colleagues "with the strength that God supplies." Whenever I feel very tired and worn out, I try to remember that if I can just hope, I will be able to keep going. The promise of hope, I like to think of as assured by the great prophet Isaiah: "Those who (hope in) wait for the Lord shall renew their strength, they shall mount up with wings like eagles, they shall run and not be weary, they shall walk and not faint" (Isaiah, 40:31). It is very encouraging to know that we, as the Israelites for whom Isaiah was prophesying, are also God's chosen people.

NURSES AS GOD'S CHOSEN ONES

Nursing servant leaders, being among God's chosen, can find great solace and joy in the beginning phrase of Chapter 3, Verse 12, of Saint Paul's letter to the Colossians. In this section of the letter Paul was speaking to the young Christian community about their new life in Christ. He began with the encouraging words: "As God's chosen ones, holy and beloved." These are indeed blessed descriptors for followers of Jesus: to not only have been "chosen" by the Lord but also to be considered both "holy" and "beloved" by Him.

The next several lines in Paul's message, however, are challenging rather than comforting. Paul first admonishes the community to "clothe" themselves "with compassion, kindness, humility, meekness, and patience" (3:12). He then goes on to command that they must "bear with one another and if anyone has a complaint against another, forgive each other" (3:13). Next Paul advises that, as Christians, the Lord's disciples must "clothe themselves with love which, binds everything together in perfect harmony" (3:14). Ultimately, the evangelist teaches that after embracing all of the above virtues the members of the community must "let the peace of Christ rule in (their) hearts" (3:15) and urges that whatever is done "in word or deed," they must do "in the name of the Lord Jesus, giving thanks to God the Father through Him" (Colossians 3:17).

One almost feels the need to take a deep breath after reading all of the above mandates that the apostle Paul not only taught but fully expected of the early Christian community. Paul identified a number of virtues that may not always be easy for a nurse servant leader to adopt — for any Christian person to adopt. To consider these attitudes and behaviors from a nursing perspective, we need to unpack the individual Christian attributes listed in Paul's letter to the Colossians.

Compassion

Compassion, it is suggested, is sometimes simply identified "with mercy, pity, and tenderness" (Downey, 1993, p. 192). This, however, Michael Downey asserts, can "obscure the depth of meaning of the word.... Though akin to these terms, the meaning of compassion is distinct. The terms refers to the very core of one's deepest feelings, much as the term *heart* does today" (1993, p. 192). Compassion essentially "may be understood as the capacity to be attracted and moved by the fragility, weakness, and suffering of another" (Downey, 1993, p. 192).

Downey's understanding of compassion is central to the vocation of the nurse servant leader; it is, in fact, the heart of a nurse's call to serve the ill and the infirm. In the book *A Sacred Covenant: The Spiritual Ministry of Nursing*, I included an entire chapter entitled "Clothed with Compassion." In the chapter, I explored the six key elements of Downey's definition of compassion as "one that can truly be embraced by nurses" (O'Brien, 2008, p. 43). Downey's characteristics of a compassionate person are:

1. The capacity to be attracted and moved by the fragility, weakness, and suffering of another
2. The ability to be vulnerable to undergo risk and loss for the good of another
3. The desire to be of assistance to the other
4. The wish to move toward participation in the experience of the other
5. A sensitivity to what is weak or wounded as well as the vulnerability to be affected by the other
6. Taking action to alleviate pain and suffering (Downey, 1993, pp. 192–193)

These characteristics, included in Downey's definition of compassion, might also appropriately be included in a definition of the nurse servant leader.

Downey's first characteristic of compassion, "the capacity to be attracted and moved by the fragility, weakness, and suffering of another," is central to the calling of any nursing leader. We may never know why we individual nurses were chosen by God for this ministry. But virtually every man or woman who has the heart of a nurse, has a heart deeply moved by the fragility and suffering of the ill and the infirm.

Annie, a head nurse in a long-term care facility, explained why she had chosen geriatric nursing over some of the more exciting specialty areas such as intensive care or the emergency department: "I know that some nurses, especially, the younger ones, think that caring for older folks, especially those who are weak and sick, is not a very exciting kind of nursing. It's true that some days it can be challenging because some older patients get grumpy if they don't feel good and some are confused. But I find that geriatric nursing is one of the most rewarding kinds of nursing you can do. These patients are very fearful about their futures. They see that a lot of their lives are over, and it's important to give them hope and keep their spirits up as well as (taking care of) their bodies. And elders are so grateful for just the littlest thing that you do for them; some are so fragile that it's almost like taking care of a little child. I love geriatric nursing because these patients really touch your heart."

Downey's second characteristic of compassion, "the ability to be vulnerable to undergo risk and loss for the good of another," is a concept also deeply embedded in the spirit of nursing. Simply look at the history and tradition of service of the profession as presented in Chapter 2. Nurse servant leaders such as Florence Nightingale, Clara Barton, Edith Cavell, Mary Breckinridge, and Geneviève de Galard risked, and in the case of Edith Cavell surrendered, their lives to care for those injured in wars of politics and of poverty.

I think one group of nurses who most powerfully exemplify Michael Downey's second characteristic of compassion are those working with patients experiencing life-threatening or terminal illnesses, especially the pediatric nurses who care for dying children. I met a group of these pediatric nurse practitioners while doing a hospital chaplaincy program. My assignment was a pediatric research oncology unit, and most of the children were on experimental treatment protocols for vicious cancer diagnoses; the majority were facing the possibility or even probability of death. The nurse practitioners on the unit became deeply attached to the children they were caring for and continually had to risk the loss they would experience when a child died.

I wrote about this group of nurses in *A Sacred Covenant: The Spiritual Ministry of Nursing* because their caring and willingness to risk so touched my heart. Whenever possible the nurses would attend a funeral or memorial service for a child who had died, but this was not always possible as some children's homes were in distant cities. It was very difficult for the nurses who were not able to say a formal good-bye to the little ones they had cared for. Thus, "the nurses asked if the hospital chaplaincy department would plan a general memorial service for the pediatric unit; this would give the staff a chance to mourn the loss of the children who had died during the past year. The pediatric nurses were aware of their personal vulnerability and deep need to grieve the loss of their precious small patients" (O'Brien, 2008, p. 43).

The "desire to be of assistance to another," Downey's third characteristic of compassion is an absolute necessity for one who is to become a professional nurse, especially a nursing servant leader. When one looks at the 10 characteristics of a servant leader, as identified by Larry Spears (2004), the desire is found to be supportive of each one: listening, empathy, healing, awareness (self and needs of others) persuasion (rather than coercion), conceptualization, foresight, stewardship, commitment (to the growth of others), and community (development) (pp. 24–26). Myriad examples of this "desire to be of assistance to another" are reflected in the nurse servant leader study participant perceptions and anecdotes reported in later chapters of this book.

Downey's characteristic of compassion that describes the wish to move "toward participation in the experience of another" is closely related to the Spears servant leadership characteristic of empathy; that is the perceptual attitude of desiring to truly cross over and understand what a suffering patient is experiencing rather than simply being sympathetic to their pain.

Megan, a team leader on a large medical surgical unit, displayed this kind of empathetic desire to understand what one of her patients was going through in her comments about Mary. Mary was a 32-year-old, 4th-stage ovarian cancer patient with two small children. Meg commented sadly:

> I'm a Mom too. I have two children like her, and I can only imagine what she's going through. To know that you're probably never going to see them grow up — to see them graduate from school, go to college, get married, have babies. All the Mom stuff you count on. I've been spending a lot of time with Mary, just sitting with her and letting her talk. I think that will help me be a better nurse for her; if I can sort of understand what she's thinking and what she's feeling right now; to put myself in her place. I know I can't really, but I can kind of try. Mary's prognosis is really poor, and she's like letting me know that, like, you know, in a lot of ways without saying "OK, I'm dying." But she's talking about writing some things for the kids or maybe making a video of things she wants to say to them. I'm trying, I know I'm not in her shoes, but still trying to put myself in her place as much as I can to help her; to be present to her when she needs me.

A nurse's "sensitivity to the weak and wounded, as well as the vulnerability to be affected by the other," Downey's fifth characteristic of compassion, flows from the concept of empathy and of wanting to participate in another's experience. This is often reflected in the attitudes and behaviors of hospice nurses and the research pediatric nurse practitioners, who risk the pain of loving and losing their patients, all of whom are at or near the end of their lives when entering the healthcare system.

Many years ago, as a young faculty member in a school of nursing, I had a brief experience in volunteer hospice care. I and another faculty member wanted the experience of hospice nursing, which was something we had not done previously. After a 10-week course in hospice nursing, we were initially assigned to care for an elderly gentleman with terminal cancer; our patient was homebound because of his deteriorating condition. We would visit the patient's home once a week, to give the family some respite, and assist with bathing, feeding, and medications and treatments. I remember that the hardest thing about the experience was becoming attached to this lovely and charming man, who was incredibly appreciative of our visits, which he always made a point of letting us know, and realizing that our interactions were limited as the disease progressed; he became weaker and weaker on each visit. We were indeed "sensitive" to his fragility but also felt personally "vulnerable" as we witnessed his impending death experience. Walking with a patient through the dying process, described by some nurses as midwifing a birth into eternal life, is a blessing and a gift. It also necessitates the nurse being able to embrace the "vulnerability to be affected" by the suffering of another.

Downey's sixth and final characteristic of compassion is taking "action to alleviate pain and suffering." This, again, is a necessary desire and central caring activity of any nurse called to serve those who are ill and infirm. It is who we are and what we are about as nurses. Nurses are definitely action-oriented professionals. We find those situations when we are, for some complicated reason(s), unable to "take action to alleviate pain and suffering" frustrating to the point of causing our own personal pain and suffering. When nurses are blocked, even for some very legitimate reason such as intractable pain, from undertaking this final characteristic of compassion, we may feel that we have failed. It is at such times that we must place our desire to embrace and practice compassion in the hands of God and seek His help, support, and guidance. There are some physical, psychosocial, and spiritual illnesses, the course and etiology of which we simply cannot fully grasp. In these situations it is only faith and trust in the mercy and the justice of an all-loving God that provides our comfort.

Ultimately, Downey observed that it was a person's "deepest inner feelings" that would "lead to outward compassionate acts of mercy and kindness" (1993, p. 192), and it is in that sense that we consider nursing not only a profession but also a vocation. "From the time of Florence Nightingale, who wrote of nursing 'A new art and science has been created . . . and with it a new profession, so they say; we say *calling*' (Widerquist, 1995, p. 4), to the contemporary practicing nurse, our profession is considered by most as a spiritual calling to serve the ill and the infirm" (O'Brien, 2008, p. 44).

Compassion Fatigue

Although not addressed in the Bible, we cannot completely leave the topic of nurses' compassion without briefly addressing the relatively new concept of compassion fatigue. We do know from scripture, however, that when Jesus needed a respite from His days of preaching and healing, and perhaps from His powerful ministry of compassion, He went away to a quiet place to heal His spirit: "In the morning, while it was still dark, He got up and went out to a deserted place, and there He prayed" (Mark 1:35).

The expression *compassion fatigue* has only come into common parlance in the past few decades, initially identifying a public image of lessening of public compassion for the poor and the sick because of an overwhelming media exposure to such suffering. Compassion fatigue is seen as a kind of overexposure to the pain of others because of the mass media attention to world problems. More recently, the nursing and healthcare literature also took up the topic of compassion fatigue as descriptive of a kind of apathy to suffering experienced by professional caregivers who may also be overexposed to their patients' pain.

Several nursing journal articles in the last decade have expressed concern about nurses' compassion fatigue related to caring for such patients as traumatized hurricane victims (Worley, 2005; Frank & Adkinson, 2007) and perioperative patients (Clark & Gioro, 1998; Schwam, 1998). Perioperative nurse Kendall Schwam points out that "compassion fatigue is not the same as burnout"; it is generally associated with the stressful experiences of "frontline troops" such as perioperative nurses, especially those working in hospitals with level-1 trauma centers (1998, p. 645). Nurses Marcia Clark and Sandra Gioro assert that perioperative nurses "who actively maintain a balanced personal and professional life" are best able to cope with trauma nursing (1998, p. 85).

Some specific suggestions for preventing or lessening compassion fatigue include:

- "Practicing good emotional health maintenance," that is, recognizing "when you are wearing down" and doing something to "replenish your spirit" (Worley, 2005, p. 416)
- Spending some quiet time alone and supporting physical health with a balanced diet and exercise (Pfifferling & Gilley, 2000)
- Seeking out one's own "inner core of peacefulness"; to "mentally pause and remember that at your core you are a peaceful, compassionate human being" (Brown, 2000, p. 24)

It would seem that perhaps the latter healing strategy was what Our Lord was doing when He withdrew to a deserted place, by Himself, to pray to His Father. This is a powerful example for nurses in all types of compassionate caring ministries.

Humility

A truly compassionate nurse servant leader is, innately, also a kind, a humble, and a patient leader. Kindness and patience directed toward the "fragility and suffering of another" are incorporated in the concept of compassion as noted above. Humility, as I have observed in the past, is a tricky virtue: once you think you've got it, you haven't (O'Brien, 2008, p. 58). Spiritual writer William Shannon points out that real humility is

> rooted in the truth of reality. Grounded in a deep awareness of our limitations and shortcomings in the presence of the divine perfection ... it leads us to a profound sense of total dependence on God and to an ardent desire to do God's will in all things. (1993, p. 516)

"It means, therefore," Shannon adds, "grasping the truth about ourselves and about God" (p. 516). "In the biblical world ... humble persons do not threaten or challenge another's rights nor do they claim more for themselves than has been duly allotted them in life" (Malina, 1985a, p. 411). Meekness is described as "the quality characteristic of humility when coupled with gentleness. The meek person not only does not threaten or challenge others but accepts others openly and confidently" (Achtemeier, 1985, p. 619). In Saint Matthew's gospel, the meek seem to be seen as those who are "patiently accepting of their status" (Coogan, 1993, p. 510).

In the beginning of Chapter 2, I observed that we stand on the shoulders of those nurses who have gone before us. One of the most obvious and blessed virtues of so many of our nursing forebears was, I believe, their true humility and meekness. We see it in all of the nurse servant leaders, from the era of Veronica of Jerusalem through leaders of the 1900s such as Geneviève de Galard, the French Air Force Nurse labeled by the media "the angel of Dien Bien Phu." When confronted by members of the media, who called her a heroine and asked about her courageous acts in caring for wounded soldiers in the midst of combat, she replied that she had only done "what any nurse would do." For centuries nurse servant leaders have quietly and unassumingly carried out a multitude of selfless, altruistic acts of caring and compassion with little or no acknowledgment or acclaim. Nurses have and still today demonstrate amazing actions of tender love and healing as part of their routine nursing practice; they are simply doing "what any nurse would do."

Forgiveness

The gift of forgiveness is described as "the removal of obstacles that lie in the way of intimate union with God and others" (Dallen, 1993, p. 406). Forgiveness includes "reconciliation with God, others, the world and even with oneself ... forgiveness of others is part of spiritual growth" (pp. 406–407) and biblically relates to "the reestablishment of an interpersonal relationship that has been disrupted through some misdeed" (Louw, 1993b, p. 232). In the New Testament it is taught that "community relations depend on members forgiving one another (Matthew 18:21–35; Luke 17:3). The Lord's Prayer makes divine forgiveness dependent on forgiveness of others" (Matthew 6:12, 14–15; Luke 11:4) (Saldarini, 1985, p. 319).

The gift of forgiveness may seem a virtue that is not all that relevant for nurse leaders, at least not in their daily practice of nursing. And yet, thinking back to my own days of hospital nursing, I believe that there are, in fact, a number of instances when nurses need to embrace the act of forgiveness: forgiveness for patients, with whom they have worked very hard, who refuse to comply with a prescribed treatment regimen; forgiveness for family members whose anger at a loved ones' terminal illness can be misdirected toward whatever nurse happens to be available at the time; or forgiveness of a healthcare facility that doesn't seem to provide adequate personnel or supplies to support the excellent care that nurses desire to give. It is only through an attitude of forgiveness that a nurse's loving care can grow and flourish.

Love

In the Lord's "great commandment" love is the primary concept. When asked which is the first commandment, Jesus replied, "You shall love the Lord your God with all your heart, and with all your soul, and with all your mind and with all your strength ... (and) you shall love your neighbor as yourself (Mark 12:28–31) (Donfried, 1985, p. 579). New Testament love "points specifically to the love of God revealed in Jesus Christ, who entered history and died out of love for creation" (Dreyer, 1993, p. 613). Love is, in fact, seen biblically as "that central quality which all other virtues, gifts, and fruit can be said to radiate and specify" (Evans, 1993a, p. 429). Some of these fruits include joy, patience, kindness, gentleness, and peace.

Love and loving care are givens for those who wish to nurse the sick, for those who are leaders in nursing the sick. Each nurse will exemplify that love in his or her own manifestation of caring, which may vary with each unique patient situation. If a nurse is truly able to practice loving care in her profession, a sense of peace will follow, despite the difficulties and challenges of the ministry.

Peace

The Hebrew word for peace "occurs more than 250 times in the Bible and its richness is shown by its many usages" (Hawthorne, 1993, p. 579). It has been suggested that "one of the most significant biblical texts highlighting the meaning of peace in a Christian context is found in the letter to the Ephesians, wherein Jesus is identified as our peace" (Jegen, 1993, p. 732). Jesus is not only our peace but, by His passion, is also a peacemaker: "Through the shedding of His blood, Jesus made peace by breaking down the barriers of hostility" (Jegen, 1993, p. 732). The term *peace* is also used in the New Testament to signify "order and concord within the Christian congregation; Paul frequently exhorts Christians to be at peace with one another "(and) ... Christians should strive for peace with all people, Christian or not" (Dewey, 1985, p. 766).

Peace, which I noted above flows from a nurse's posture of loving care, may seem an attribute rather difficult to maintain within the hustle and bustle of the contemporary healthcare system. Real peace, however, is a gift of the soul, of the inner spirit of a person. Nurses who are truly at peace in their calling and their ministry can find themselves in the midst of a proverbial healthcare "madhouse" and yet never lose their composure. While external activities of the day may briefly ruffle a nurse leader's sense of well-being, the associated stress ultimately dissipates for the nurse whose heart is at peace. This sense of inner peace for the nurse servant leader is a very precious gift as it is a gift which he or she shares with others in the caregiving environment. As Paul exhorted the early Christians, peace should be embraced for "order and concord" within the community, as well as within oneself.

This chapter, exploring the biblical roots of the nurse's call to serve, reflects through both the literature and nursing narratives, how both Old and New Testament calls to serve others are lived out in the lives of contemporary practicing nurses. Nurses embrace the concept of servanthood as a grace and a gift of God with which He has blessed the practice of professional nursing. Nursing is the one ministry that receives its mandate to serve directly from the recorded words of Jesus in the New Testament: "For I was hungry and you gave me food, I was thirsty and you gave me something to drink, I was a stranger and you welcomed me, I was naked and you gave me clothing, I was sick and you took care of me, I was in prison and you visited me ... just as you did it to one of the least of these who are members of my family, you did it to me" (Matthew 25:35–36, 40).

REFERENCES

Achtemeier, P. J. (Ed.). (1985). *Harper's bible dictionary.* San Francisco: Harper & Row.

American Red Cross Bulletin. (1922). The vision of service. *Trained Nurse and Hospital Review, LXVIII*(1), 33.

A private duty nurse. (1922). *American Journal of Nursing, 22*(11), 900–902.

Billroth, T. (1895). *The care of the sick at home and in the hospital* (4th ed.). London: Samson, Low, Marston & Co.

Booth, J. C. (1929). The faithful nurse. *American Journal of Nursing, 29*(4), 380.

Brown, C. (2000). Healing healers. *Nursing Standard, 14*(48), 24.

Callahan, A. (1993). Heart. In M. Downey (Ed.), *The new dictionary of Catholic spirituality* (pp. 468–469). Collegeville, MN: Liturgical Press.

Catherine De Jesus-Christ. (1938). *At the bedside of the sick: Precepts and counsels for hospital nurses.* London: Burns, Oates & Washbourne.

Clark, M. L., & Gioro, S. (1998). Nurses, indirect trauma, and prevention. *Image, the Journal of Nursing Scholarship, 30*(1), 85–87.

Coogan, M. D. (1993). Meek. In B. M. Metzger & M. D. Coogan (Eds.), *The Oxford companion to the bible* (p. 510). New York: Oxford University Press.

Dallen, J. (1993). Forgiveness. In M. Downey (Ed.), *The new dictionary of Catholic spirituality* (pp. 406–407). Collegeville, MN: Liturgical Press.

Dewey, J. (1985). Peace. In P. J. Achtemeier (Ed.), *Harper's bible dictionary* (pp. 766–767). San Francisco: Harper & Row.

Donfried, K. P. (1985). Love. In P. J. Achtemeier (Ed.), *Harper's bible dictionary* (pp. 578–581). San Francisco: Harper & Row.

Doohan, H. (1993). Service. In M. Downey (Ed.), *The new dictionary of Catholic spirituality* (pp. 875–877). Collegeville, MN: Liturgical Press.

Downey, M. (1993). Compassion. In M. Downey (Ed.), *The new dictionary of Catholic spirituality* (pp. 192–193). Collegeville, MN: Liturgical Press.

Dreyer, E. (1993). Love. In M. Downey (Ed.), *The new dictionary of Catholic spirituality* (pp. 612–622). Collegeville, MN: Liturgical Press.

Edwards, D. R. (1985). Heart. In P. J. Achtemeier (Ed.), *Harper's bible dictionary* (p. 377). San Francisco: Harper & Row.

Evans, G. P. (1993a). Fruits of the Holy Spirit. In M. Downey (Ed.), *The new Catholic dictionary of spirituality* (pp. 429–431). Collegeville, MN: Liturgical Press.

Evans, G. P. (1993b). Gifts of the Holy Spirit. In M. Downey (Ed.), *The new Catholic dictionary of spirituality* (pp. 436–439). Collegeville, MN: Liturgical Press.

Fraga, C. (1927). A real vocation. *American Journal of Nursing, 27*(5), 351–354.

Frank, D. I., & Adkinson, L. F. (2007). A developmental perspective on risk for compassion fatigue in middle-aged nurses caring for hurricane victims in Florida. *Holistic Nursing Practice, 21*(2), 55–62.

Fredriksen, P. (1993). Love. In B. M. Metzger & M. D. Coogan (Eds.), *The Oxford companion to the bible* (pp. 467–469). New York: Oxford University Press.

Gunn, G. E. (1926). Only a nurse. *Trained Nurse and Hospital Review, LXXVI*(3), 300.

Habel, M. L., & Milton, H. D. (1939). *The graduate nurse in the home: Meeting community needs.* Philadelphia: J.B. Lippincott.

Harmer, B. (1925). *Textbook of the principles and practice of nursing.* New York: Macmillan.

Hawthorne, G. F. (1993). Peace. In B. M. Metzger & M. D. Coogan (Eds.), *The Oxford companion to the bible* (p. 579). New York: Oxford University Press.

Hayward, D. R. (1929). Hands. *American Journal of Nursing, 29*(5), 536.

Homans, V. D. (1929). A nurse's prayer. *American Journal of Nursing, 29*(8), 1028.

Humphry, L. (1919). *The nurse's service digest: A manual of nursing.* New York: Orsamus, Turner, Harris.

Imeldine, M. (1926). The nurse's recompense. *American Journal of Nursing, XXVL*(3), 192.

In the hospital. (1922). *Trained Nurse and Hospital Review, LXVIII*(3), 213.

Jegen, C. F. (1993). Peace. In M. Downey (Ed.), *The new Catholic dictionary of spirituality* (pp. 732–734). Collegeville, MN: Liturgical Press.

Johns Hopkins Nurses' Alumnae Magazine. (1929). Any nurse, 1929. *American Journal of Nursing, 29*(7), 786.

Kohlenberger, J. R. (1993). *The concise concordance to the New Revised Standard Version.* New York: Oxford University Press.

Louw, J. P. (1993a). Fear. In B. M. Metzger & M. D. Coogan (Eds.), *The Oxford companion to the bible* (p. 225). New York: Oxford University Press.

Louw, J. P. (1993b). Forgiveness. In B. M. Metzger & M. D. Coogan (Eds.), *The Oxford companion to the bible* (p. 232). New York: Oxford University Press.

Lumpkin, G. T. (1926). The Christ spirit which makes the hospital great. *Trained Nurse and Hospital Review, 77*(6), 628–629.

Maas, R. (1993). Obedience. In M. Downey (Ed.), *The new dictionary of Catholic spirituality* (pp. 709–712). Collegeville, MN: Liturgical Press.

Malina, B. J. (1985a). Humility. In P. J. Achtemeier (Ed.), *Harper's bible dictionary* (pp. 411–412). New York: Harper & Row.

Malina, B. J. (1985b). Service. In P. J. Achtemeier (Ed.), *Harper's bible dictionary* (p. 930). New York: Harper & Row.

Mascot, B. M. (1921). The spirit of service. *Public Health Nurse, 13*(4), 20.

Matera, F. J. (1985). Servant. In P. J. Achtemeier (Ed.), *Harper's bible dictionary* (pp. 929–930). New York: Harper & Row.

McQuhae, A. (1927). Ah, Mother, if our lamps have failed. *Trained Nurse and Hospital Review, LXXVIII*(4), 386.

Modern Hospital. (1930). The dedication of the nurse. *American Journal of Nursing,* *30*(10), 1234.

Muddiman, J. (1993). Word of God. In B. M. Metzger & M. D. Coogan (Eds.), *The Oxford companion to the bible* (p. 818). New York: Oxford University Press.

Neyrey, J. H. (1985). Soul. In P. J. Achtemeier (Ed.), *Harper's bible dictionary* (pp. 982–983). New York: Harper & Row.

Noffke, S. (1993). Soul. In M. Downey (Ed.), *The new dictionary of Catholic spirituality* (pp. 908–910). Collegeville, MN: Liturgical Press.

O'Brien, M. E. (2008). *A sacred covenant: The spiritual ministry of nursing.* Sudbury, MA: Jones and Bartlett.

Perry, J. D. (1925). Christmas greeting. *Trained Nurse and Hospital Review, LXXV*(6), 581.

Pfifferling, J. H., & Gilley, K. (2000). Overcoming compassion fatigue. *Family Practice Management, 7*(4), 1–6.

Pope, F. E. (1898). What it is to be a nurse. In J. Hodson (Ed.), *How to become a trained nurse: A manual of information in detail* (pp. 11–14). New York: William Abbatt.

Rothweiler, E. L. (1937). *The science and art of nursing.* Philadelphia: F.A. Davis.

Saldarini, A. J. (1985). Forgiveness. In P. J. Achtemeier (Ed.), *Harper's bible dictionary* (p. 319). New York: Harper & Row.

Sanders, G. J. (1914). *Modern methods in nursing.* Philadelphia: W.B. Saunders.

Satyer, A. (1922). The daily psalm. *Trained Nurse and Hospital Review, LXIX*(5), 235.

Schoonover-Shoffner, K. (1997). A call to servanthood. *Journal of Christian Nursing, 14*(4), 13–27, 37.

Schwam, K. (1998). The phenomenon of compassion fatigue in perioperative nurses. *AORN Journal, 68*(4), 642–648.

Service. (1993). *Zondervan's compact bible dictionary.* Grand Rapids, MI: Zondervan.

Shannon, W. H. (1993). Humility. In M. Downey (Ed.), *The new dictionary of Catholic spirituality* (pp. 516–518). Collegeville, MN: Liturgical Press.

Shelly, J. A., & Miller, A. B. (2006). *Called to care: A Christian world view for nursing* (2nd ed.). Downers Grove, IL: InterVarsity Press.

Smith, D. M. (1985). Word. In P. J. Achtemeier (Ed.), *Harper's bible dictionary* (p. 1141). New York: Harper & Row.

Spears, L. C. (2004). Prescription for organizational health. *Reflections on Nursing Leadership, 30*(4), 24–26.

Unterman, J. (1985). Commandment. In P. J. Achtemeier (Ed.), *Harper's bible dictionary* (p. 176). New York: Harper & Row.

Wead, C. B. (1926). The lighting of the seven candles. *American Journal of Nursing, 26*(12), 933–934.

Wead, C. B. (1927). The Christmas attitude. *Trained Nurse and Hospital Review, LXXIX*(6), 642–643.

Widerquist, J. (1995). Called to serve. *Christian Nurse International, 11*(1), 4–6.

Widerquist, J., & Davidhizar, R. (1994). The ministry of nursing. *Journal of Advanced Nursing, 19*(4), 647–652.

Window in English Cathedral. (1926). *The Trained Nurse and Hospital Review, LXXVI*(3), 279–280.

Woods, C. S. (1922). The vision. *The Trained Nurse and Hospital Review, LXIX*(6), 494.

Worley, C. A. (2005). The art of caring: Compassion fatigue. *Dermatology Nursing, 17*(6), 416.

4 Nursing's Call to Servant Leadership

Here is my servant whom I uphold, my chosen in whom my soul delights.

—Isaiah 42:1

As a nursing leader, I believe every leader has a call to service. It is our duty as leaders to first be servants. Working the ICU (intensive care unit) as a charge nurse, I am a servant to my patients, to my team, to the physician, and to the entire nursing staff. Being a leader takes a lot of discipline. One of the compelling characteristics is first to be humble. . . . be a humble servant. Each day we deal with patients who need our service. Each day we deal with staff who need our service. Being a leader takes compassion, takes caring; it takes listening. When I'm in charge, I have to be very, very vigilant to listen to every sound around me. To listen to every nurse who has problems, who has concerns, to every patient who has concerns. . . . I listen with my heart and listen to the energies around me. The positive energy, the negative energy — this is what drives me.

—Regina, nurse practitioner serving as an ICU
(intensive care unit) charge nurse

During the past decade there has been significant discussion in the nursing literature as to whether contemporary nursing can be considered a respected professional occupation and also a spiritual vocation, that is, a calling to serve, as originally described by Florence Nightingale, following Jesus' mandate to care for the sick (Matthew 25:36). It is clear that nursing, as practiced in the third millennium, is a professional endeavor. To explore the current vocational identity of nursing, a study was initiated among 35 professional nurse leaders, employing the phenomenological method of Max van Manen (1990). The primary aim of the initial study (phase 1) entitled, Called to Serve: The Lived Experience of the Nursing Vocation, was to "explore and describe the lived experience of nursing as a spiritual calling, as understood by contemporary practicing nurse leaders." The term *spiritual* could be understood by the nurses in a religious or a humanitarian sense.

An overarching concept that emerged from analysis of the data, elicited in the phase 1 interviews, was that of service. The attributes of service or servanthood, as described in the published characteristics of servant leadership, were frequently reflected in the documented perceptions and experiences of the nurse leader study participants.

Building on initial analysis of the comments shared by the 35 phase 1 participants, a second group of 40 nursing leaders was added to the project sample; this effort was labeled study phase 2. The purpose of the study's second phase was to validate the nursing leaders' perceptions of the lived experience of servant leadership, as a concept, as identified in the literature by such scholars of servant leadership as Robert K. Greenleaf (1977), Larry C. Spears (2004), and Robert F. Russell and A. Gregory Stone (2002). Focused interviews were directed to explore how individual nurse leaders understand and demonstrate characteristics of servant leadership in their day-to-day practice of nursing. The purposive nursing sample included in study phases 1 and 2 was drawn from the population of nursing leaders who consider nursing to be a spiritual calling as well as a profession.

The ultimate goal of the project was to use the data elicited in the practicing nurse leaders' interviews to support development of a model of servant leadership for nursing. This model may be incorporated in curricula of schools of nursing, as well as in continuing education programs in medical care centers such as hospitals, clinics, nursing homes, hospices, home health agencies, and churches (where parish or congregational nursing programs exist).

CALLED TO SERVE—THE LIVED EXPERIENCE OF A NURSING VOCATION

Specific Aims

The purpose of the project was, as noted, twofold. In phase 1, the nursing leaders' perception of nursing as a vocation or calling to care for the sick was initially explored broadly, employing the hermeneutic phenomenological method of van Manen. Following identification of the concept of service as an overarching theme in the initial analysis, a secondary analysis of the phase 1 data was carried out to determine if relationships existed between nurse study participants' perceptions and experiences of their vocation of service and the servant leader characteristics and attributes identified in the literature. Through this analysis a number of nursing servant leadership characteristics and attributes specific to nursing were identified; these were described as nursing servant leadership themes and subthemes.

The nursing servant leader themes and subthemes identified in phase 1 were then further explored and validated in phase 2 through the method of focused probing.

Following analysis of the qualitative data elicited from nursing leaders in phases 1 and 2 of the study, the detailed model of servant leadership for nursing was developed, which can be disseminated to the larger nursing community. The model's purpose is to elucidate the meaning and parameters of servant leadership as understood by practicing nurses.

Conceptual Definitions of Terms

Nursing Vocation or Calling to Serve

The nursing vocation or calling to serve, for the purpose of this study, was defined as a felt spiritual call to serve the ill and the infirm, in the spirit of Florence Nightingale, following the Christian mandate to care for the sick. For nonreligiously affiliated nurses the calling to serve was understood as a humanitarian call to serve one's fellow man and woman.

Servant Leadership

> The servant-leader is servant first.... It begins with the natural feeling that one wants to serve, to serve first.... The best test (of servant leadership) is: Do those served grow as persons? Do they, while being served, become healthier, wiser, freer, more autonomous, and more likely themselves to become servants? (Greenleaf, 1977, p. 27)

Nursing Servant Leadership

It is important to point out a significant difference between nurse servant leaders and those servant leaders in business and industrial organizations. In the latter settings, the servant leader is responsible only for staff providing the workforce of the organization. In the nursing arena, however, servant leaders, from the highest level nursing administrator in a medical center to the team leader of a small nursing subspecialty area, are responsible not only for the healthcare staff members they supervise but also for the well-being of the patients and families for whom those staff members care. Thus, there is, in a sense a dual leadership role for nursing leaders in the contemporary healthcare system.

Methodology

The Called to Serve study design was that of hermeneutic phenomenological inquiry employing the method of exploration and analysis as articulated by van Manen (1984, 1990). *Phenomenology* is defined by van Manen as "the study of the lifeworld—the world as we immediately experience it prereflectively rather than as we conceptualize, categorize, or reflect on it. Phenomenology aims at getting a deeper understanding of the nature or meaning of the everyday experience" (1990, p. 9). He notes additionally that phenomenology posits an approach that must be "presuppositionless," meaning without predetermined biases, concepts, or ideas that would "govern the research project" (p. 29). Phenomenological research, understood as the study of "the significant world of the human being" (p. 9), is then an appropriate method for the study of nurses' understanding and lived experience of nursing as a calling to serve and as an opportunity to practice servant leadership.

The use of a hermeneutic phenomenological approach has been described as a marriage of interpretation and essence of a phenomenon; the research "tries to be attentive to both terms of its methodology: it is a descriptive (phenomenological) methodology because it wants to be attentive to how things appear, it wants to let things speak for themselves; it is an interpretive (hermeneutic) methodology because it claims that there are no such things as uninterpreted phenomena" (van Manen, 1990, p. 180). "Heideggerian hermeneutics locates the unit of analysis in the transaction between the participant and the interpreter" (Koch, 1995, p. 834). Van Manen observes that phenomenological analysis "is not introspective but retrospective. Reflection on lived experience is always recollective; it is reflection on experience that has already passed or been lived through" (1990, p. 10).

Overall van Manen understands hermeneutic phenomenological research as encompassing six significant activities:

1. Turning to a phenomenon that seriously interests us and commits us to the world
2. Investigating experience as we live it rather than as we conceptualize it
3. Reflecting on the essential themes that characterize the phenomenon
4. Describing the phenomenon through the art of writing and rewriting

5. Manipulating a strong and oriented pedagogical relation to the phenomenon

6. Balancing the research context by considering parts and whole (1990, pp. 30–31).

Van Manen's explanation of these activities was interpreted for the Called to Serve study in the following ways:

- Have a deep and "abiding" interest in the topic, citing Heidegger's words: "To think is to confine yourself to a single thought that one day stands still like a star in the world's sky" (Heidegger, 1974, p. 4, cited in van Manen, 1990, p. 31). The investigator in the presently proposed study has, for many years, had a "deep and abiding" interest in the phenomenon of nursing as a vocation. This is witnessed by the author's numerous nursing studies and publications either centrally or tangentially discussing the concept (and during the past decade eight individually authored books have focused on the topic of spirituality in nursing, including the concept of nursing as a vocation).

- Explore a phenomenon as a lived experience by "reawakening the basic experience of the world" (van Manen, p. 31). The specific aim of the present study was to "reawaken" the concept of nursing as a vocation of service by exploring the "lived experience of nursing as a calling among a population of contemporary professional nursing leaders."

- "Reflective grasping of what it is that renders this or that particular experience its special significance" (van Manen, p. 32). A focused interview guide, possessing both content and construct validity was developed to guide the phenomenological interviews with the nursing sample. Following transcription of the interviews, the texts were read and reread reflectively to identify key themes that emerged from the lifeworld data elicited from nurses who considered nursing to be a vocation of service. Thematic analysis (as described by van Manen) condensed the themes to arrive at a higher level of abstraction.

- "Thoughtfully bringing (the phenomenon) to speech" through the activity of writing or to again quote Heidegger "To let that which shows itself be seen from itself in the very way in which it shows itself from itself" (1962, p. 58, cited in van Manen, p. 33). Through the thematic analysis, themes reflective of nursing as a vocation of service were explored and described in thematic statements in order to bring to life the concept of nursing as a vocation among contemporary nurses.

- "To be oriented to an object means that we are animated by the object in a full and human sense. To be strong in our orientation means that we will not settle for superficialities and falsities—not allow ourselves to be sidetracked" (van Manen, p. 33). It was determined that for this particular study only nurses who perceived nursing as a vocation of service would be included as study participants. To that end a final question was included on the demographic data form asking if the potential study participant viewed nursing as a vocation. If the response was negative, that individual was not included in the research.

- "At several points (in the research) it is necessary to step back and look at the total, at the contextual givens and how each of the parts need to contribute toward the total. Is the study properly grounded in a laying open of the question?" (van Manen, pp. 33–34). Following each hermeneutic phenomenological interview with a professional nurse leader, the data generated was evaluated both individually and in relation to the overall aim of the study. Selected serendipitous findings were pursued in subsequent interviews if these data were considered relevant to the overall study aim and did not sidetrack the purpose of the research.

Study Sample

It is suggested that "purposeful sampling is used most commonly in phenomenological inquiry. This method of sampling selects individuals for study participation based on their particular knowledge of a phenomenon for the purpose of sharing that knowledge" (Speziale & Carpenter, 2003, p. 67). "The logic and power of purposeful sampling lies in selecting information-rich cases for study in depth. Information-rich cases are those from which one can learn a great deal about issues of central importance to the purpose of the research" (Patton, 1990, p. 169).

The purposive sample for the overall study (phases 1 and 2) consisted of a total of 75 professional nursing leaders who admitted to perceiving nursing as a calling to care for the sick; 35 nurses participated in the first of the two study phases described earlier; 40 nurse leaders were added to phase 2. All study participants were registered nurses, with leadership experience, currently employed in a variety of settings including nursing administration, management, education, research, and practice. Nurses engaged in practice represented myriad settings such as the hospital, clinic, rehabilitation center, long-term care, and home care. Nurse participants practiced in differing specialty areas such as: medical-surgical nursing, critical care, pediatrics, psych-mental health care, obstetrics and gynecology, community health, school health, and rehabilitation nursing. Nurse respondents had the credentials: RN (diploma registered nurse), ADN (associate degree in nursing), BSN (baccalaureate degree in nursing), MSN (masters degree in nursing), DNSc (doctorate in nursing science) or PhD, RN (doctor of philosophy in nursing) and reflected a variety of religious faith traditions.

Nursing leader project participants were both male and female. No age criteria were specified; however, study respondents must have practiced nursing for at least 1 year prior to the interview; most, being nursing leaders, had practiced for much longer periods of time. An attempt was made to include nurses from a variety of age categories and representing varied lengths of time in nursing.

Study Setting

Interviews were conducted at a location of the study participant's choosing, such as the home or workplace, and were audio-recorded to preserve integrity of the data. Privacy was assured for the interview.

Bracketing of Presuppositions (Phenomenological Reduction)

Prior to conducting study interviews, the investigator's biases and presuppositions were identified and bracketed as appropriate to van Manen's requirement that hermeneutic phenomenological research be "presuppositionless" (1990, p. 29). Bracketing is described by van Manen as "the act of suspending one's various beliefs in the reality of the natural world in order to study the essential structures of the world" (p. 175).

The term *bracketing* was originally derived from the work of Husserl. Husserl conceived bracketing as being "done so that what is essential in the phenomenon of consciousness can be understood without prejudice ... Husserl's use of the three terms—phenomenological reduction, *epoche*, and bracketing ... all refer to a reflective process by which opinion and prejudice are suspended to focus attention on what is essential in the phenomenon" (LeVasseur, 2003, p. 411). Husserl's student, Heidegger, however, differed on the point, believing that it was not possible to completely bracket presuppositions and biases. Heidegger essentially believed that it was impossible to obtain naive descriptions of phenomena, suggesting that when we interact with another person we must necessarily interpret his or her story in light of our own knowledge, experience, and preconceptions. Thus, these need to be identified and admitted and ultimately incorporated into a hermeneutic phenomenological analysis.

[Heidegger] held that consciousness could not be separated from 'being in the world'. Because of this we are unable to completely bracket prior conceptions and knowledge — we are necessarily embedded in a historical context…. For Heidegger and others we are already 'thrown' into the world, and all thinking, even the most general and reflective, is embedded within projects and interests that constitute practical worldly involvement. (LeVasseur, p. 415)

LeVasseur believes, however, that a more "sympathetic interpretation of Husserl's notion of bracketing can bridge the seemingly irreconcilable viewpoints of interpretive and descriptive phenomenology" (p. 417). LeVasseur points out that we do bracket our understanding, in a way, when we become curious. We assume we do not understand a phenomenon fully and also that Husserl's "notion of bracketing emphasized a temporary suspension of our theories and prior knowledge and not a permanent denial of them" (p. 417). LeVasseur also noted that while "phenomenology has become a popular approach for nursing inquiry," a "precise description of *bracketing* has sometimes been overlooked" (p. 408).

To respond to LeVasseur's latter concern, the present study employed steps included in the three phases of reflective bracketing as identified by Robin Edward Gearing (2004) as follows:

- "Abstract formulation," or articulation of the researcher's theoretical approach to the study, that of hermeneutic phenomenology, as presented in the phenomenological research method of van Manen
- "Research praxis," the process of setting aside, suspending, or holding in abeyance presuppositions about the phenomenon, and explicitly stating the phenomenon to be studied. The suppositions to be set aside are both internal ("personal knowledge, history, culture, experiences and values") and external ("suppositions based on academic or scientific ideas (e.g., orientations, theories").
- Temporal structure, "the starting point, where the bracketing begins, duration, the length of time it occurs and the end point, where it ends"
- Reintegration, "or unbracketing, and subsequent reinvestment of the bracketed data into the larger investigation. This process refers to the folding of the bracketing technique back into the research … generally the reinvestment of data derived through bracketing emerges in the analysis section of the investigation" (Gearing, 2004, pp. 1433–1435).

The first step in reflective bracketing, identified by Gearing, that of "abstract formulation," was carried out through identifying the hermeneutic phenomenological approach to the study of nursing as a vocation. The first phase of Gearing's second step, research praxis, was initiated through an explicit statement and description of the phenomenon to be studied, that of nursing lived as a vocation of service. A "nursing vocation journal" was created by the investigator with notes on the following:

- "Internal suppositions" including personal knowledge (literature review) and experience (personal history) of nursing as a calling
- Nursing culture and values as understood by the investigator
- "External suppositions" including "academic or scientific" ideas (nursing theories including the concept of the nurse's vocation was identified
- "Temporal structure," a statement of starting and ending points of the bracketing

In this study of nursing as a vocation or calling to serve, the bracketing began at the time data collection (nursing leader interviews) was initiated and ended as the investigator moved into the final stages of thematic analysis and phenomenological writing. At this point, according to Heidegger's hermeneutic approach, the investigator's preknowledge of the nursing vocation lifeworld will interact with interpretation of the study participant's understanding of nursing as a vocation.

The nursing vocation journal documented the investigator's personal history of a nursing vocation, perceived as a spiritual calling, through identifying and reflecting on such experiences as both "capping" and "graduation" ceremonies carried out in a local church, yearly religious retreats held by the investigator's school of nursing, and suggested religious readings related to the nursing vocation.

Gearing's final stage of bracketing, identified as "reintegration," was carried out when, as noted above, the analytic process moved into the last phase of "folding" the investigator's bracketed presuppositions on the topic of nursing as a calling to care for the sick back into the research.

Study Instruments

It was observed by van Manen that in hermeneutic phenomenological research the "interview serves two very specific purposes":

(1) It may be used as a means for exploring and gathering experiential narrative material that may serve as a resource

for developing a richer and deeper understanding of a human phenomenon, and (2) the interview may be used as a vehicle to develop a conversational relation with a partner (interviewee) about the meaning of an experience. (p. 66)

Additionally van Manen points out, "It is important to realize that the interview process needs to be disciplined by the fundamental question that prompted the need for the interview in the first place" (p. 66).

For the first phase of the study, two instruments were used. First, study participants were asked to complete a demographic data form from which a demographic study subject profile of nursing leaders was created. Demographic items included the study participant's age, gender, nursing education, religion, nursing leadership role, nursing area of specialization, work setting, and length of time in nursing.

Next, an investigator-developed focused interview guide, exploring the lived experience of nursing as a vocation or spiritual call to care for the sick, was employed to direct questioning. The Nursing Vocation Interview Guide (NVIG) contained one broad phenomenological question addressing the meaning of nursing as a vocation or calling to care for the sick, followed by a number of probes that explored such topics as the meaning of a nurse's personal spiritual call to care for the sick, how one's call to care for the sick attracted the person to nursing, how the vocation is lived out in one's nursing practice, whether one's perception of nursing as a vocation had changed over time, and whether any specific patient care interactions could be cited that were supported by the nurse's perception of his or her vocation to care for the sick.

The NVIG was submitted to a panel of experts in the area of nursing leadership in order to obtain content validity of the instrument (phenomenological question and probe items); construct validity was obtained through review of the nursing vocation and servant leadership literature.

Phase 2 of the study consisted of an exploration and validation of the nursing servant leadership themes that had been identified in the secondary analysis of data obtained in phase 1. This was done through repetition of the broad phenomenological question about the meaning of one's vocation to care for the sick and a number of probing questions related to the nursing servant leadership themes and subthemes identified in phase 1.

Phase 2 study participants also completed the demographic data form used in study phase 1.

Procedure

Nurse leader study participants were initially accessed through the investigator's contacts within the nursing administration, management, education, research, and practice communities; purposive "snowball" sampling was also employed in order to obtain referrals for additional project respondents. After appropriate informed consent procedures were carried out, qualitative study interviews of approximately 1 hour were conducted; all interviews were audio-recorded to preserve the purity of the data. For confidentiality, recordings were destroyed following transcription.

Protection of Human Subjects

Study participants who had read and signed the informed consent form were reminded that they could refuse to answer or discuss any question and that they could withdraw from the study at any time. It was not anticipated, nor did it happen, that the study question or probes would cause (caused) emotional discomfort; however, should this have occurred, an interview would have been terminated and appropriate supportive intervention provided by the investigator. The principal investigator and all interviewers involved in phases 1 and 2 of the project completed the NIH Human Participant Protection for Research Education Tutorial.

Data Analysis

Recorded interviews were transcribed verbatim. Qualitative data analysis was carried out according to the guidelines for phenomenological-hermeneutical analysis as articulated by van Manen. The analytic stages of the van Manen method included phenomenological reflection (reading and rereading the interview texts), thematic analysis (aimed at identifying underlying themes in the lifeworld descriptions), composing thematic statements (descriptions of key themes that emerge in data analysis), and phenomenological writing (summarizing study findings related to the phenomena of interest) (Speziale & Carpenter, 2003, p. 59).

Initially, as noted earlier, one overarching concept, that of service, was identified as undergirding the practice of professional nursing among the sample population of nursing leaders. This led initially to development of 5 nursing vocation attitudinal themes and 1 subtheme describing nurse leaders' perceptions of nursing as a spiritual calling to serve the sick. In secondary analysis of phase 1 data and analysis of phase 2 study data, 9 nursing servant leadership themes and 16 subthemes were identified and validated.

These broad existential categories "form the overall unity of one's lifeworld or lived experience of the world" (Van der Zalm & Bergum, 2000, p. 212). The goal of the phenomenologist is "to provide an understanding of the internal meanings or essences of a person's experience in the lived world by careful description of that experience, striving to understand the experience, rather than provide causal explanations of that experience" (Van der Zalm & Bergum, p. 212). That is, the concept of servant leadership in nursing is described and explained according to the lived experiences of nursing leaders as reflected in the empirical data elicited in study interviews.

In carrying out the analytic methodology for data analysis in hermeneutic phenomenology, the concept of the "hermeneutic circle" must be understood. That is, the circle of interpretation that posits that one cannot understand the whole of a phenomenon without understanding the individual parts, yet one cannot understand individual parts without some overall understanding of the whole. Thus the interpretive analysis is continually moving back and forth from the parts to the whole. This concept also refers to Heidegger's conceptualization that one brings his or her own presuppositions to any study and then looks at the world as already lived to seek new understanding. The hermeneutic circle has been described for text analysis:

> We understand the parts of a text first in view of our preunderstanding of the whole which is challenged in the act of understanding itself. Hans-Georg Gadamer emphasized the productive role of these preunderstandings for the process or interpretation. Without perspectives we do not see at all, yet through perspectives we see only as far as they allow us. Gadamer calls the condition and the perspectives of interpreters their "horizons" and the act of understanding a text's sense the "fusion of horizons" (Jeanrond, 1990, p. 463).

In the Called to Serve study, individual themes and subthemes were identified, explored, and analyzed individually, in relation to each other, and in relation to the overall understanding of nursing servant leadership.

The final phase of the data analysis as identified in van Manen's conceptualization of hermeneutic phenomenological research is the written recording of study data to create rich phenomenological descriptions. The present research on nursing's call to servanthood included many nursing leaders' reports of the lived experience of the nursing vocation identifying and describing the behavioral characteristics of servant leadership. Although a sample size of 75 study participants is large for a qualitative phenomenological study, it was felt that the breadth as well as the depth of the interview data would add validity to the descriptions of the lived experience of servant leadership in nursing.

The trustworthiness and authenticity of the phenomenological study data is supported through following the suggestions of Speziale and Carpenter (2003) who assert: (a) "the trustworthiness of the questions put to study participants depends on the extent to which they tap the participant's experiences" (p. 70). This is assured through the establishment of both construct and content validity of the Nursing Vocation Interview Guide; and (b) "consistent use of the method and bracketing prior knowledge helps to ensure pure description" (p. 70). Also, as earlier described, the investigator created a nursing vocation journal to document bracketing of presuppositions and knowledge according to the methodology identified by Gearing (2004).

Following analysis of the phase 1 and phase 2 study data, elicited from practicing nurse leaders, a model of servant leadership for nursing was developed. The model incorporates nurse leader vocational perceptions and the attitudes and experiences of nursing leaders whose philosophy of nursing reflects an overall understanding of the concept of servant leadership as identified in the contemporary servant leader literature. The defining characteristics of servant leadership, as described broadly for organizations and institutions, are in the nursing model defined and operationalized as appropriate to a variety of leadership roles within professional nursing.

Study Sample: Phase 1

The 35 nurse leader participants interviewed for phase 1 of the Called to Serve study ranged in age from 26 to 69 years; the largest number, 14 or 40%, were in the 51–60 year age group. The next largest group were from 41–50 years with 10 nurses or 29% of the sample population. Only 1 nurse was in the youngest (21–30 year) age range; this was probably because nurse leaders were specifically sought for the purposive sample.

Fifteen nurses had master's degrees and 11 had BSN degrees; 4 had diplomas or associate degrees; and 5 had doctoral preparation. Sixty-three percent or 22 of the nurses were Roman Catholic, 12 were Protestant, and 1 nurse was a member of the Jewish faith. Twenty nurse leaders practiced in a hospital setting; 10 in schools or universities, and 4 in clinics. Twenty-seven or 77% of the group had been in nursing for a range of 11 to 40 years, with five having practiced between 41 and 50 years.

The most frequently identified area of specialization was medical-surgical nursing (13 or 37%); pediatrics was next, capturing 7 nurses. Four nurses specialized in the critical care areas, two in maternal-child, two in oncology-research, and one each in the areas of emergency nursing, public health, OB/GYN, recovery room, quality management, preoperative nursing, and perinatology.

Leadership roles among the phase 1 study sample of 35 nurse leaders included the following categories:

- Administrator—2
- Manager—3
- Supervisor—1
- Head nurse—8
- Charge nurse—9
- Team leader—4
- Nurse practitioner—1
- Nurse educator—5
- Nurse researcher—2

None of the phase 1 study group identified themselves as clinical specialists. Specific nursing leadership roles within these categories included:

- Administrator (vice-president for nursing in a hospital and administrator of critical care areas)
- Manager (manager of a high-risk pregnancy unit, quality management compliance officer, public health case manager)
- Supervisor (supervisor of an outpatient diabetic clinic)
- Head nurse (head nurse of a medical-surgical unit, head nurse of a medical-surgical clinic, head nurse of a critical care unit)
- Charge nurse (charge nurse of medical-surgical unit; pediatric clinic; OB/GYN unit, recovery room, and emergency room)
- Team leader (team leader on a medical-surgical unit, pediatric/family-centered care unit, psychiatric/mental health unit)
- Nurse practitioner (adult health nurse practitioner)
- Educator (nursing educator in pediatrics, critical care, and medical-surgical nursing)
- Researcher (oncology research nurse)

The demographic profile of phase 2 study participants is presented in Chapter 5.

PHASE 1 FINDINGS: NURSING VOCATION ATTITUDINAL THEMES

The five attitudinal themes reflecting nursing leaders' perceptions of the meaning of a nursing vocation or nursing's call to serve included: A Blessed Calling (subtheme: A Christian Mandate), Passionate Caring, Ingrained in the Spirit, the Extra Mile, and A Privilege. All of the attitudinal themes were labeled using the exact wording of one or more of the nurse leader study participants. Other nurse study participants were identified with possessing a particular vocational attitude or perception if his or her comments reflected the theme either directly or with related thoughts. For example, for the theme A Blessed Calling, while a number of nurses used the words *blessed calling*, some described nursing itself as a blessing, a blessed vocation, or stated that they felt blessed to be a nurse, as the sample responses reflect. The five nursing vocation attitudinal themes provided the basis for the perceptual dimension of the nursing servant leadership model presented in Chapter 5.

To further explicate the perceptual dimension of the lived experience of a nursing call to serve, the following presentation of nurse leaders' comments, describing each of the five vocational attitude themes, is followed by a case example reflective of the overall theme—the nursing vocation as a call to serve.

A Blessed Calling

Join with me in . . . relying on the power of God who saved us and called us with a holy calling, not according to our works but according to his own purpose and grace.

—2 Timothy 1:8–9

A Blessed Calling and the other four nursing vocation attitudinal concepts were categorized as themes when more than half of the phase 1 study participants verbalized the perception as central to their understanding of the nursing vocation. While not all nurse leaders use similar wording, the meaning of the theme was inherent in their responses. As noted, the nurses' perception that nursing is a blessed calling was described in precisely those words by a number of nursing leaders; some other nurses used the terms *blessed* or *blessing* and *calling to serve* in the same paragraph as the nursing leader study participant examples demonstrate.

Essentially what the nurse leaders conveyed in their responses was the fact that, for them, the profession of nursing was a calling with a unique and spiritual dimension undergirding the vocation. It was a calling that they felt blessed and gifted to have received, and many did indeed use the term *gift* in describing their nursing call.

"Nursing Care as a Calling" was the title of a journal article that described the nurse's calling as "a deep desire to devote oneself to serving people according to the high values of the profession" (Raatikainen, 1997, p. 1111). In studying the perceptions of 179 practicing nurses in five hospitals, the investigator concluded that "the calling experience is not in conflict with professional principles" (Raatikainen, 1997, p. 1111). Similarly in discussing "Hearing the Call to Nursing," Elizabeth Jeffries concluded that nurses are hungry "for meaning in our work . . . (and that) the word *work* comes from the Greek word meaning *to worship*. Our work is a means of worship" (1998, p. 35).

Nurse leader comments, elicited in the study Called to Serve, which described nursing as a blessed calling included the following:*

> "Nursing is a blessed calling; a spiritual calling to serve the sick" (64, DNSc, educator, community health).
> "I am truly blessed (to be a nurse). It's a blessed calling. I am blessed to love my job so much" (57, ADN, head nurse, medical-surgical).
> "If I didn't think nursing was a blessed calling or ministry and felt like it was just a job, I would not be here presently as a nurse" (54, MSN, supervisor, outpatient clinic).
> "For me nursing is a blessing; how I do good also happens to be the way I make a living" (59, PhD, RN, educator, pediatrics).

> From the very beginning of my practice of nursing, I saw it as a calling. . . . Because I thought I was called to be a nurse. I always thought it was a blessing to be called to nursing because it is easy to serve; it is easy to wash people's feet, to feed the poor, to clothe those who aren't clothed, to visit prisoners. It's easy to do all those things when you are a nurse. (57, ADN, head nurse, medical-surgical)

> To help a dying patient maintain the dignity that obviously he or she deserves ... is a tremendous blessing. I feel that

---

* Nurse leader study participants are identified by age, degree (diploma registered nurse— Diploma RN, associate degree in nursing—ADN, baccalaureate degree in nursing—BSN, master's degree in nursing—MSN, or doctoral degree in nursing—DNSc or PhD, RN), leadership role, and nursing specialty.

I am blessed to be able to do that, to be able to be a part of that. (59, PhD, RN, educator, pediatrics)

When I think of nursing as a vocation or a calling to serve the sick, I think it goes back to the days of Florence Nightingale, which might be a little sappy, but it does go back there. My mother was a nurse, and it was really a blessed vocation for her and certainly a calling because she was very good at what she did. My friends today who have stayed in the field are very dedicated and believe in what they are doing. They are changing lives for the better for their patients and clients. I think it takes a certain personality to be a nurse. I guess that is where the calling comes in. (66, BSN, head nurse, school health)

Still other nurses, while not specifically using the words *blessed* or *blessing*, identified their nursing vocation as a call from God as the following comments reflect:

God called me to do nursing, and brought me to it, and He will take me through it … He uses me as a vessel through which He works. Nurses are something beautiful that God has His hand on . . . we are here to serve . . . for God as well as for humanity. (43, BSN, head nurse, critical care)

Nursing is the opportunity to be God's hands and His feet and His voice in caring for those people that He has entrusted to me. (70, MSN, educator, medical-surgical)

I (sometimes) think of exploring the purpose in my life; doing some self investigation in deciding what direction I need to go and what God has for my life. And I think to myself "I need to be a nurse." (45, MSN, head nurse, critical care)

The essence of nursing is our ministry, that we see God in our patients. (54, MSN, head nurse, medical-surgical and critical care)

Most nurses I know see nursing as a calling; maybe not in sense of hearing God 'Thou shalt be a nurse.' I don't think many people experience that. Maybe some do, but I think there is sort of a quiet, deep inside knowing that this is what I am supposed to do. This feels right, and it is nourishing to me and others so maybe this is the spiritual calling, that inner voice that says you've found it. (58, BSN, research nurse, oncology)

And a community health nurse spoke of the blessing of her calling to serve the "underserved":

> Most of my patients are underprivileged or underserved, and when I go talk to them or visit them at home, I see myself as being of service. . . . I'm trying to find the right words, being as a servant to point them in the right direction. . . . I see (nursing) as a blessed call to serve, especially those who are not as fortunate as I am. I see it as a way of helping people to understand that they can live healthier and better lives. (40, MSN, head nurse, public health clinic)

The theme of A Blessed Calling may be described as reflecting the study group of nurse leaders' firmly held perception that professional nursing is not simply a job but rather a sacred or holy calling from God to commit one's life career to serving the ill and the infirm. As a dimension of living out that blessed calling, nurses repeatedly identified their caring as modified by a deep sense of love and even a passion for ministering to the sick.

Subtheme of A Blessed Calling: A Christian Mandate

Because the phase 1 study sample group was, with one exception, Christian, many of the nurse leaders identified nursing as a Christian ministry when describing their vocation; a number of the respondents quoted Jesus' mandate to care for the sick as reflected in New Testament passages.

In describing a Christian nursing vocation, Judith Allen Shelly identified several characteristics that included: "the motivation for Christian nursing comes primarily from a sense of gratitude to God"; "the Christian nurse functions as part of the body of Christ"; and "Christian nursing views the person, created in the image of God, as having infinite worth, regardless of the contribution the person can make" (1994, pp. 3, 11). Shelly also observed "As Christian nurses we continue to be Christ's heart and hands in today's hurting world" (2004, pp. 3). And, nurse and philosopher Bart Cusveller asserted, "The principal stake of Christians in nursing, the principal significance of Christian commitment to nursing care, is to be faithful" (1999, p. 6).

Study nursing leaders' comments reflected the above concepts:

> My whole nursing is based in the New Testament: "in so much as you have done it unto me, with the least of these you have done it unto me." So I always think I am giving service to God

through taking care of His people. I think that (the nursing vocation) is our commission from Christ that we take care of His people. That we do for them and take care of them. There have been nurses ever since the Crusades ... knowing that I am being a dutiful servant to my Lord reinforces me. (69, MSN, clinical educator, medical-surgical)

When I think of nursing as a vocation, as a call to serve the sick, I immediately think of Matthew 26:36: "I was ill and you cared for me." I also think of "I was hungry and you gave me food; I was thirsty and you gave me drink; I was naked and you clothed me; I was in prison and you visited me." Because nurses do all these things. Yes, we take care of the sick as our primary role, but in the process we give a drink of water to a thirsty patient, feed a post-op who can't feed himself, put a clean gown on a feverish and perspiring patient, and visit elders imprisoned in their homes or nursing homes — especially nurses who do home care or parish nurses. (65, PhD RN, educator, adult health nursing)

Nursing, as a Christian vocation, is doing what Jesus would do. . . . sometimes when I am battered and beat, I place myself in His hands and ask Him to help me . . . and then I think about being of service, about doing unto others as you would have them do unto you. (40, MSN, public health case manager)

I think that our commission is from Christ, that we take care of His people; there have been nurses ever since the Crusades. . . . knowing that I am being a dutiful servant to my Lord reinforces me. I believe that if I did not perceive nursing as a spiritual call to serve, I would have chosen another field. I think central to nursing's spiritual vocation is the concept of service. I keep remembering the scripture that reminds us that "Jesus came not to be served but to serve." And, as Jesus' follower, as a Christian nurse, that should be and is the joy and the satisfaction and the excitement of my nursing: that I can, as Jesus did, serve rather than be served. (65, PhD, RN, educator, adult health)

We are the hands of Christ. That's what comes to me right away when I think of nursing. There's a song: 'Christ Has No Hands But Ours,' you know. We must show the care and compassion of Christ. (64, DNSc, educator, community health)

(As a new nurse) I was just so glad to get up everyday. I was so happy I was a nurse. I wanted to be there. I was learning; I was enjoying patient care. So much to learn and so much to make an impact on people's lives and families; it was very important to me. I was just so glad to be a nurse. . . . People on the very edge of life, it just conveyed to me how powerful God was and that He performs miracles. I would always go back to how Jesus healed the sick and the lame. I could no way compare any power I have as a human to that, but I believe that Christ works through us to effect change at all levels. It is God's will that somebody goes to the very brink of death so that he can appreciate life ... you can have a small part in it. . . . If you are a witness to that you are also a vessel through which He works in order to cause that miracle. I wanted to be part of that. (43, BSN, school health nurse)

My first place of employment was a nursing home. And what better opportunity to put your faith and your belief to work than with the elderly many of whom, actually, don't have the opportunity to speak for themselves. So, definitely, compassion and caring and the sharing of Jesus' love that you have within yourself can be given to others. (50, MSN, quality management compliance officer)

When I think of nursing as a vocation, I think of our lives being called by God to serve our neighbor and to live as Christ, loving and helping where we can as He loved and helped us. So specifically in nursing we have chances to do hands on with physical comfort and relief from pain and healing medicines. You have a chance to help the patient with any emotional anxiety and education and also (touch) their soul; especially a person who really sees his or her need for a relationship with God and spiritual healing when they are in this situation where they have lost control of the health of their body or the control they thought they had over the future. . . . I realized, as a Christian, what an opportunity to serve people this way. . . . You know, I am Christ and I want to be His hands and His feet and His mouth. So whatever I am doing, especially in this setting with people who have so many needs, that is underneath and through all my nursing. (38, charge nurse, team leader, maternal-child/family nursing)

My faith tells me that I should go out and heal the sick; that is what the Bible says. I believe that since I am a Christian I have the calling to go out and heal the sick. It's what I am called to do as a Christian, and so it is a part of what my nursing is. Sometimes I cannot go out and preach (but) I can do it in my profession. I can pray with patients. (37, ADN, charge nurse, emergency room)

When you see nursing as service, you see it as your calling, then I ask God every day to bless me in my work and (tell Him) that He is in charge of my day. I feel like I take God with me into my classroom when I lecture every day. I ask Him to guard my words and let Him shine through me to the students. When I go with the students into the clinical setting, I do the same. At least I always try to wrap my days in prayer so that I am following God's path for me and His light will shine through me. So that nursing is just so much more than a job; it is my calling, it is service. Everything I do is service to Christ. (52, PhD, RN, educator, psych-mental health nursing)

As reflected in the above nurse leaders' comments, many study participants perceived their nurse ministry as guided, supported, and strengthened by a Christian philosophy of love, caring, and commitment for and to those in need. The nurses' comments also reflected the fact that they understood their call to serve as coming from Jesus to be both a blessing and a privilege. As reflected in the overall theme A Blessed Calling, nursing leaders derived from their sacred calling a passionate desire to care for those who were fragile and in need.

Passionate Caring

By this everyone will know that you are my disciples, if you have love for one another.

—John 13:35

Passion may seem like a strong word to describe a nurse's ministry to care for the sick, yet in discussing the topic of home nursing care "as a calling," nurse Elizabeth Jeffries asserts "Home care professionals need to possess a passion for their work especially if they are to thrive in the current environment. They must believe that, at some level, they have been called to do this work" (1999, p. 6). Jeffries adds: "A calling causes a desire and a passion for doing something that cannot be suppressed"

(p. 6). And, in discussing how the spirit of nursing influenced her practice, nurse Jennifer Bridges observed: "As Florence Nightingale once said: 'Nursing is an art,' and one must have a passion to create masterpieces. The passion and dedication to helping others had motivated me to seek numerous opportunities to make a difference" (2005, p. 22).

A related concept to passionate caring is that of compassion. Compassion has been described as "the heart and soul of deep caring, and goes well beyond the common usage of the word to express empathy, concern, and kindness" (Dunaway, 2006, p. 60). Although a nurse's compassion may sometimes be challenged by continual exposure to pain and suffering (compassion fatigue), compassion is "a renewable resource" (Lamendola, 1996, p. 16). That is, one's passion for the nursing vocation, and associated compassion for those who are suffering, may be strengthened and renewed by experiencing the joy and fulfillment of serving another in need; this is demonstrated well in the nurse leader study participants' comments:

> Nursing is about serving another human being … if that's not your sole purpose … you won't be happy and you won't do a good job. You have to be passionate about caring for others. (59, PhD, RN, educator, pediatrics)

> I always wanted to be a nurse from the time I was very small … I always saw nursing as a calling. I think it is a calling, and you have to truly want to do it passionately, and if you don't want to do it, you are not going to be good as being a nurse. (51, MSN, educator, medical-surgical and critical care)

> My employer now definitely has a really good view of nursing as a vocation because at several of our meetings, my boss will say to us: "It's a really good thing you all really love what you do, and really have a passion for helping people. Because if you didn't, I mean, why would you put up with the things you put up with? And you wouldn't get the results that you get if you didn't think that it was your passion or your calling or your vocation." (32, BSN, charge nurse, medical surgical)

While other nurses did not use the expression *passion*, they did speak of their "love," even "deep love" for nursing:

> I think if I didn't feel a deep love for what I do as a currently practicing nurse, then I don't think I would have stayed in nursing. I personally wanted much more than just a job. (62, MSN, medical-surgical clinic head nurse)

I went into nursing because I can't imagine anything else. I love people. I love working with people. I love dealing with their problems. I love nursing! (57, ADN, head nurse, medical-surgical)

For me, nursing is a caring vocation that needs to have a lot of love and understanding by the nurse to do the best job possible, along with the technical skills and the management skills; you have to do it with love. Without love, the good works of nursing mean nothing. I personally could survive on minimal as long as I could care for others; then I will be a happy soul. (50, MSN, educator, health care management)

Nursing is something you really have to want to do; to love doing. (45, MSN, clinical specialist, patient education)

Nursing, as a vocation, is something that you embrace, you love and it is a part of you. . . . A profession you become educated in but a vocation you embrace. (57, ADN, head nurse, medical-surgical)

I love what I do; I love the field I'm in. I love dealing with new parents and new life. Many times that is wonderful, and the times when it's not, that's when the vocational part of my nursing comes in; the vocational part of it is really put to the test in the bad times. Like how do I go in that day when I know that a baby has passed away? That is when I draw from the inner strength that I get from the feeling that nursing is a vocation and not just a job. (47, BSN, head nurse, obstetrics/gynecology)

As the above study participants' comments demonstrate, nurses who understood their profession as a blessed or higher calling also felt compelled to carry out their nursing ministry with both passion and compassion for those who are suffering. To be able to care for the sick with such a deeply spiritual commitment, nurses also expressed the fact that, for them, nursing was a ministry ingrained in the spirit of who they were as persons.

Ingrained in the Spirit

There are varieties of gifts but the same Spirit ... to one is given ... the utterance of wisdom ... to another, gifts of healing.

—1 Corinthians 2:4, 8, 9

The point can be made that "each calling is unique to each individual" (Jeffries, 1999, p. 6). A calling is also something that is deeply centered in an individual's spirit. Jeffries gave the example of a nurse case manager who felt that she was called to help others through the nursing profession. "Grounded in values of serving others," Jeffries observed, the nurse is "as passionate about nursing now as she was 30 years ago" (p. 6).

Nurse theorist Margaret Newman, in a discussion of the spirit of nursing, supports the concept of nursing being ingrained in the heart of a nurse. Newman asserts that "The essence of nursing is not doing or manipulating but is being open to whatever arises in the interaction with the client. It is being fully present, with an unconditional acceptance of the client's experience. The nurse offers his or her self" in the nurse-patient interaction (1989, p. 6). The latter point is clearly reflected in the following nursing leaders' perceptions:

> Nursing is something that has been ingrained in the spirit; you just know that you are called to do it. Not every person can do it. I think that some people may start out wanting to do nursing but realize later on that there is a void there. Nursing is something that is a part of you. It is ingrained in the spirit and everything that is you. It is wanting to serve the needy, wanting to serve humanity, and wanting to extend yourself in a service-oriented profession. I think that in that sense you have to be more a giver than a taker and willing to just extend yourself, and sometimes it is exhausting, but that is what we do as nurses. (43, BSN, charge nurse, critical care)

> Nursing's concept of service is embedded in you; being called to serve people is embedded as an essential dimension of your nursing practice. (52, MSN, team leader, cardiac rehabilitation)

> Because I see nursing as a vocation, I embrace it as a way of life, just as much as getting up and taking a shower and eating breakfast is a part of me. Nursing is not something I do on the side; it's every day all of me. Just as I will always be a mommy no matter what, I will always be a nurse. It's in me, who I am, a part of me, and I try to improve on the vocation … to the best of my ability. (50, MSN, manager, quality management)

> I know I am called to serve. Nursing is in the very fiber of my being. I experience it like I see the police do; they are never off duty. When they see crime, they get involved…. When I see

something like a fellow (train) passenger who looks like he is having a cardiac event I try to intervene using the essentials of my nursing practice. (50, MSN, educator, psych-mental health)

(As time goes on) I feel stronger about nursing; more appreciative of it, more aware how satisfying it is; how truly deep down in my bone marrow it is just satisfying. I could stay (on duty) for hours until I get exhausted. It takes a lot for me to say I need to go home. (58, DNSc, oncology research nurse and patient educator)

I think of Florence Nightingale when she went out to serve the soldiers, and I think nursing is something that comes from within you; it is a desire to do good and help others. (40, MSN, case manager, public health)

Nursing is not what I do; it is who I am. (26, BSN, pediatrics clinic charge nurse)

I was born to be a nurse. (64, DNSc, educator, community health)

I have always wanted to be a nurse; it was just something that was born in me I guess. (60, diploma RN, charge nurse, pediatrics)

Nursing is all encompassing. You don't just walk away at the end of 8 hours; it is part of your being. (45, MSN, clinical educator, critical care)

Nursing is not separated out; its just a part of who you are. You can't turn it on and off. You have something to give and you want to continue doing this. If you feel it is a calling then you are able to continue and get up every morning with a good feeling and being about to give because it does take a lot of giving. . . . I stay (in nursing) because I love it. I feel that that's the way it's supposed to be. (58, DNSc, oncology research nurse)

Considering the fact that nursing is a vocation, it just helps me accept the little aggravations that go along with it. To me it is part of the job, but it is not really a job; it is something that I love doing, and I would not be happy if I was not doing it. Nursing is a part of me and a part of my life, and as I just said

I wouldn't be happy if I wasn't doing it. So therefore it obviously is something that gives me great fulfillment and great pleasure. I can't imagine doing nursing with just considering it as a job. There are too many things, too many frustrations. I cannot see how anybody could go into nursing and just consider it a job. I am sure that there are people who do, but I cannot see how you can do nursing and do it well without it being a major part of your personality and your being. (60, diploma RN, charge nurse, pediatrics)

I look at nursing as a way of giving back. I had a wonderful life even at a young age. I was always a caring, giving person. When everybody finished their chores I would go around and ask "Can I help anyone else?" It comes natural for me to want to be a nurse. I had an aunt who was a nurse and I had a first cousin who was an RN, and I admired them tremendously. My grandmother was a midwife. It is probably in my genes. It's very natural, very easy. I don't consider nursing a job; it was a natural route for me to take. (49, BSN, team leader, medical-surgical)

(Choosing nursing) it's sort of like an intuitive thing, like I knew. I've always been a nurturing kind of person. When I was younger, with my family, with animals. It's sort of like I never had to think about it. I always knew. It's kind of like I don't know if it was a message from God or what it was. But I always knew; there was never a doubt in my mind…. I never swayed from what I wanted to do and that was to become a nurse. And so that was it … sort of like intuitive. I knew it, like you just know. I knew! (51, BSN, head nurse medical-surgical)

My mother told me, a long time ago, I was attracted to nursing at age 3. It is because when she was sick, my attention to her as a daughter, feeling her head, asking how she was, and I was only 3 years old. Was there anything she needed? I was always at her side when she was feeling ill. That is how I began to feel inside of me; it was part of me and I have never let go of that vocation or that feeling that I wanted to be a nurse. When I saw the nurses in the hospital how professional they were and how caring, wearing their starched white uniforms, it made me feel that I was connected to that role of nursing. (54, MSN, charge nurse, medical-surgical clinic)

In describing nursing as central to their personalities, nurse leaders used expressions such as "ingrained in the spirit," "embedded in you," "who I am, a part of me," "in the very fiber of my being," and "something that comes from within." Nurses also admitted to feelings such as "I was born to be a nurse," "nursing is not what I do; it is who I am," and "nursing is . . . just a part of who you are." The theme Ingrained in the Spirit can be defined as a deeply felt confidence that the choice of nursing as one's profession is absolutely the correct response to God's call for a life career.

To live out the blessed calling, with a passionate sense of caring, in a work ingrained in one's spirit, a nurse will often go "the extra mile" in his or her professional activities of caring for the sick.

The Extra Mile

Bear one another's burdens and in this way you will fulfill the law of Christ.

—Galatians 6:2

Perhaps the most frequently identified theme related to nursing leaders' perception of their profession as a calling to serve was that of going "the extra mile" in order to provide excellent patient-centered care. A few nurses used expressions such as: going the "extra step," "doing above and beyond," not being "bound by a time clock," but many actually verbalized the words *the extra mile* in describing their service to their staff, patients, families, and students.

In a message to her organization members entitled "Service and Excellence: Going the Extra Mile," president-elect of the Society of Urologic Nurses Tamara Dickinson described nursing as a service possessed of "a sense of compassion and empathy that sets nursing apart" (2007, p. 354). The concept of nurses achieving a doctoral degree was described as going "the extra mile" (Andalo, 2005, p. 20). "Going the extra mile" was identified as the catalyst for nurse managers conducting a Delphi technique study to allow staff input prior to instituting change on a unit (Beech, 1999, p. 281). A key theme revealed in an ethnographic study of the nurse–patient relationship was that of patients' applause for nurses who go the extra mile (Fosbinder, 1991, p. 1).

The relevance of nurses going the extra mile is demonstrated in the study nurse leaders comments:

(Viewing nursing as a vocation) helps me go the extra mile. I think if I did not see nursing as a calling I would just go about my day, you know, think of it more as a job than a vocation.

I probably wouldn't go the extra mile. (32, BSN, team leader, medical-surgical)

One example (of the nursing vocation) was working in the school setting, which has its challenges in that you are the only healthcare professional there. We had a particular situation of a young boy who was an immigrant who came to the United States who was not legal and not eligible for any type of health insurance. And he had just been here a few weeks and it appeared that he had a severe hearing loss. One thing I realized, that particularly in school nursing, you have to go above and beyond trying to find resources and not take "no" for an answer. I think I was successful in spearheading what we needed to do for that young boy. Many times (in nursing), you have to go the extra mile.... I think sometimes you can really put your heart and your soul into trying to help a family deal with a situation that is challenging and get them health care and the resources they need. (49, MSN, educator, community health)

I find a great deal of accomplishment and self-worth in taking care of patients. People have often said to me, my patients in particular: "You give so much, you go the extra mile." I have heard that frequently. I think maybe I don't know any other way to do it, but it makes me feel good to take care of patients that way. It makes me feel good to help patients, to know that I have met their needs and made them comfortable and made their day better. Yes, I am doing it for them, but I am also doing it for myself because it makes me feel good. (55, MSN, manager, high-risk perinatal clinic)

I think you see it (the concept of service) in people who view nursing as a vocation versus just a job. What are the characteristics of these nurses versus the others? I think, with vocation, nurses connect with patients and families; not that people who view it as a job don't, but it is more difficult. Vocation is the ability to do the extra 10% or 20% for the patient, even though you may not be getting paid for it, or it's your break. You go the extra step. Nurses who view nursing as a vocation do that. (58, PhD, RN, educator, women's health)

If I were just in a job right now and didn't have a calling for nursing, I'm pretty sure I would just do the bare minimum.

I would make sure I have all my reports in on time, you know, but I wouldn't come in early to meet with clients, wouldn't stay late to help a parent get to their specialty clinic on time, or make sure they know how to get there, or things like that. I mean going the extra mile, I guess. (32, BSN, charge nurse, medical-surgical and critical care)

My nursing practice is influenced by my perception of nursing as a vocation in that I always liked to do the extra things, the extra mile. I always liked to volunteer for extra time at work even as a student if there was a need; it seemed to me that that's what I really felt serving others was about. I can remember volunteering for a number of holidays in the hospital, especially Christmases, because I felt the hospital was a blessed place to be on the feast days celebrating Jesus's birth such as Christmas. (69, PhD, RN, educator, adult health)

Finally, a hospital team leader described the "extra mile" behavior of a nursing colleague:

I know a nurse practitioner who definitely goes the extra mile, goes out of her way for people. Like, today for example, we had a patient that needed to go to the hospital for an X-ray, and they had no transportation and didn't speak English. It happened that it was at the end of her shift, so she just decided that she would go ahead and drive them there. They were a Spanish speaking family so, before they left, the nurse wrote everything out for them in English in case they got to a point in the hospital where they didn't know where to go for the test. So, they could just hand somebody the card with the directions: need to go to X-ray, need to go here or there, and need to see this doctor. She really goes out of her way. (33, BSN, team leader, med-surgical nursing)

The expression going the extra mile was used so frequently by nurse leaders that it might also be defined as a central theme to the nurses' understanding of their vocation of service. Nurses do not consider a caring activity complete until the need of a staff member, patient, or family member had been resolved to the best of the nurse's ability. If that takes extra time, extra energy, extra dedication, and extra caring, so be it; this is simply what is meant by the vocation of nursing. This is a part of the privilege of being called to be a nurse.

A Privilege

As I can testify, they voluntarily gave according to their means and even beyond their means, begging us earnestly for the privilege of sharing in this ministry to the saints.

—2 Corinthians 8:3–4

Consistent with the four previously identified themes that reflect the study group members' perception of their vocation as being A Blessed Calling that is Ingrained in the Spirit and that involves Passionate Caring and going The Extra Mile, nurse leaders also considered their ministry of caring for the sick to be A Privilege. Some nurses described their call to serve as a gift, others as a privilege.

Carole Anderson described nursing as a privilege in a *Nursing Outlook* editorial:

Nurses are privileged; by virtue of our profession, patients give us the right/privilege to share with them their most intimate, joyful, painful, and fearful moments.... We are allowed the privilege of sharing in some of the most significant times in people's lives. (1998, p. 101)

As witness of Anderson's comments, Julia Thomas described how, as a student nurse on a pediatric ward, she had been present for the death of a child. She reported: "Helping parents to grieve was a privilege I will never forget" (2006, p. 27). Nurse Helen Britton defended hands-on patient care with the observation, "I consider assisting patients with their hygiene needs to be a privilege ... I have never considered those activities to be menial tasks" (2003, p. 31).

"Called to Serve" nurse study participants reflected similar attitudes:

I didn't have an insight into why I was doing it (entering nursing), but I knew that it felt right. I knew that there was something that was leading me. It was something I was doing good. It was pretty awesome. . . . I realized during my nursing education that my being able to serve as a nurse was a privilege. Nursing is a privilege . . . I am doing what I was called to do. I realized it was a gift to be shared, and I felt good about it. And that was what kept me going. (52, MSN, rehabilitation unit head nurse)

I learned from my faculty members in school that nursing was a privilege. They talked about nursing being a gift in their lives and not as being a burden, not as something they had to be doing. I never remember nursing being referred to as work, it was just a part of them, and I think that is significant. (45, MSN, educator, critical care)

I was brought up with the understanding that helping others was among the highest goods . . . doing that . . . makes me feel fulfilled. It's a privilege to be able to help others in nursing. (58, BSN, charge nurse, oncology)

I was told over 10 years ago that your vocation should be your vacation. It truly is. . . . I think the vocational part of nursing is really key as opposed to a nurse who considers the profession a job. It is not a job; it is a privilege. . . . "I think (it's necessary) really picking and choosing the best and brightest nurses for mentoring and precepting (new nurses). I think that (perceiving nursing as a vocation) is really the key as really opposed to a nurse who really considers the profession just a job. It's not a job, it's a privilege. (52, BSN, charge nurse/team leader, perioperative nursing)

I'm very, very proud of my decision to become a nurse. I'm proud to tell people I'm a nurse. I am proud to say I enjoy what I do. It's the perfect profession for me. No matter what I did I would still seek to be a caring, giving person, but I would never have achieved the fulfillment that I have received by being a nurse in any other field. Nursing defines me. (55, MSN, manager, high-risk perinatology clinic)

In nursing I believe that the sense of accomplishment pays me back in dividends much greater than any job ever could. This comes from viewing nursing as a vocation rather than just a profession or job. . . . I believe that I gain certainly equal, if not more, grace and happiness from my patients as I give to them. I realize that in meeting another person's needs I am fulfilling my own need. . . . I honestly embrace the day I walked into the school of nursing and have never once regretted the decision to make nursing my profession. The vocation or calling to serve that I have followed has given me so much happiness. (54, MSN, educator, critical care and pediatrics)

And, a nurse educator shared a privileged patient interaction:

Working with a lot of them (patients) is a privilege and supports (my perception of) nursing as a vocation. I had this patient . . . an older man with prostate cancer, and I did counseling with him before surgery. I saw him off to surgery, spent time with his wife, and got her settled in the waiting room. So I saw him about 7 a.m. and then again at about 6 or 7 p.m. after the surgery. He was in the recovery room and had just been told that he had cancer. I said his name . . . he looked up . . . he put his hand out and touched my cheek. It was just the most tender thing. His eyes just said, "Thank you for being here." Very few words were exchanged, and at first I thought that he was reaching out to shake my hand but then he was reaching for my face. That touch was a privilege and a gift. (58, DNSc, oncology research nurse and patient educator)

The theme of A Privilege describes the nurse study participants' verbalized gratitude for their calling and their gift of being allowed to serve the ill and the infirm, the suffering and the sorrowful, the lonely and the fearful. Nurses' greatest joys, the activities in which they find the most satisfaction and the deepest fulfillment, are those caring activities in which they respond to their calling, act with love and passion, recognize the inherent nature of their gift of nursing, and go the extra mile for those they serve. It is in this committed, caring, precious ministry of nursing, of serving those who are frail and in need, that nurses recognize the great privilege they have been given; they recognize that it is truly in giving that one receives.

The following case example shared by a nurse leader study participant well sums up the nurse's vocation of caring presented in the five nursing vocation attitudinal themes described above.

CASE EXAMPLE: THE NURSING VOCATION AS A CALL TO SERVE

I had a patient who was an AIDS patient, and he was dying. . . . Those patients feel isolated because they are on isolation, and they feel not enough nurses pay attention to them. Some are difficult. I had this patient who was like that, but I thought to myself "Well, I have to expect patients to be that way ... they are ill and stressed, and their life is being torn apart." It is a stressor on all ends: financially they are not able to feed their families, and they may be hospitalized for a long time. But the nursing vocation of caring and compassion in me, this strong voice in me, says "Something has happened to cause this in this person . . . and it's incumbent on me to explore a little farther their suffering. . . . Just give me the opportunity to help; tell me what you need or what you need me to do. And my patient in isolation, he broke down and said he was fed up, . . . he cried and was fearful that nobody wanted to come into his room. He said, "You can ring the bell, and they never come. The meals are cold because people leave them outside the door, and when anyone does come in they do what they have to do and are gone." People were treating him like he had leprosy or the plague. So he was angry and the human tendency is that when someone lashes out, you want to lash back. But you, as a nurse called to serve, can't do that. I think that is the higher calling of the nursing vocation, the blessed calling and the compassion that you have precludes you from lashing out; it's assuming a higher level of assisting humanity. (43, BSN, team leader, medical-surgical and critical care)

This chapter has presented the methodology for a nursing study entitled Called to Serve: the Lived Experience of a Nursing Vocation, as well as five nursing vocation attitudinal themes, and one subtheme, as identified in the initial analysis of the phase 1 study data. These themes reflect the nurse leaders' perceptions of their vocation as a spiritual calling to care for the ill and the infirm. The five themes — A Blessed Calling (and subtheme A Christian Mandate), Passionate Caring, Ingrained in the Spirit, The Extra Mile, and A Privilege — are related and together form a philosophy of nursing that might be summarized under the broad concept of servanthood.

Because the concepts of service and servanthood emerged so frequently in the qualitative data elicited from the initial 35 nurse leader study participants, a secondary analysis of the phase 1 data was carried out, broadly guided by the conceptualizations of servant leadership as identified by Greenleaf (1977), Spears (2004), and Russell and Stone (2002). Phase 1 findings were also validated in phase 2 phenomenological interviews, with an additional 40 nursing leaders. The focused interview probes were guided by the nursing servant leadership framework identified in phase 1 of the study.

Some examples of the phase 1 nurse leaders' specific comments regarding service included:

I see nursing as a call to serve, to serve others, especially those who are not as fortunate as I am. And I also see it as a way of helping people to understand that they can live healthier and better lives. (40, MSN, case manager, public health)

The nursing vocation brings to mind the chance to help others through difficult situations in their lives and to be of service in some way to help them grow through their suffering and their situation…. The entire (nursing) education was geared toward serving others, to help others to meet their full potential…. (Viewing nursing as a vocation) became the bedrock of my practice. That I am there to help the people that I meet in my daily practice. That the most important thing in my practice is to serve them, to teach them, and to help them meet their health challenges and possibly overcome them and continue to grow as individuals. (60, Diploma RN, charge nurse, emergency room)

When you see nursing as a vocation it is just a part of who you are. You can't turn it on and off. You have something to offer, to give, and you want to continue doing this. And I think if you feel nursing is a calling to serve, then you are able to continue to get up every morning and feel good about it. Being able to give, because it does take a lot of giving. Especially with the job I am in now, which I think is emotionally taxing; working with cancer patients and hearing their stories of crisis and to try to intervene with the right (balance) of lightness and seriousness. To give them the information that they need and try to detect what they are saying, my head and heart get pretty full. I think I keep coming back because I love it; I feel like that is what I am supposed to do. (58, DNSc, research nurse, oncology)

I can't imagine just going in (to the unit) and saying "I'm here from 8 to 4. Good-bye. See you later," and just leaving the patients. I don't know what it would be like to take that piece of serving and caring away. I think it would be really bad. It's not just the money part of the job; nursing is something you must really feel in your heart and soul, that you want to help people. You have to embrace that, and you have to be able to do it. If you don't have that I think you will leave the profession; I don't think you will stay in nursing. (51, MSN, supervisor, medical-surgical/critical care)

I prioritize now when I am working. I take it very seriously. I do what I need to, do but at the same time I feel like I'm not just here to give shots and pass pills. These patients are depending on me…. I think people who look at this (nursing) just as a job quickly move on and do other things. I think if you want to be in this field for any length of time and have that longevity be a part of you, then you have to see nursing as a vocation, as a calling to serve. You are not just there for the money; you are not there for glamour. I take this very seriously. I come here (to the hospital) in the morning, and I really feel that it is what I was called to do. (33, BSN, team leader, medical-surgical)

In terms of how my nursing practice has been influenced by my perception of nursing as a vocation or calling to serve the sick, I think I have always wanted to work with patients who really did have a great many needs that had to be met. My perception of nursing as a vocation is the framework from which I do all my work that could be defined as nursing, whether it be working in acute care, working in cancer nursing, working as an educator. The calling to serve, that word *serve*, to meet the needs of another, is the essence of the branch I call nursing.... that transcends something one might call a job. (54, MSN, head nurse, critical care)

I remember always hearing about nursing as a helping profession. That's basically what attracted me to it. I knew that by being a nurse I wouldn't just be serving myself, I would be serving others, helping others. It's kind of something bigger than yourself, doing something that will have an impact on people. And you may affect their lives, temporarily, or you may even have a greater impact on them. (51, BSN, team leader, medical-surgical)

Many of us in the nursing department I work in are similar in age ... but a number of them who are younger look at nursing differently, and that's important to keep in mind. I think it is just a generation type thing that younger people tend to look at things differently. But basically, anyone who becomes a nurse, whether it be last year, next year, or 35 years ago, you have to have the sense of serving and caring, or you are not going to be happy as a nurse. (53, Diploma RN, head nurse, medical-surgical/critical care)

The concept of service is essential to nursing practice. There is so much joy in giving and serving. And I'm thankful I get to do it. . . . That's what it (nursing) is about; great joy in being able to help someone else. (38, BSN, charge nurse, maternal-child)

Nursing and service are part of the whole of nursing. I was educated to the model of … nursing being how really you serve God through your nursing practice. (59, PhD, RN, educator, pediatrics)

Findings from the secondary analysis of phase 1 data and analysis of phase 2 data, as well as development of a nursing servant leadership model, are presented in Chapter 5, "A Model of Servant Leadership for Nursing."

REFERENCES

Andalo, D. (2005). Going the extra mile. *Nursing Management, 12*(7), 20–22.

Anderson, C. A. (1998). Nursing: A privilege. *Nursing Outlook, 46*(3), 101.

Beech, B. (1999). Go the extra mile: Use the Delphi technique. *Journal of Nursing Management, 7*(5), 281–288.

Bridges, J. (2005). How is the spirit of nursing evident in your practice? *Arkansas Nursing News, 1*(5), 22.

Britton, H. (2003). Hands-on nursing is a privilege not a chore. *Nursing Standard, 17*(19), 31.

Cusveller, B. (1999). Does Christian nursing make a difference? *Christian Nurse International, 15*(2), 4–6.

Dickinson, T. (2007). Service and excellence: Going the extra mile. *Urology Nursing, 27*(5), 354.

Dunaway, M. T. (2006). Compassionate caring. *Caring, 25*(12), 60–61.

Fosbinder, D. M. (1991). *Nursing care through the eyes of the patient.* Unpublished doctoral dissertation, University of San Diego, California.

Gearing, R. E. (2004). Bracketing in research: A typology. *Qualitative Health Research, 14*(10), 1429–1452.

Greenleaf, R. K. (1977). *Servant leadership: A journey into the nature of legitimate power and greatness.* New York: Paulist Press.

Jeanrond, W. G. (1990). Hermeneutics. In J. A. Komonchak, M. Collins, & D. A. Lane (Eds.), *The new dictionary of theology* (pp. 462–464). Collegeville, MN: Liturgical Press.

Jeffries, E. (1998). Hearing the call to nursing. *Nursing 1998, 28*(7), 34–35.

Jeffries, E. (1999). Home care as a calling. *Caring, 18*(1), 6–7.

Koch, T. (1995). Interpretive approaches in nursing research: The influence of Husserl and Heidegger. *Journal of Advanced Nursing, 21*(5), 827–836.

Lamendola, F. P. (1996). Keeping your compassion alive. *American Journal of Nursing, 96*(11), 16R–16T.

LeVasseur, J. J. (2003). The problem of bracketing in phenomenology. *Qualitative Health Research, 13*(3), 408–420.

Newman, M. (1989). The spirit of nursing. *Holistic Nursing Practice, 3*(3), 1–6.

Patton, M. Q. (1990). *Qualitative research & evaluation methods.* Thousand Oaks, CA: Sage.

Raatikainen, R. (1997). Nursing care as a calling. *Journal of Advanced Nursing, 25*(6), 1111–1115.

Russell, R. F., & Stone, A. G. (2002). A review of servant leadership attributes: Developing a practical model. *Leadership & Organization Development Journal, 23*(3), 145–157.

Shelly, J. A. (1994). What is Christian nursing? *Christian Nurse International, 10*(3), 3, 11.

Shelly, J. A. (2004). Outcomes of Christian nursing. *Journal of Christian Nursing, 21*(2), 3.

Spears, L. C. (2004). Prescription for organizational health. *Reflections on Nursing Leadership, 30*(4), 24–26.

Speziale, H. J., & Carpenter, D. R. (2003). *Qualitative research in nursing: Advancing the human perspective.* Philadelphia: Lippincott Williams & Wilkins.

Thomas, J. (2006). Student experiences in the real world of nursing: Starting out. *Nursing Standard, 21*(7), 27.

Van der Zalm, J. E., & Bergum, V. (2000). Hermeneutic phenomenology: Providing living knowledge for nursing practice. *Journal of Advanced Nursing, 31*(1), 211–218.

van Manen, M. (1984). Practicing phenomenological writing. *Phenomenology and Pedagogy, 2*(1), 36–69.

van Manen, M. (1990). *Researching lived experience: Human science for an action sensitive pedagogy.* New York: State University of New York Press.

5 A Model of Servant Leadership for Nursing

Serve one another with whatever gift each of you has received.
—1 Peter 4:10

I think of service in its entirety, as a leader; service is the foundation of my role as a nursing leader. Because, if I didn't place myself to be available and to serve others than I would not consider myself a good leader. I think of the many times when I have been in charge. It is always about serving the group and what I can do to help you make your day a better day. In that respect I am pretty much putting myself in the hands of others. What is it that I can do to serve you so that you can have a better day, so that we can work together as a team. And you are not putting yourself just in the service of your coworkers, but you are putting yourself in the service of other staff, of patients, and families. I think especially in nursing, it is a profession that is based on helping others in service. That is what it means to be a good nurse servant leader. I think that service is the foundation of leadership in nursing.
—Alice, charge nurse, medical-surgical

In this chapter the findings from the secondary analysis of the Called to Serve phase 1 study data, elicited from 35 nurse leaders, and the findings from analysis of the phase 2 study data, generated in interviews with 40 additional nursing leaders, are combined. First a detailed demographic profile of the phase 2 study participants, as well as a summary demographic profile of all 75 nursing leader study participants, is presented. Following that, empirical examples of the 75 nursing leader perceptions and experiences, reflecting nine key nursing servant leader behavioral themes and 16 subthemes emerging from the phase 1 and phase 2 analyses, are identified and described. The relationship of the nursing servant leadership themes to the 10 characteristics of servant leadership in general, as posited by Larry C. Spears (2004, pp. 24–26), as well as to the 9 functional attributes and 11 accompanying attributes of servant leadership identified by Robert F. Russell and A. Gregory Stone (2002, pp. 145–157) is demonstrated in a categorical table.

Finally, an overall conceptualization of the lived experience of servant leadership in nursing is presented in both textual and diagrammatic forms. As well as a written description of a model of servant leadership for nursing, a symbolic representation of the conceptualization presents, in graphic form, the pathways between and among the nursing vocation attitudinal themes (presented in the preceding chapter) and the nurse servant leadership themes and subthemes, displaying the overall concept of servant leadership in nursing.

CALLED TO SERVE: PHASE 2

After preliminary analysis of the data elicited from the initial 35 nursing leaders in study phase 1, the additional 40 nurse leaders were added to the project constituting a second study phase (phase 2). The rationale for interviewing the additional (phase 2) nursing leaders was to further explore and elucidate the philosophy and behavioral characteristics of servant leadership in nursing following emergence of the overarching concept of service in phase 1 study interviews. The ultimate goal was development of a model of servant leadership for professional nursing.

Study Sample — Phase 2: Demographic Profile*

The 40 nurse leader study participants interviewed for phase 2 of the research ranged in age from 23 to 69 years. The age ranges were fairly evenly distributed with 11 (27.5%) of the nurses in the 31–40 age group; 9 (22.5%) in the 41–50 age group; and 11 (27.5%) in the 51–60 age group. Six nurses were under 30 years of age, and only three were older than 60. As with phase 1 of the study, the nurses tended to be older as nursing leaders were solicited for participation in phase 2.

Twelve or 30% of the sample were master's-prepared nurses; 17 (42.5%) had achieved a BSN degree, and only 3 nurses were diploma graduates. Six nurse leaders had doctoral degrees, five nurses had earned the PhD, and one a DNSc degree.

Fifty-five percent or 22 of the nurses were Roman Catholic, 15 were Protestant, 1 nurse was a member of the Jewish faith, and 1 nurse was Muslim. Two other study participant nurses identified themselves, one

---

*Demographic data describing the 35 phase 1 nursing leader study participants are presented in Chapter 4, "Nursing's Call to Servant Leadership."

each, with the labels "spiritual" and "agnostic" respectively; one nurse stated "none" (no religion) in regard to the demographic category of religion, and one nurse responded "NA" (not applicable) on the religion classification category.

Twenty-seven (67.5%) nurse leaders practiced in a hospital setting, five in schools or universities, five in clinics, and three nurses worked in private medical or legal offices. Fourteen or 35% of the group had been in nursing for from 1 to 10 years; 10 nurses had practiced for 11 to 20 years, and 9 had practiced from 21 to 30 years. Six members of the group had been in nursing for 31 to 40 years, and one nurse had practiced for over 40 years.

The most frequently identified areas of specialization were medical-surgical nursing (13 or 32.5%) and critical care nursing (12 or 30%). Three nurses were involved in trauma nursing and/or postanesthesia care nursing, and two were psych-mental health nurses. Other categories of nursing specialization identified by study group participants included home health care, maternal-child and family nursing, occupational health, palliative care, renal nursing, health policy, perioperative nursing, pain management, emergency department nursing, women's health, oncology, and community health.

Leadership roles among the phase 2 study sample of 40 nurse leaders included the following categories:

- Administrator—5
- Manager—6
- Supervisor—3
- Head nurse—2
- Charge nurse—9
- Team leader—6
- Nurse practitioner—5
- Nurse educator—4

Specific nursing leadership roles within these categories include:

- Administrator—Vice-president for nursing in a hospital, administrator of critical care areas, administrator/director of occupational health, assistant department head of medical-surgical nursing, and director of palliative care
- Manager—Nurse manager of a critical care area, nurse manager of surgical services, nurse manager of a renal department, nurse manager health policy law; division officer ambulatory care and division officer medical-surgical nursing
- Supervisor—Supervisor of home health care, supervisor of intermediate care and postanesthesia care, and supervisor of perioperative care

- Head nurse—Head nurse of a medical-surgical unit and senior CRNA (certified registered nurse anesthetist) in a trauma unit
- Charge nurse—Four nurses were identified as charge nurse of medical-surgical units, two of maternal-child units, one nurse was charge nurse on a critical care unit, one was charge nurse on a trauma unit, and one nurse was charge nurse on a chemotherapy treatment unit.
- Team leader—Three nurses were team leaders on critical care units: one nurse was team leader on a medical-surgical unit, one nurse was team leader on a trauma unit, and one nurse on an oncology unit.
- Nurse practitioner—Five nurses were identified as nurse practitioners: Two were adult health nurse practitioners; one was a family nurse practitioner, one was a community health nurse practitioner, and one was a psychiatric-mental health nurse practitioner.
- Educator—Three nurses were university-based nursing educators: one in medical-surgical nursing; one was in psych-mental health nursing, and one in nursing theory and research; and one study participant was a nurse educator in a hospital emergency department.

Summary Demographic Profile of 75 Nurse Leader Study Participants

The combined sample group of 75 nurse leaders who participated in phase 1 and phase 2 of the study Called to Serve were, in the main, between the ages of 30 and 60 years; baccalaureate, masters, or doctorally prepared; predominantly Christian; practiced nursing in hospitals, clinics, or universities; and represented a wide variety of nursing specialty areas with medical-surgical nursing and critical care as the leading categories. The total sample of 75 nursing leaders included 7 administrators, 9 managers, 4 supervisors, 10 head nurses, 18 charge nurses, 10 team leaders, 6 nurse practitioners, 9 nurse educators, and 2 nurse researchers.

NURSING SERVANT LEADER BEHAVIORAL THEMES

Whoever serves, let it be with the strength that God supplies, so that God may be glorified in all things.

—1 Peter 4:11

Analysis of interview data from the study sample population of 75 nursing leaders revealed the following 9 key nursing servant leadership behavioral themes and 16 related concepts or subthemes. The key themes and related concepts are:

1. Listening with the Heart: The Sounds of Silence, the Mystery Behind the Visit
2. Giving of Yourself: Crossing Over, Compassionate Care
3. Doing Ministry: Making Connections, the Wounded Healer, a Sacred Trust
4. Assessing Needs: Being Grounded, Taking Time Out
5. Becoming an Advocate: To Protect and Defend
6. Discerning Decisions: Staying Focused
7. Making a Difference: Doing Your Best, Generating Excitement, a Nurturing Environment
8. Being There to Serve: Beyond the Ordinary
9. Embracing a Higher Purpose: A Caring Vocation

These nursing servant leadership themes, derived from the study group's perceptions of a lived experience of a nursing vocation, are supported by the general servant leadership literature as reflected in Table 5-1.

Table 5-1 demonstrates the relationship of the 9 key nurse servant leader themes to 10 servant leader characteristics described by Spears (2004, pp. 24–26) and 9 functional and 11 accompanying attributes of servant leadership identified from a review of the servant leadership literature carried out by Russell and Stone (2002, pp. 145–157).

The questions asked of the 35 nurse leaders who participated in phase 1 of the Called to Serve study focused broadly on the lived experience of nursing as a vocation of caring, exploring such topics as:

- The meaning of a nurse's spiritual call to care for the sick
- How one's call to care for the sick attracted the person to nursing
- How the vocation was lived out in one's nursing practice
- Whether one's perception of nursing as a vocation had changed over time
- What specific patient care interactions could be cited that were supported by the nurse's perception of his or her vocation to care for the sick?

From these data the nursing vocation attitudinal themes, described in Chapter 4, were derived. At this point in the analytic process it was also recognized that the concepts of servant, serving, and service were emerging repeatedly in nursing leader descriptions of their attitudes and experiences.

TABLE 5-1 Relationship of Nurse Servant Leader Behavioral Themes to Spears' Characteristics of the Servant Leader, and Russell and Stone's Functional and Accompanying Attributes of Servant Leadership

Nurse Servant Leader Behavioral Themes	Spears' Characteristics of a Servant Leader	Russell and Stone's Attributes of Servant Leadership	
		Functional	Accompanying
Listening with the Heart (Listening)	Listening	Trust	Listening
Giving of Yourself (Giving)	Empathy	Honesty Integrity	Encouragement
Doing Ministry (Ministering)	Healing		Visibility
Assessing Needs (Assessing)	Awareness	Appreciation of others	Competence
Becoming an Advocate (Advocating)	Persuasion	Modeling	Persuasion Influencing
Discerning a Decision (Discerning)	Foresight	Vision Pioneering	Communication
Making a Difference (Intervening)	Commitment to the growth of others Building community	Empowerment	Teaching Delegation
Being There to Serve (Serving)	Stewardship	Service	Stewardship
Embracing a Higher Purpose (Caring)	Conceptualization		Credibility

Sources: Russell, R. F., & Stone, A. G. (2002). A review of servant leadership attributes: Developing a practical model. *Leadership and Organization Development Journal, 3*(4), 145–157. Spears, L. C. (2004). Prescription for organizational health: Servant leadership. *Reflections on Nursing Leadership, 30*(4), 24–26.

Thus, a secondary analysis of phase 1 data was carried out in an attempt to determine if relationships existed between the nurse study participants' perceptions and experiences of leadership and the servant leader characteristics and attributes identified by scholars of servant leadership such as Spears and Russell and Stone. Through this analysis a number of servant leader characteristics and attributes were identified in the guise of nursing leadership themes and subthemes. To validate these findings, as described earlier, phase 2 of the study was initiated adding 40 more nurse leaders to the study sample. During data collection with the latter group, the nursing servant leader themes and subthemes identified in study phase 1 were explored through the method of focused probes.

As demonstrated in Table 5-1, many of the nursing servant leadership key themes were closely related to those of servant leadership in general, notably the characteristics and attributes identified by Spears and Russell and Stone. For example, the nursing theme of Listening with the Heart was supported by both Spears' and Russell and Stone's servant leader characteristic/attribute of listening, and the nursing theme of Giving of Yourself was closely allied, in the nurses' own words, with the concept of empathy, Spears' second characteristic of a servant leader. Spears' characteristic of healing was only infrequently identified, by that terminology, by the nursing leaders; this may be because physical healing is so central to nursing practice as to simply be considered a given by nurses. Spiritual and psychological healing might, however, be considered a part of nurses' Doing Ministry. Assessing Needs is related to Spears' concept of awareness (self-awareness and awareness of others' needs), and the nurses' descriptions of their roles as patients' advocates could be associated with Spears' characteristic of using persuasion rather than coercion in working with another. Persuasion was also identified by Russell and Stone as an accompanying attribute of servant leadership.

The nursing leaders understood nursing as having a "higher" purpose that could be associated with conceptualization, and Discerning Decisions might be included as a dimension of foresight. While the term *stewardship* was not prevalent in the interview data, the concepts of caring and serving were ubiquitous, as was that of Making a Difference, which reflected the nurse's commitment to a vocation of stewardship.

A number of the nurse servant leader subthemes also might be identified with established servant leadership characteristics and attributes. Some examples include:

- Crossing Over—Spears' servant leader (SL) characteristic of empathy
- A Wounded Healer—Spears' SL characteristic of healing
- Beyond the Ordinary—Spears' SL characteristic of stewardship and Russell and Stone's servant leadership accompanying attribute of stewardship
- Taking Time Out—Spears' SL characteristic of awareness, especially self-awareness, and Russell and Stone's accompanying SL attribute of competence

The following pages present the Called to Serve study data that supported identification of the 9 key nursing servant leadership themes and 16 nursing servant leadership subthemes. At the end of each of the nine thematic subsections a case example reflective of the overall key theme is presented. All case examples are drawn directly from the interviews with nursing leader study participants.

Listening with the Heart

"The Sounds of Silence"
"The Mystery Behind the Visit"

> *If you love to listen you will gain knowledge, and if you pay attention you will become wise.*
>
> —Sirach 6:33

Nurse theorist Verna Benner Carson explained that "The ability to listen is both an art and a learned skill. It requires that the nurse completely attend to the client with open ears, eyes, and mind" (1989, p. 165). Listening to staff, patients, or family members "is something that nurses, by nature, do well. It is part of the caring ethic of our profession. The art lies in listening with the heart as well as with the ears….The ability to listen with the heart is a gift for the listener as well as for the one being listened to" (O'Brien, 2001, pp. 42–43). The gift is the privilege of being entrusted with the knowledge of another's pain and suffering and of being acknowledged as one who will handle that knowledge with care and compassion.

In a study exploring the kind of nurses patients want, one of the three key themes, which included "teaching (patients) about their conditions" and "relieving pain," was "listening to patients' worries" (Webb & Hope, 1995, p. 101). Listening to new patients can help "avoid distress on admission and preserve dignity" (Gray, 2005, p. 31); and nurse leaders can "enhance their leadership skills" by listening to patients and staff members (Bulley, 2001, p. 24).

Listening to staff was identified as a "key for hospitals on *Fortune*'s list of top employers" (Mathias, 2004, p. 1). In a national study of home care agency nurses, it was found that "listening to staff concerns" was one of the most valued nursing leadership characteristics (Smith-Stoner, 2004, p. 536). Listening to patients' families was identified as a critically important nursing leadership characteristic both for hospital patients (Britto, Kotagal, & Boat, 2005, p. 187), and those receiving home care (Caserta, 1989, p. 3) and psychiatric services (Jensen, 2004, p. 33).

It has been found that nurses have sometimes not picked up on the fact that a patient needed a caring listener (Barrere, 2007, p. 114); this relates particularly to the kind of compassionate listening that occurs when a nurse listens with his or her heart to a patient's problems. In a poignant article on "Listening with the Heart," William Rankin poses the rhetorical question "What does it take to listen with the heart?"; his response is that it is a "willingness to regard (an individual) as a human being" (1988, p. 127). Nurse Donna Trimm, in discussing "a listening heart," observed that especially in dealing with people who are grieving, "there is no need to say the right words. We only have to listen with our hearts" (2003, p. 19).

The Called to Serve study nurse leaders spoke repeatedly of the importance of listening in an attentive and caring manner to the needs and concerns of staff, patients, and family members for whom they were responsible. The nursing leaders expressed the feeling that, through listening, they would not only be able to keep their finger on the pulse of the daily problems and pressures of the healthcare area they managed, but would also gain insight into what needed to be done for the future success of the organization and its services.

It is important to point out that, as with the nursing vocation attitudinal themes presented in the previous chapter, nursing leaders are in a somewhat unique position in that, in a leadership role, they are responsible not only for the staff members who serve under their guidance but also for the ultimate welfare of the patients and family members for whom those staff member care.

The Called to Serve study nursing leaders described the listening inherent in their role as being a true listening with the heart to the concerns of those they serve:*

> I learned as a nurse that just listening to patients, really listening with the heart, was one of greatest healers for many kinds of suffering. Listening with a caring heart can heal loneliness, fear, anger, grief, and so many of painful emotions that a patient may be suffering from. Listening is one of the key activities of nurses seeking to heal hurting patients. But it's a special kind of listening—not just listening for the words they are saying, but listening with your heart because you really care and the patient knows that you care. That's the kind of listening that makes

---

*Nurse leader study participants are identified by age, license (diploma RN) or degree (associate degree in nursing—ADN, baccalaureate degree in nursing—BSN, master's degree in nursing—MSN, or doctoral degree in nursing—DNSc or PhD, RN), leadership role, and nursing specialty.

all the difference; that's the kind of listening that is healing to someone who is hurting. They know you want to share and understand their pain. (69, PhD, RN, educator, adult health)

As a caring nurse, I think that it is my job when somebody is suffering emotionally to listen with my heart, to lend an ear. It's part of the whole package of nursing; it comes with the job….this is for when I'm at work and even outside of work, I am perceived as a nurse. I am called to help people, to listen to them who are friends and relatives outside of work. I think listening is definitely important for those suffering emotionally or spiritually. (33, BSN, team leader, medical-surgical)

I worked in oncology for a number of years, and that area has many people who are quite ill and truly suffering physically and emotionally with their illness. I have seen how being a calm, listening heart [with a] caring presence can be very helpful to people. While some people try to be upbeat, positive, and funny with patients, there are times when the patient just needs a calm, caring, quiet, listening presence. That is what I try to do. (49, MSN, head nurse, school health)

There is a way of having a caring presence with your patients. This is the time you spend with the patients listening with your heart to what they reflect in their attitude, their tone of voice, their facial concern. The patient knows "The nurse is concerned about me." There is a feeling of trust, a feeling of presence in being there for them. (54, MSN, supervisor, medical outpatient clinic)

(Working with staff) I wanted them to be more conscious, to be better able to relate and listen to find out where patients were and to meet those needs rather than just working on the body, like a car taking care of the parts….They (nurses) may be very good at assessing needs physically and meeting those; they may be very good at dressing changes and back rubs. But I think you need to see the whole person. If they don't listen and see their nurse's calling as spiritual, how can they be aware of some kind of void in a patient? Or how can they meet needs in that area? At least if they are trained to think of a patient as a whole person, to listen, they could call a chaplain for a person if needed. (38, MSN, charge nurse, maternal-child)

The Sounds of Silence

In a discussion on "learning to understand a patient's silence," Brian Lomax suggests that "gaps in a conversation may provide almost as many clues to the health of the patient as the dialogue itself" (1997, p. 48). Lomax points out that silence may indicate resistance or stubbornness or may simply be "a way of using time to think" on the part of the patient (p. 49). A nurse can support a silent patient by "simply sitting with the patient until he or she is ready to talk" (p. 49). Silence, on the part of a patient, may also be a cultural variable (Davidhizar & Giger, 1994, p. 703); or can be a self-protective measure for "relatives, medical and nursing staff" in working with a dying patient (Youll, 1989, p. 88).

Listening to silence was a frequently identified concept, related to the nursing servant leader theme of Listening with the Heart described by the Called to Serve nursing leaders. As one nurse manager put it: "I always tell my staff to listen to what is not being said." Often it is a patient's (or a staff member's) silence that speaks eloquently of a particular problem or anxiety that the individual is not able to immediately verbalize at the time.

> Listening to the things patients don't say to you can be as important as listening to what they do say, what they verbalize. Sometimes you have to just listen to the "sounds of silence" to see what the patient is trying to tell you. Maybe he or she is so afraid about an illness, or even dying, that they can't talk about it. Sometimes you just have to sit and be quietly present with them and allow the silence. And try to understand why they are silent. What does the silence really mean? What is it that they are not saying or that they can't say right now but maybe really need to? (69, PhD, RN, educator, adult health)

Several other nurse leaders commented:

> (As supervisor) one of the things I say to the (staff) nurses all the time is "What is the message you are not hearing from the patient? What is it that that patient is trying to communicate by his or her silence? There is a message that you are not hearing." You have to look behind an angry response or complaining and look for the silent message you are not hearing. (49, MSN, supervisor, medical-surgical/critical care)

> Sometimes it's so important just to be there (with a patient) without any magical words. Words are less important to me.

Just being there and listening and seeing if a patient has something to say or not say. It's not what I have to say; it's what
the patient has to say or not say. And if I am here, you don't
have to say anything, you can be silent now, and I will see you
tomorrow and we will get through this. (58, DNSc, research
nurse, oncology)

Silence goes back to the very early concepts and ideas that you
learn in school. And some of those things that you were taught
you don't understand them in their application at that time.
You can try to use psychotherapeutic communication when
sometimes it is just being there. The patient doesn't have to
say anything, and you don't have to say anything. You might
just be at the bedside holding the patient's hand. There have
been many times when I've done that. (43, BSN, head nurse,
school health)

There was a time when I walked into the room (of a dying
child) and the mother looks at me, and I look at her and I know
why I am there. It was just silence. And she starts crying and
I do too. I put my arms around her. She doesn't say anything,
and we just sob because we both know what I am there to tell
her. I feel fine being able to cry with that mother and hold her
and hold her child who is dying. They have been a great gift
to me, and it has been a great gift to care for them; just moving
through to the end. (59, PhD, RN, educator, pediatrics)

I cared for cancer patients who have passed away and learned
the importance of silence. To this day I teach my students the
importance of silence. I would say to my cancer patients, "I
am going to sit with you for 15 minutes and you can talk if
you like, or I'll just be with you if you don't feel like talking."
I told them it was my time to be with them, if they wanted to
hold hands or have a back rub. But even if they wanted nothing they knew that this was my time for them. I remember
a particular patient, after a couple of days of silence, finally
breaking down and sharing some angry thoughts. He said
"Why don't you give up on me?" I explained that I realized
that even if he didn't want to talk, knowing that somebody
cared enough to just be with him was important. Frankly, he
was comforted that he was finally able to get the anger out.
He said, "You listened. You actually allowed me to say these

things that have been building up inside." It was a lesson for me. I knew in my heart that being with a patient, even though it seemed silent on the surface, like I may be wasting time, it was an important service. I knew it was not wasted time. And, even if that patient had never spoken to me, I still knew I was giving him my time, and he was worthy of it. (54, MSN, head nurse, critical care)

The Mystery Behind the Visit

One of the most difficult areas of communication related to listening on the part of a nursing leader, involves the individual who speaks but is not able to actually say what it is that they want or need to say during an interaction. This leaves a leader attempting to guess or intuit what the person is trying to convey. Such cloudy interactions between a nurse leader and staff or a nurse leader and a patient may be the result of "deficient interpersonal skills" that can result in a destructive "culture of silence" in a healthcare institution (Thornby, 2006, p. 266).

This second nursing servant leadership concept related to a listening heart, which emerged in study interviews, was labeled by one head nurse as "the mystery behind the visit." Most of us, as nurses, have had the experience of being approached by a student, a staff member, or a patient with a question or a perception that seems to not quite fit the occasion or situation at hand. It often takes some time and perhaps some careful probing by a leader in order to determine exactly what information it is that an individual is seeking to share or to obtain.

Nurse study participants shared perceptions and anecdotes descriptive of "the mystery behind the visit":

I think it's really important to listen to patients and to see patients as, you know, not a disease entity — whether they have a disease or they don't. I think a lot of times patients come in (ostensibly) for something like a cold, but actually they are really depressed, and you have to try to read into what's bothering them that day. And so, sometimes that's the mystery behind the visit. (51, BSN, team leader, medical-surgical)

I think as a leader you have to listen very carefully not only to patients but to staff or to students if you're working with them. You have to really try and find out what they're saying. What I mean by that is that they may ask to talk to you for some ordinary reason or even something that doesn't seem to make sense. I've had staff come to my office and say something like, "Can I talk to you about the unit's staffing for the Christmas holiday?" And you think it's a mystery why they are here because the schedule's been posted for about 3 weeks. And maybe you do talk about that for a little while, and you're kind of wondering why the staff member even had to ask you about it. And then next thing you know the conversation moves to a much different, more personal level, like "Well, I've been having this problem in my family, and it's hard to keep coming to work and not bring it with me, and I wonder if I should keep working or take a leave of absence." And so "What do you think?" And you realize that that topic was the real reason for the visit, not the staffing of the unit but the nurse's worries about her personal problems. You have to listen to sort out the mystery, to find out the real meaning of the visit or meeting that may be very different than what was initially proposed for discussion. (69, PhD, RN, educator, adult health)

I think realizing that patients are more than physical beings you need to let them talk about how they are feeling mentally, emotionally, spiritually. Possibly referring them for medication or to talk to their pastor or priest, their church. You listen for all those kinds of things so that you can try to pull in all their (possible) resources. You listen for what they are trying to communicate but maybe not saying directly. Sometimes you have to be a detective. (51, BSN, team leader, medical-surgical)

Sometimes a routine visit to a patient turns out to have unexpected and important outcomes. I mean you might drop in a room for a quick check to make sure a patient did take the meds that you left because he was still eating breakfast when you passed them. And you find out he did take the pills, but just as you are about to leave something about the way he looks catches your eye, the look on his face. And so you come back to the bedside and say: "Is something wrong? Are you hurting somewhere?" And he says that yes, he's having a lot of pain and feels really weak, and you might find out that he's doing some unexpected bleeding and needs to go back to surgery. So the routine visit could have an important outcome; it could even save his life. (69, PhD, RN, educator, adult health)

I had a patient who was not talking. I love my patients and try to help them deal with whatever they are going through. I was trying to get her to talk and cheer her up. I was trying to find out what was really going on. At last she admitted she was not worried about herself, she was worried about her son because he didn't know she was in the hospital. I asked her if she was a Christian, and she said yes and I quoted something from the Bible to help her know that God would take care of her and her son. She was really happy at the end of our meeting. (37, ADN, charge nurse, emergency room)

We sometimes get emotionally involved with our patients, and our listening can be healing. There was a family whose little girl had leukemia that I got very, very close to. I cared for her for probably 5 or 6 years before she finally passed away. It was physical care, but it was also emotional support for her parents. I was the person her parents could talk to about their feelings and how hard it was for them to stay positive when they were around her. There were things that they needed to say but couldn't. I feel that I was able to give them support through listening and was able to help them continue through the process of healing. After she died, I was able to listen to their grief and understand their grief and participate in their grief. We all had a chance to heal through that. (60, Diploma RN, charge nurse, emergency room)

There was a man...who had a pretty serious kind of cancer. And I was working the night shift and went in to check on his vitals as I went through each room. And he was up pacing the floor in the middle of the night. And I said, "What's wrong?" And he replied that everything was OK. But I said, "Do you want to talk?" At first he said no. And then he said "Well, OK." And he had never been an expressive, communicative type of person before, but he wanted to talk now. So good. We sat down...I had like 15 or 20 minutes at that point. He shared that he had been away from God for many years and that he was seriously concerned about where his soul was going because his cancer wasn't looking good. I could comfort him with the story of the thief on the Cross (and other Christian beliefs)....He did listen to that kind of spiritual talk and he did better....he seemed to be having some peace and something he could cling to in God's word. (38, MSN, charge nurse, medical-surgical)

Case Example: Listening with the Heart

One of the things that I find in my role as a nursing supervisor is that nurses often don't listen to patients enough; they may find it difficult and they call me....One particular day there was a woman patient who had a psychiatric history but who was also physically ill. She was a patient in the hospital and was complaining about a number of things. The nurses felt somewhat exasperated and weren't able to deal with whatever all she was complaining about. So, I went in and sat down with the patient and said "Tell me what is going on here." I could tell in an instant that the woman felt neglected; that she had not had a chance to really connect with any of the nurses who she thought didn't want to pay any attention to her. I let her talk for 20 minutes or so. She told a story about how someone had come in to her room and washed the floor while her clothes were still there. And that now her clothes were all wet, and they were the only clothes she had. I said "I will make sure your clothes are washed perfectly the way you want them washed, and we will bring them to you so they will be clean and ready for when you go home." And her demeanor immediately changed. She was like the nicest, sweetest lady after that. And part of it was just spending a little time listening to her and understanding that she had this problem and needed someone to take care of it. It was just really listening to her with my heart and getting to know her. (50, MSN, supervisor, medical-surgical/critical care)

Giving of Yourself

"Crossing Over"
"Compassionate Care"

> *As God's chosen ones, holy and beloved, clothe yourselves with compassion, kindness, humility, meekness, and patience.*
> —Colossians 3:12

While the concepts of giving of yourself or self-sacrifice may not be considered politically correct in some professional circles, they were cited frequently by study nurses as key dimensions of their nursing vocation of service. In research on "medical-surgical nurses' self-perceptions as healers,"

Jackson identified a dominant theme among study nurses as self-sacrifice "at the expense of self-care" (2003, p. 1). In discussing nurses' professional identity, E. J. Pask argued that nurses embrace self-sacrifice "in their inclination to work for the good of their patients, at the expense of themselves" (2005, p. 247). Self-sacrifice or the offering of oneself for the good of others was described as central to the vocation of military nurses who may, in fact, be called to lay down their lives in the line of duty (O'Brien, 2003).

When study nurse leaders spoke about nursing as a vocation of service, a spiritual call to serve, they frequently voiced the need and even the desire to give of themselves, to make personal sacrifices when needed, to achieve a needed healing. Nurses spoke about going the "extra mile," as described in the previous chapter, in terms of placing the needs of others before their own. Nurse leaders felt that the greatest satisfaction and joy in practicing their profession occurred during times of giving of themselves for the sake of those they served.

When nurse leader study participants spoke of giving of themselves in the course of their professional practice they often identified the concepts of understanding and compassionate care as critical elements of such behavior. A few nurses used the term *empathy* in describing their ministry of giving of themselves, others spoke of "crossing over," or attempting to stand with their staff, patients, or family members in their pain and suffering. Related to this "crossing over," nurse leaders frequently asserted the importance of "compassionate care." Compassion and crossing over were revealed as important dimensions of the nursing group's servant leadership theme Giving of Yourself.

As a behavior within the theme Giving of Yourself, the characteristic of empathy or attempting to truly understand what another person is experiencing is an attribute that is dear to the hearts of nurses. Often one will hear a nursing comment, perhaps concerning a patient with a newly diagnosed terminal illness, such as "I try to put myself in his or her situation and imagine how I would feel." Because nurses continually witness a variety of kinds of suffering related to illness and infirmity, they naturally move beyond sympathizing with another's pain to a real empathy for the person's condition.

There is a significant amount of literature that addresses the concept of empathy in nursing. Some of the topics addressed by nurse authors include:

- The nature and evolution of empathy in nursing (Sutherland, 1993)
- A conceptual analysis of empathy in nursing (Greiner, 1989)

- Empathy in the nurse–patient relationship (Baillie, 1995; Ramos, 1990)
- The relationship between professionalism, work ethic, and empathy in nursing (Dagenais & Meleis, 1982)
- A discussion of two types of empathy: basic empathy and trained empathy (Alligood, 1992)
- The distinction between the concepts of empathy and sympathy (Yegdich, 1999)

Although several of the nurses in the Called to Serve study did, in fact, use the word *empathy* in describing their self-giving related to the problems of staff, patients, patients' family members, and students, the more frequently used phrases were "giving of yourself," "crossing over," and providing "compassionate care." Compassion served, at times, to be understood as a synonym for empathy. Interestingly the Hebrew word for compassion (*rahamin*) is described as expressing "the empathic attachment of one being to another" (Downey, 1993, p. 193). Downey explains that the term *compassion* "refers to the very core of one's deepest feelings, much as the term *heart* does today" (p. 193). In empathizing with another's suffering a compassionate nurse can often "use his or her own wounds as a source of understanding" (O'Brien, 2001, p. 63).

The Called to Serve nurse leaders spoke eloquently of giving of themselves in their nursing.

> Nursing is much more than just going to work and having a job. You really are giving yourself, giving of yourself to help other people....My job is more than just a job. It is a vocation that I give myself every day....When you view nursing as a vocation, it helps you to see the patient as a whole. You really think about what their needs are physically, mentally, and spiritually....You really try to make them comfortable and do everything you can to help them. (36, BSN, team leader, pediatrics)

> Nurses know that spiritual care can have the ability to translate into healing. It may not be in words; it could be a touch or a look. When I go in to see a patient, I don't stand at the foot of the bed with a clipboard, I sit down, I hold their hands, I touch them, we make eye contact, we talk, we share, we laugh, we cry. Patients appreciate that. Giving of yourself is nothing more than holding their hand, maybe. My spirituality enables me to do that...your spirituality and what that means in your life. Some people, it doesn't mean anything to. They take it for

granted. But in the nursing vocation or profession, I think you have a unique position to experience spirituality at a different level. I was raised in a religious family...therefore religion and spirituality played a role in my ability to what I believe is my service to humanity. There are many ways we serve, and everyone has to find their way. Nursing gave me the ability to meet that goal and make me feel fulfilled [so] that I can care for sick individuals and help them meet their goals. I think that knowing yourself and how you feel about spirituality enables you to give of yourself and meet the needs of your patients. (55, MSN, manager, perinatology)

Nursing is really giving a part of yourself...opening myself up to my patients...being a cheerleader for them. It's a demonstration of caring about them as individuals that makes the difference. (52, PhD, RN, educator, critical care)

I think if you consider nursing a vocation, you give a part of yourself, a dimension of yourself, to the practice. It is doing more and going beyond and actually caring about what you are doing. Sometimes that means taking the initiative to do maybe a little bit more in a creative way—to feel like at the end of the day the job has been done well and correctly. Not just kind of going through the motions. (45, MSN, head nurse, school health)

I look at nursing definitely as a calling to serve the sick. Because I think any nurse has to give 100% of herself or himself into the profession, and to truly be a professional, they have to look at it beyond being an ordinary type of job. I think it is truly a caring profession; nurses need to give of themselves sometimes when they are not feeling up to giving of themselves. I think I recognized from the time I became a nurse that in order to find it a satisfying and fulfilling career, you have to look at nursing and see it as much more than just an ordinary job. (49, MSN, head nurse, school health)

Nursing is a contribution of yourself to the well-being of humanity. (You) constantly explore what your gifts are and what do you need to be doing and what are you going to do with this desire to care for the sick....I did a lot of community outreach down in Mexico and Jamaica. This was not perceived as work, I did it...for exploration of my vocation of nursing, and I enjoyed it. I did it because I felt it was my obligation to share my talent and gift of taking care of sick people and people who were disadvantaged and less fortunate than myself. (45, MSN, head nurse, school health)

Crossing Over

In a discussion of empathy and transcendence, Davis (2003) highlighted one aspect of empathy that she identified as "the crossing over stage," which can result in a deep sense of "understanding and compassion" for those we care for (p. 273). The concept of crossing over was also the focus of an article discussing interaction with patients and families from different cultural backgrounds (Tripp-Reimer, 1994). One way of potentially crossing over boundaries to the world of an ill person and allowing the individual to cross into the world of the caregiver was suggested by Carol Edwards (2002) who proposed that patients be considered "honorary members of the healthcare team" and thus contribute to their own care (p. 340).

The theme of actually attempting to cross over emotionally and stand with a staff member, patient, or family member who is suffering in some way was described by a number of the Called to Serve nursing leader study participants. Such behavior seemed, to nursing leaders, to be an expected attribute of their nursing role:

In nursing you need to try and understand what the patients are going through....By that I mean that you need to try to cross over to that place where they are lonely and afraid in their illness and to try and truly understand. You know most patients don't want you to feel sorry for them. They want you to try and really understand what they're going through, as much as you can, and just be there for them. (69, PhD, RN, educator, adult health)

Nursing is the God-given ability to go out and meet people where they are, with all their disabilities and inabilities, and to understand their suffering and to communicate—to try and go over to their place of suffering. (66, BSN, head nurse, school health)

Since I started out as a hospital nurse, I have felt that there was a calling there not only for the patients but the patients' families. I just felt a sorrow for them in dealing with a loved one who was ill. I always look at the situation as if that were me in the bed; how would I like to be treated? (70, MSN, educator, medical-surgical)

When you view nursing as a vocation, it helps you see the patient as a whole person and try to put yourself in their place. You know, to really think about what their needs are physically, mentally, spiritually. (26, BSN, charge nurse, pediatric clinic)

When I think of nursing as a vocation, I think of it as an occupation that involves self-sacrifice; it involves long days and long hours. To be a good, good nurse you have to ultimately put yourself in the place of the patient. You have to learn from them. They know their needs; they are the ones who can teach us. It is like the essence of humanity. (63, DNSc, nurse educator, community)

I think it's really important to see the patient's point of view. I think it's important because no matter how tired you are, you are up walking around while the person you are caring for has a million problems or they are in bed and can't walk around and care for themselves. Nothing that you are experiencing can ever be as bad usually as what the patient is going through. I think it helps patients to know that you look at it that way. Then you have something to give them. (66, MSN, team leader, mental health)

When I am having a bad day, you know, one of the days I want to throw in the towel, go home early. Those are the days, when I think, you know, what if I were the one here at the hospital. I could be the one seeking treatment. I could be the one feeling vulnerable. I could be the one who doesn't know what is going on. I could be the one who is frightened and unsure. (26, BSN, charge nurse, pediatric clinic)

The nursing vocation helps you put yourself in others' place. I can remember (a long time ago) in particular an evening where the supervisor came in and found several of us (staff nurses) crying with the family member of a patient who had just died of cancer. And she (supervisor) pulled us aside and scolded us and told us that we were not helping the family by crying with them; that we needed to be strong.... I never agreed with that supervisor. Many of us thought that she really was incorrect in her approach, and I probably have cried since then with many patients or family members who have touched me and who, I hope, were touched by my willingness to try and be with them, to share in a little way what they were experiencing, trying to help them with their load. (54, MSN, head nurse, critical care)

The vocational aspect of nursing helps me to be more empathetic. And put myself in my patients' shoes, whether they are suffering mentally or physically or spiritually. It helps me put myself in their shoes and really find out what their needs are. (35, BSN, team leader, community health)

Compassionate Care

Compassion has been described as a *sine qua non* for nursing practice (Shantz, 2007, p. 48). Compassionate care "depends on showing empathy for a patient's illness experience no matter what his or her background" (Sanghavi, 2006, p. 283), and an environment of compassionate care, where "patients feel that their emotional and spiritual needs are met, is at the heart of holistic care" (Nussbaum, 2003, p. 214). Whenever a nurse reaches out with compassion to a patient, it can make his or her "burden a little lighter and the pain a little more bearable" (Parachin, 2003, p. 9).

Over and over, in interviews with nursing leaders, the concepts of compassion and compassionate care were described as important dimensions of living ones' nursing profession as a call to serve, that is, as a ministry identified under the mantle of servanthood. Compassion for those served was considered central to the vocation of nursing the sick; this compassion was extended to staff members, family members, and, for educators, to students for whom they were responsible:

Seeing nursing as a calling, I think, makes me more compassionate as a nurse. I empathize with my patients. I can be more filled with compassionate care. I'm with them, and it's not just the tasks I do for them but also for their emotional needs; I'm there for the whole self....These people are depending on me. (33, BSN, team leader, medical-surgical)

I was attracted to nursing out of a deep compassion for human beings and to be able to alleviate suffering in some way. If I can just...give someone a hand because we all go through this—whatever suffering the patient go through. And nursing is a form of reconnecting with humanity because we're all part of the human family. They say that sorrow shared is divided, and joy shared is multiplied. And that is what really happens in nursing. (50, BSN, charge nurse, medical-surgical/critical care)

Nurses are just plain people with some insights and, it is hoped, a lot of compassion that carries over into care and is communicated to the patient. I think they pick up on it; if it is there they pick up on it. I think that is where the calling to serve comes from. It comes from inside, and you do the best you can to understand what they (patients) are going through....The more you listen to people, the more the ideas expand....The vocation to serve is a call in terms of kindness or compassion or being good to other people....It is important to take care of one another and nourish one another and be there for them if you can in whatever sense that they need, whether it's physical needs or spiritual needs or emotional support. Just your presence. You are there with some understanding of what they are going through...that is our responsibility. We have that gift, that insight, or that desire to give what you can to make (patients') path a little bit easier, their loads a little lighter. (58, DNSc, research nurse, oncology)

Sometimes we have to bend the rules a little bit so we make sure we are allowing compassion and kindness to be evident.... I have to really be compassionate in my vocation of nursing. I hope that even when I teach students, I am imparting to them that nursing is a caring compassionate service profession. And it is more than just a job. And that is the first step in their education, and they need to know and continue that. I hope I am giving them that...to help them understand. I hope that they see that in me....I think that over time my perception of nursing has changed...you just evolve as a person, as a nurse over time, the things that you see and the things that you learn... just become a part of you but...the caring compassion part of (nursing) hasn't changed. (51, MSN, supervisor, critical care)

In the vocation of nursing you need to meet the patients' needs in all aspects of patient care. You have to have compassion, empathy, and spirituality; this enables you to be a good nurse. (55, MSN, charge nurse, perioperative)

If I did not see nursing as a vocation every day I would be stressed out. Not seeing it as a vocation or calling is dreadful. It is only when you see it as a calling, that you have been called to help people, that it is less stressful. The most important thing in the nursing vocation is not to come into it for the money. Be compassionate, be there to help people, and answer the calling to serve. (37, ADN, charge nurse, emergency room/critical care)

For your patients who are suffering physically, you have to give compassion; trying to empathize how they are feeling and not viewing it as "Oh, I just have 15 minutes to see you...you're talking too long." You just sort of have to try to look at how things are for them, how they're feeling and try to empathize with them. And always wanting to do the right thing for the patient, relieve their pain or discomfort, or try to, if you can't do anything else, just listen to them. Because that's probably what they need also. I think that aspect of empathy and compassion sets nurses apart from other healthcare providers—the caring aspect. (51, BSN, team leader, medical-surgical)

There is a patient who will always be with me; who really needed our compassion, our compassionate care....she was 28 years old, married, she had two young boys, 3 and 4, and after the second child was born she found out that she had stage 4 breast cancer. They did a mastectomy, and she was told never to get pregnant again, but 2 years later she was pregnant. At about 24 weeks gestation she was admitted to the hospital because she was having difficulty breathing. They...found she had metastasis to the lungs, and the tumors were so large they were pressing on the thorax. She insisted on her ability to stay alive so she could give birth to the baby. She made it to 30 weeks and they did a C-section and delivered the baby. The baby went to NICU, and I prayed with her and her husband and her children. She eventually passed away but entering into her strength, her belief, her love for her family, gave me the strength that I could go on; her strength gave me strength. (55, MSN, manager, perinatology)

Case Example: Giving of Yourself

I'll tell you about a nurse who really gives of herself and one of our chronic AIDS patients who passed away recently. The nurse had worked a night shift, and (after she got off) she drove out to the patient's home, bathed him, took him to McDonald's, and took him home. (The patient) he had CMV retinopathy, was almost blind, neurologically not here, yet he knew that she was there. He passed away shortly after, but, you know, that is living nursing as a vocation. (26, BSN, charge nurse, medical-surgical/critical care)

Doing Ministry

"Making Connections"
"The Wounded Healer"
"A Sacred Trust"

> *And whenever the evil spirit...came upon Saul, David took the lyre and played it and Saul would be relieved and feel better.*
>
> —1 Samuel 16:23

In a study conducted a decade ago, exploring broadly the spiritual care provided by 66 practicing nurses, I learned that nursing did indeed consist of a "ministry" for the majority of study participants. Because that sense of ministry was often not reported on end-of-shift reports or charted on formal hospital records, I described the nurses as "anonymous ministers" (O'Brien, 2008a, pp. 98–125). I have also identified nursing as consisting of a "hidden ministry" (O'Brien, 2008b, pp. 89–98) and as having a "tender ministry" (O'Brien, 2001, p. 21).

In their article entitled "The Ministry of Nursing," historians Widerquist and Davidhizar pointed out that "historically the nursing profession has roots in the Christian concept of ministry" (1994, p. 647). Their assertion is supported by the vast amount of early nursing literature, especially that authored by nurse historians, documenting the perception and experience of nursing as ministry as carried out by early practitioners of our profession.

The term *ministry* is derived from "the Greek word for serving or attending upon someone" (O'Meara, 1990, p. 657) and has been described as "the service of the kingdom of God that flows from the call and empowerment of the Holy Spirit" (McGonigle, 1993, p. 658). Many of the Called to Serve nurse leaders, who described their nursing as consisting of an experience of "doing ministry," related that perception to having a vocation of service to God and to the Gospel message of caring:

> When I do nursing, when I care for someone who is sick, I have a real feeling that I'm ministering to that person; that I am doing ministry. That goes back to the idea that the gospel

tell us, as Christians, to care for the sick and that when we care for them we care for the Lord. Nursing is definitely a ministry, and when you do nursing you have a sense of doing ministry. (64, DNSc, nurse practitioner, community health)

If I did not experience nursing as a vocation, as doing ministry, it would not work. Nursing is too difficult. It doesn't always support you economically and socially. You are not being taken out to lunch every day by the company. I think nursing is too difficult to pursue if it's not a vocation (for you). I think you need that understanding that it is a vocation to do it and to stick with it and to do it well. (45, MSN, head nurse, school health)

The use of self in my nursing vocation, knowing that I do it differently than anyone else, that it has my fingerprint, my imprint, the way I approach a patient in my ministry. And hopefully learning from my patients, I believe that I gain much more than I give. And this experience of ministering to another makes me a better person, a fuller person, and a bigger person. (54, MSN, head nurse, critical care)

I really think, especially when I was younger, that if I didn't have the feeling that nursing was a calling to serve, a ministry to the sick, I would just say, "I don't want to work nights, I don't want to work weekends, I don't what to get my hands dirty. Why do I have to deal with difficult patients for little money…Why would I want to do that?"….I could go to some other job where I could work when I wanted to and have nice clothes. But that is not really what I wanted. I really wanted to be a nurse. I think that is the difference between a job and a vocation. I like people…I give them something of myself, and it makes me feel good….I think nursing is a great profession, a great vocation. (50, ADN, charge nurse, recovery room)

I will call a friend; we touch base frequently….she was the first person that told me that nursing was not a job to her, it was a vocation. It took me by surprise. I had never thought of that before. But I loved working with her. I loved her dedication. We had the same goals. It made me think that I do think of nursing as a vocation; it is not just a job. It is a ministry. I have never labeled it before. (52, MSN, charge nurse, cardiac unit)

(Regarding nursing as a vocation) The first thing that comes to mind is having a caring presence for your patients and even toward your staff members. We are a special profession that has been founded by religious organizations. Because of that I feel that nursing in itself is a type of ministry to the sick. We have a special bond (with patients) that is unique…I feel that we are called to a higher calling as we are a spiritual profession in a way that we understand the whole person, as he is, his whole psycho, social, and spiritual feeling toward his health and toward his own responsibility toward that health. We, are in fact, an instrument in helping him meet those goals by addressing the area….I see God in my patients—everyone! That is the ministry of nursing. Even from a Judeo-Christian perspective, yes, you do see God in your patients. In different cultures they may have a different understanding of God, but I still see God in them. There is the presence of a higher being in that person. I think God has given each of us a special blessing, whether you are the patient or the nurse. Of course, as a Christian we are taught to see Jesus in our patients. I see God. Definitely. (54, MSN, supervisor, outpatient clinic)

I've been doing a supervisory job.. Every time I take on a new role I have to rethink how this (seeing nursing as a vocation) works for me. It's really not a change in the role as vocation but a change in the execution of that idea. How do I do that now? How do I maintain this idea of vocation? What is my ministry now that I am in this different position than I was before? Because my idea that nursing is a vocation for me doesn't change. The execution of it does change though: how I live a nursing vocation in this supervisory job versus a bedside job. (49, MSN, supervisor, critical care)

I don't think the concept of nursing as a ministry of service has really changed over time. I think there has been a lot of influence and factors out there that change our perspectives of nursing theory and basic nursing practice due to new science and technology. But actually the essence of nursing as our ministry has not really changed; the nurse and her whole being as a presence to the patient population. I don't think it has really changed. The essence of nursing has not changed. (54, MSN, head nurse, medical-surgical clinic)

I do ministry in my nursing. I see God in my patients. I see a poor soul in need of love and compassion. The Bible tells us to care for those less fortunate. I always try to put that in practice in caring for patients. (At night) I have walked into a patient's room and sometimes see elderly patients who are just lying there, open their eyes, and I will gently touch them. Not just touch them, but hold their hand, and you can see and feel such a peace happen. At the same time I'm doing a nursing assessment, it is an automatic response but it is that additional touch that gives me peace, and I know it gives the patient peace. I can sense it. (50, MSN, manager, quality management)

Making Connections

It has been observed that the nurse–patient relationship, the venue within which the nurse is able to make connections with his or her patients, is "the foundation of nursing care, the context in which the nurse practices" (Hagerty & Patusky, 2003, p. 145). It is through the communication that occurs in the nurse–patient relationship that healing connections are made and that both nurses and patients view the interaction as reflecting a satisfying and caring bonding (McGilton, Robinson, & Boscart, 2006).

Making Connections was an important theme related to ministry, as understood by the group of nursing leaders participating in the Called to Serve study. For these nurses, the concept of making a connection with a staff member, patient, family member, or student meant entering his or her life and having an impact related to the healing process. The concept of making a personal connection with an individual in need gave life to the themes of Listening with the Heart and Giving of Yourself.

I think when you make a connection with people who are sick, as a nurse, it becomes personal. And you begin to realize that you have a real impact on their lives. When you value this interpersonal connection…it enhances the relationship between nurse and patient….You can't help but know that you are in a relationship that is something beyond the client and the person serving. You can say…I helped (the patient). You walk away in awe of the healing, caring impact that you have on patients. (49, MSN, supervisor, critical care)

The vocational aspect of nursing supports my caring for patients because I think I can connect easier. It's like I have an insight. I can walk in to a patient's room, and the nurse they

had before didn't connect with them or they were angry....
But I can walk in and I always have a smile on my face, and
I can connect with them. And sometimes me touching their
arm to get their attention or just giving them a gentle back
rub. Making sure to put an IV in as painlessly as possible.
Patients appreciate those small kinds of things, and they give
a positive response back. (52, MSN, charge nurse, cardiac
rehabilitation)

You make connections with the families of patients. I think of
the patients especially when I was in the ICU environment; the
families really support you. I think they actually see that you
are or believe that you are there because you want to be there.
I think I get the most support from the families. (50, ADN,
charge nurse, recovery room)

Where I really saw the connection was in the ICU burn unit,
which I loved. It was a different ball game, and you have a lot
of closeness with the family because they were there so long.
And I felt that it was a vocation—a calling, because you had to
be so nurturing to the family member that would be there for
three months, six months during grafting and surgery. They
were there so long that you became very close with the family
as well as the patient if the patient was not comatose and was
awake. A lot of the patients were on ventilators and noncom-
municative. But I love the primary care nursing where you
get to know the family and the patients with smaller burns
that were awake....It's a very close knit, warm atmosphere,
which is a professional, vocational, calling kind of atmosphere.
(49, BSN, charge nurse, medical-surgical/burn unit)

Nursing as a vocation extends to some of the rituals; you go
through the moral decisions of people who are sick and people
kind of tend to connect the illness to us. They connect a lot of
decisions to people who are nurses. They do that in a way that
tends to help them to look for answers. It's kind of strange
because it's often not about how soon does Johnny's leg get
better. It is about how does Mom feel about (the problem) with
Johnny's leg. We all sort of fit in (the picture) as nurses because
people are looking for the spiritual support that we provide
and that is part of the connection that we have with people
when we are nurses. (49, MSN, supervisor, critical care)

You can't always take away the physical suffering of patients... but sometimes there are things you can do in terms of spending some time with people. I start to see people as souls, as the other person being connected to you...I have this idea of how we are all connected...so you do whatever you can to help people in their suffering....Presence is helpful, talking with patients is helpful, giving them the opportunity for others to be with them is helpful. There are things that you can do, and I think knowing that for me helps me know that I am connected to that person. (49, MSN, supervisor, critical care)

I don't think I realized, when I first started working, how much of an impact it would make on my personal life. You know, I don't think I realized how much my patients would affect the way I took care of other patients. You develop such solid relationships with patients; you connect with them. And I never realized how much a part of your nursing that would be. As you get to know them (patients) so well, they make you a better nurse and help you understand how to care for other people better than you did when you were a brand new nurse. (36, BSN, team leader, pediatrics)

The Wounded Healer

With the advent of holistic health care and holistic nursing, it has been recognized that "the nurse, standing as he or she does on the holy ground of caring for the sick, is well situated to be the instrument of God's healing" (O'Brien, 2008, p. 10). In the forward to the book *Healing Presence: The Essence of Nursing,* nurse Julie MacDonald observed that "all nurses...have at one time or another enjoyed the privilege of sharing our healing presence with patients" (2007, p. xvii). MacDonald adds that in employing this healing presence with those who are ill, nurses use "compassion and empathy" (p. xvii).

Nursing theorist Jean Watson suggests that nurses lead through caring and healing (2000, p. 1); this thought is supported by Richard Cowling, who argues that the "clinicalization" of health care has sometimes excluded attention to a patient's wholeness and proposes "a unitary conceptualization of healing" that appreciates and accepts the individual as whole person (2006, p. 155). The concepts of healing touch and natural healing in nursing are described by Wright (1995) and Legge (1995) respectively, and the importance of providing a healing environment for patients is advocated by nurses Lucia Thornton (2005) and Jayne Felgen (2004) respectively.

The idea of an individual engaged in ministering to others being a "wounded healer" received significant attention following the 1979 publication of Henri Nouwen's book *The Wounded Healer: Ministry in Contemporary Society*. Nouwen's based his interpretation of the concept on a Talmudic passage describing the awaited Messiah:

> He is sitting among the poor covered with wounds. The others unbind all their wounds at the same time and bind them up again. But he unbinds one at a time...saying to himself, "Perhaps I shall be needed: if so I must always be ready." (Tractate Sanhedren, as cited in Nouwen, 1979, p. 82)

Nursing leaders can use personal wounds, when not completely unbound, as "a source of strength, understanding, and empathy when addressing the suffering of others. The nurse as a wounded healer caring for a wounded patient can relate his or her own painful experiences to those of the ill person, thus providing a common ground of experience" to support their caring (O'Brien, 2008, p. 11). The wounded healer concept is relevant in a variety of general nursing arenas (Hall, 1996), as well as in settings such as hospice or palliative care (Laskowski & Pellicore, 2002).

The servant leadership subtheme of being a wounded healer was generally verbalized indirectly rather than directly by the Called to Serve study group of nursing leaders. Healing is so central to what nurses seek to do in their day-to-day activities of caregiving that it was inherent in the many anecdotes and nurse–patient interaction examples that the study participants shared. Sometimes a ministry of healing occurred for their staff members, patients, or families through the nurse leader "making connections" with those he or she served. At times, the nurse leaders admitted that having been wounded themselves was helpful in bringing about healing in their patients.

> Sometimes, you know, you can really empathize with your patients, with whatever it is they are going through. And that's because maybe you've been through it yourself or something like what they are going through. You know, you've been hurt and suffering also. You've been wounded like the patient or family or even one of your staff members, and to help them you can lean on that experience. You can use your own woundedness to help heal someone else who is wounded. You can become a wounded healer. (69, PhD, RN, educator, adult health)

I chose to work in pediatrics because I really feel a sense of empathy for the children that I care for. I remember how scared I was when I was little and went to visit the doctor. I try to remember that when I take care of patients. I have never been chronically ill. I have never had a long hospital stay. I can't put myself there. But I can remember, even now, how timid I would feel even going to my primary doctor and how certain approaches were threatening or scary. That is why I try, in caring for kids, to be sensitive, nonthreatening, and to try to find some component that I can relate to. (26, BSN, charge nurse, pediatrics)

It's important for patients knowing that someone is there, that cares for them, that understands. Having had my husband who died, being able to just say something like, "I understand because my husband died." It's not such a pat answer because I really know what it's like. And knowing what it is like to have a loved one in critical care, I'm more sensitive to (the needs) of family members in that situation. (52, PhD, RN, educator, critical care)

Thirty some years ago I was diagnosed with cancer and had a couple of surgeries, and I think that brought me a little bit closer to the need for nurses' understanding more than just coming in and giving medication or taking my temperature. It was the need to have somebody share that really bad news and understand. I think that influenced my giving more than just basic care....when you become a patient you have a different view of patient needs. My feeling is that every nurse should be a patient, and they would approach their job as a vocation. (69, MSN, educator, medical-surgical)

In all honesty, what we in the nursing field face, the suffering of human beings is also our suffering, and it's really hard to embrace if we don't embrace our own suffering; to watch others in their suffering and watching family members asks us for empathy and compassion. It invites us to be compassionate with full mercy, mercy that cannot be measured in dollars and cents. (50, BSN, charge nurse, medical-surgical/critical care)

My calling to serve in nursing helps me serve others with emotional losses. There's other than being in (physical) pain. We have a lot of patients who have to deal with miscarriages or full-term babies that have died in utero and then they had to go through labor. Very few get C-sectioned unless they are hemorrhaging or something emergent in going on. They go through labor just like everyone else. That's very emotional and stressful for all of us involved, to deliver a dead fetus. I've had two miscarriages, so I empathize with those women, and I tell them that. That's makes a difference. I tell them that I had two losses in my life, and you never forget that. You will always remember the pain. "I certainly empathize with you, I tell them, but you will be OK." A lot of them find that very comforting. (49, BSN, charge nurse, obstetrics and gynecology)

A Sacred Trust

The work of the nurse "involves aspects of human life that are both sacred and profane" wrote school of nursing professor Zane Wolf (1986, p. 29). In describing the "sacred work" of nurses, Wolf pointed out that "nurses listen to the tears and expressions of dying patients, rejoice at the birth of new babies...counsel the families of the elderly, feed the 'do not resuscitate' patients, pray with suffering families" (p. 33). The nurse's role, she added is "closely enmeshed in moral and ethical dilemmas" (p. 33). Wolf's perception of the sacredness of nursing is supported by other authors such as hospice nurse Kate Reid, who asserted that "sacred moments, the essence of the human-to-human encounter between pallia-tive care nurses and dying people, are important and intimate moments in our nursing practice" (2006, p. 55). Nurses Martin Hemsley and Nel Glass who described the "sacred journeys of nurse healers" identified in a phenomenological study of nurses' healing experiences (2006, p. 256).

Rather than considering certain nursing therapeutics as painful procedures, Biley and Chiocchi suggest that we place these activities in the context of a "a sacred healing dance" in which the nurse and patient are working together to achieve a healthful outcome (2007, p. 2). This can also be a way of viewing painful or difficult emotional patient interac-tions as described by Lois Gerber who related the heartbreak of seeing one of her troubled patients discharged. A thank-you note from the patient, however, led Gerber to realize that "nursing lets me enter another's sacred space, sometimes without knowing it" (2007, p. 43). She added, "I'm more convinced than ever that nursing is a divine way to connect to others" (p. 43).

Nurse leader Called to Serve study participants repeatedly spoke of the sacredness or holiness or gift of having been called to the vocation of nursing. While nursing was viewed as a humanitarian endeavor, in terms of caring for the physical and psychosocial needs of the ill and the injured, there was a strong spiritual theme running through the majority of data elicited in the open-ended interviews. The spirituality of nursing was envisioned, by a number of nurses, as related to a "sacred trust" they had been given to care for God's people who were in need.

In writing about the spirituality of trust, Robert Schreiter defines trust as "denoting a confidence or a sense of security in the reliability of someone else. It results in a state of being certain or secure" (1993, p. 982). Schreiter adds, further, that "the term is a relational one, describing the quality of a relationship among two or more persons" (p. 982). Schreiter's understanding of trust is appropriate to explaining the nursing leaders' embracing of the concept. Nurses felt that they had been given a gift from God in being called to nursing: the Lord was trusting them with the care of his fragile sons and daughters in need of health and healing; they responded to the sacredness of that calling.

Comments of study participant nurses reflect their perception of their gratitude and sense of blessing in the sacred trust placed in them in their profession:

> The nursing vocation goes hand in hand with being servants. I think that nursing is a sacred trust. That caring for those that God has given to us as truly gifts is really being a servant. I think that holding something sacred demands an awareness of the sacredness of what it is and also a commitment to reverence and respect and real care for them. I think that for me, as a nurse, it is truly cradling in each of the patients the face of God. That is a sacred trust that we have been given. It is our responsibility and also our call to continue to live out that legacy as faithful servants. (48, MSN, administrator, palliative care)

> I see the nursing vocation itself as a sacred trust, a blessing, and a gift from God. I also see my nursing research activities as being a sacred trust. First, I have to establish trusting relationships with healthcare givers and members of the research team with whom I will be working. Then, most important, I have to establish trust with the patients, and sometimes their families, who will participate in my research studies. This is especially sacred because I have to be very careful, ethically, to never violate the confidentiality of a study participant that is promised in the "informed consent" form that they and I (or someone working with me) signs.

Research is also a sacred trust because I have to handle the research data with care and then try and get it to publication as soon as possible—to get the information that we learned from the study into the hands of practicing nurses. This is very important so that we will not have wasted the time the study participants gave us by being in the study. And also that we don't waste the financial award that was given to support the research.

All of nursing is a sacred trust, whether it be involved in direct patient care, administration, education, or research. As I said, nursing is a blessing to be held in trust as a gift from God. (68, PhD, RN, educator/researcher, chronic and life-threatening illness)

I see my nursing as sacred, a holy gift from God. It's a trust also; I think I could even call it a "sacred trust" or a "holy trust." It's God trusting me to care for his poor and sick people and trusting that I will do it with love and care and compassion. It's me holding these people in trust. They trust me to take care of them to the best of my ability. Their families trust me as a nurse. So there is a lot of trust going on, and it is definitely sacred because what nurses do has to do, often, with the sacredness of life, with life and death. It's such a gift to be a nurse. It's such a gift to say that I have a sacred ministry. (64, PhD, RN, parish nurse, faith community nursing)

Taking care of dying patients is really about the most sacred thing you can do; it's really sacred, that time in the nurse–patient relationship. The patient and their families are trusting you to accompany them on the final journey to the unknown—from physical life to eternal life—that transition which is sacred in itself. I remember one young woman with ALS (amyotrophic lateral sclerosis); it's a horrible disease. She had been on the vent for weeks, and her family didn't want to let her go, but finally they said OK, it's time. They were at her bedside along with her physician and chaplain and several of us nurses who had cared for her a lot. The chaplain said a beautiful prayer, and the doctor de'd the vent. We all just sort of prayed quietly, and she passed very peacefully. It hurt a lot to see her go, but I was blessed to be there; it was definitely a sacred moment. (52, doctorally prepared nurse consultant in intensive care nursing)

Case Example: Doing Ministry

> One patient care interaction that reflects my seeing nursing as
> ministry that comes to mind, was when I was a young nurse.
> There was this fairly young man (dying) with lymphoma, and
> he and his wife and family were very close. I don't know what
> it is, but there are particular people that you connect with. I
> felt very connected to him. Maybe it was because he was the
> first person that I was ever involved with that was dying. And
> obviously as a new nurse I felt so inadequate. I thought "How
> can I help heal this family and this individual?" and just spent
> time with them, listening, more than anything. I found out that
> listening was probably the biggest gift of ministry that I could
> give to this critically ill patient and his family. I didn't have
> to "fix" things, I just had to be with them. I remember that
> so vividly, and here is it 30 some years later. I remember the
> emotions, not the details, but I remember the emotion and the
> connection. (58, PhD, RN, educator, maternal-child)

Assessing Needs

"Being Grounded"
"Taking Time Out"

> *Immediately aware that power had gone forth from him, Jesus turned*
> *about in the crowd and said, "Who touched my clothes?"*
> —Mark 5:30

One significant dimension of assessing staff, student, patient, or family needs, important for contemporary nursing leaders, is that of cultural
awareness. This is related to the myriad multicultural communities now
populating many urban hospitals and clinics. A model of "culturally com-
petent health care" was developed by one transcultural team to assist nursing educators in teaching cultural awareness (Campinha-Bacote, Yahle, &
Langenkamp, 1996), and a faculty group developed a "program to promote
multicultural awareness among faculty and students" at their institution
(Rew, Becker, Cookston, Khosropour, & Martinez, 2003, p. 249).

To help nursing students develop a sensitivity to the needs in their
caregiving environment, a study was carried out employing photographs
that the students scored for complexity and aesthetics (Decker & Blecke,
1999). Environmental awareness in a healthcare facility is an important
dimension of the practice of patient centered care.

The servant leader theme of Assessing Needs, one's own as well as those of staff, patients, families and/or students, was central to most of the Called to Serve nursing leaders' perceptions of nursing as a vocation to serve.

Assessing the needs of staff members is an important attribute for nursing leaders. Nurse administrator Ann Haggard suggests "a house-wide educational needs assessment for staff" as one way of attending to staff nurses needs (2007, p. 193). A similar concern for staff nurses continuing education needs, related to acute and long-term care, was described by nurse educator Nancy Claflin. Claflin carried out a study in a Veteran's Affairs Medical Center to "identify nurses' priorities for con-tinued learning and to examine the priorities related to age, educational level, location in the organization, experience, position in the organiza-tion, and shift worked" (2005, p. 263). Attention to individual staff needs, related to cultural diversity in the nursing workforce, was identified in two nursing articles as being a nurse leader's responsibility (Chang, Chou, & Cheng, 2006; Hunt, 2007).

Obviously the assessment of patients' needs is of grave concern to nursing leaders both for themselves and among the staff nurses they supervise. Interestingly several nursing articles admit to lacunae in this area on the part of practicing nurses. An emergency department study, which compared patients' needs and patients perceptions of how they were met, revealed that "nurses may not always accurately perceive patients' needs or the strength of those needs" (Hostutler, Taft, & Snyder, 1999, p. 43), and an ethnographic exploration of nurse–patient communication in a hospital setting found that "nurses often missed cues that patients needed someone to listen to their concerns" (Barrere, 2007, p. 114). A cur-rent evaluation of nursing practice pointed out the importance of assess-ing patients' changing as well as consistent needs: "As a profession we must keep our fingers on the pulse of society and be ready to respond to the changes of society's needs" (Wilson, 2005, p. 116).

Assessing the needs of those they served, a key theme among the nurse leaders, supported understanding of their nursing vocation. Nurses told stories, some from their early careers or even prior to entering nurs-ing, that revealed their initial and continued consciousness of the needs of those around them. This awareness of another's problem or need was also related to a strong desire to do something to help alleviate the pain or discomfort of the situation. For some nurses a recognition of others' healthcare needs was the beginning of their attraction to nursing as both a vocation and a profession.

Nursing leaders described "assessing needs" as being related to "being grounded" in their nursing related to their commitment to excellent practice and "taking time out" when personal needs demanded.

> I grew up in a spiritual environment, my granddad was a minister, and my brother is a minister now. (In nursing) you don't have to be a minister, but what you do is ministering. I think that you are there spiritually and emotionally for whatever [the] patient needs. And if someone wants (spiritual ministry) and appreciates that, that is OK. But you have to be aware that there are other patients that may not want that. I think it is knowing what the patient needs. Then you give them what they need; it's assessing needs. (51, MSN, supervisor, critical care)

> I have to be supportive and be aware of what the patients' needs are. I feel like that is my job; if they are in pain, assess the pain immediately. That is my first priority…that is just how I operate. (33, BSN, team leader, medical-surgical)

> In nursing you are there to take care of the patients. The patients' needs come first all the time. And that goes along with the calling because you can't be selfish if you have a calling….In so many cases, I see the care is being fragmented. Which then makes me even more determined not to fragment the care. I look to see what is going on in a (patient) room, assess the environment—like the room needs to be straightened up, the patient needs to be shaved or whatever. I look to see that the physical needs, as well as the environment of care and other needs of the patient and family, are met. (45, MSN, team leader, medical-surgical/critical care)

> Patients have so many different needs for caring, nurturing…I am using adjectives that I think are appropriate to nursing. Soothing, comforting, educating, healing, helping, assisting, promoting, encouraging, rewarding, fulfilling. Those are the things that come first in my mind when I think of the nursing profession and what nurses do. (55, MSN, manager, perinatology)

> When you view nursing as a vocation, it helps you to assess the patient as a whole. You know and to really think about what their needs are both physically, mentally, and spiritually. You sort of see the whole person and are able to help them better by doing that, by assessing everything that's going on,

and not just what's physically going on. (36, BSN, team leader, pediatrics)

The vocational aspect of nursing) that is when you try to make sure you are meeting patients' comfort needs. You are an advocate to make sure their needs are met. Whether it is pain medication...or just giving emotional support. Sometimes it is just the little old lady who needs somebody to hold her hand.... just assessing what the patient needs physically or emotionally and dealing with it. Whether it is pain medication or you need to leave them alone so they can sleep; or whether you need to sit there and hold their hand. (45, MSN, team leader, medical-surgical/critical care)

As a young nurse...everything is new; you are a novice. You are learning things and experiencing things for the first time. Some of the patient needs you hadn't ever experienced in nursing school. Some of the needs you experience on your own because you didn't see those while you were under the tutelage of a preceptor. I remember the first death that I experienced with a patient. I was out of orientation at the time. I realized that people, clients, or patients, had different needs that they go through in the dying process. I could see in the process of death that some began to work on letting go and passing on and doing what they needed to do at the end. But others were not yet ready to pass on; their need was to hold on to life....Nurses play an active role in helping patients and families get where they need to be. (43, BSN, head nurse, school health)

Being Grounded

A nurse's enthusiasm for and commitment to his or her nursing specialty area greatly supported a careful "assessment" of the needs of staff, patients, and patients' families. The ability to remain committed to a particular career path in nursing is considered important for a nurse's groundedness in the profession. A British nursing author suggested that "creating a flexible career path will benefit patients, service, and staff alike" (Duffin, 2007, p. 22). Nurse Tina Marelli pointed out that currently "there are more opportunities than ever (for nurses), more work setting choices, more specialties and certification areas, and a range of geographic locations" (Marelli, 2006, p. 19).

As well as the vast array of professional opportunities for nurses, a spiritual and emotional grounding, however, still holds an important place in job satisfaction and general groundedness in the profession of nursing. In a "manifesto for the profession," nursing consultants asserted that "the profession must behave with pride, compassion, and fortitude. This is a career for big hearts, not faint hearts…(nurses are)…for 'best patient care' and against 'unloved, uncaringness, and fear'" (Nursing is the most emotionally rewarding career, 2005, p. 26).

The Called to Serve study group of nursing leaders recognized the fact that being personally grounded was important in terms of leadership style and ability. A number of the nurses verbalized a concern about being and staying "grounded," especially when encountering stressful work situations. Personal groundedness was frequently associated with a nurse leader's spirituality and perception of nursing as a vocation of service; this, he or she felt, provided the support and the strength to remain steady and secure in the profession of caregiving, as well as being continually alert to assessing and attempting to meet the needs of those for whom the nurse was responsible.

> On those days when I am really tired or having a difficult day, or really stressed, it is the fact of knowing that nursing is a vocation, and not just a job that grounds me, that helps me be grounded, to redefine my place in that day. That helps me focus on what is important and place things perspective.…I'm seldom in a situation where things happening are so totally overwhelming that I cannot actually do my job. Being stressed, being tired, having things difficult, are all things that are annoyances and don't compare to the importance of the patients whom I am serving. (54, MSN, head nurse, critical care)

> I am a very sensitive person, so I try to differentiate what my feelings are from the care I am providing when I am feeling something negative. I try to be self-aware, to stay grounded, to prevent my own feelings from getting in the way of my care. (55, MSN, nurse practitioner, mental health)

> I was young and naive when I started nursing. I was very much into Florence Nightingale and the lamp.…I saw (nursing) more as having an immediate impact instead of really, at times, what you do is not recognized, and it is not appreciated, and the only person who understand the impact

of what you are doing is yourself. You have to be grounded in your vocation. You have to be comfortable with that in order to be a good nurse. (26, BSN, charge nurse, pediatric clinic)

Certainly I have had many days when I'm tired and have been stressed and just feel like "What am I doing here?" I have to say I look and I have always thought that there is a reason why I am in this place (hospital) with the people that I'm serving and doing what I'm doing. I feel a calling from God to do the best job I can possibly do. And there are moments when it's extremely frustrating, and I just say to myself "You have to stop for a minute and realize that you need to put the needs of others before your own needs." You know, recognizing that I, myself, am a very fortunate person in being able to live a comfortable life, and not everyone has that. I also have been very healthy and not everyone has that. It's thinking of the Beatitudes, and just kind of drawing on my religious and spiritual side has given me the strength to deal with some of the frustrations on a daily basis, to keep myself grounded in my calling to serve. (49, MSN, head nurse, school health)

Prayer, God helps me get through the (nursing) day. When you have a patient in ICU that is crashing, that is when I think about that it just all seems like too much. It seems like "Wow, if I could just take the stimulation away for a minute and sit quietly." But you know that you have walked into a day where that is not going to happen. So, you just say to yourself, "You know what, I just need to be a nurse today." That is all I need to do and just rely on your (inner) strength in knowing that that is what you need to be doing. (45, MSN, head nurse, school health)

Viewing nursing as a vocation impacts day-to-day practice because I think it keeps you grounded, keeps you in place—in place when the day has lots and lots of difficulties. When I first went to work at an AIDS agency in [large urban area], I was feeling overwhelmed because I didn't know that much about AIDS. I had to quickly educate myself and everyone around me, and learn how to teach. That was my first teaching job. It was difficult to do that, but my sense was that this was for a greater good. I was piloting a new program where we would have nurses in this AIDS agency and nursing students come.

So my sense of vocation overcame the difficulty of trying to learn a new job and the demands....This is where the vocation comes in; this is what I am called to do. So you don't just say "I have just too much work to do here, and so I am going to quit and find an easier job." (66, MSN, team leader, mental health)

Taking Time Out

Interestingly, a number of nursing journal articles discussed the value and importance of nurse leaders "taking time out" from nursing responsibilities when personal needs dictated. Some of the positive benefits of taking time out from one's usual routine identified include:

- Appreciation of "what really matters when it's time to come back to reality" (Watts, 2007, p. 34)
- Learning what tasks one can say no to and what tasks are important (Rigolosi, 2005, p. 241)
- Protecting personal health (Arif, 2006, p. 26)
- Promoting spiritual well-being and job satisfaction (Irvine, 2004)
- Supporting staff working relationships through taking time for coworker recreational activities (Gray, 2002)

The study nurse leaders were uniformly pragmatic about how they assessed their own needs related to servant leadership roles. Although, as noted in the earlier themes, nursing leaders desired and sought to listen with their hearts to others' needs, to be compassionate, to give of themselves, and to recognize the needs of those they served, they also realized that there were and would continue to be occasions when it was appropriate to take time to feed their own spirits. Many nurses spoke of the need, sometimes for a few minutes, sometimes for a few days, to take time out to refresh themselves. This kind of self-healing was considered critical in order for the nurses to continue to function as creative servant leaders in the nursing profession.

One of the things that I do (when there are problems needing to be resolved on the unit) is I have to take time out. When I'm really, really stressed out, I basically take time out, and I sit in a quiet place and sort of center myself because I know that I have to do that; to think about it. I know that I have to do that because if I don't then something will be left out that I don't want to miss. It could be something intangible: somebody is doing something they shouldn't or whatever. But when I'm really stressed out, I will spend 10 minutes sitting at my desk or just 10 minutes in the cafeteria closing my eyes and trying to refocus. Realizing it is not all about what is going wrong, but it is about refocusing. (49, MSN, supervisor, critical care)

(On difficult days teamwork helps). You try to just keep going. You pull away and take some time out if you realize you are off sync, letting things get to you. I usually go and talk to one of my colleagues here and try to figure out what is really going on. It is usually just fatigue and trying to do so much in a limited time—being pulled in a couple of different directions. We have a full clinic schedule and have another life as well. I need to pull back. Talking to other nurses helps. I'm so ticked off because of this or I'm so sad because (my patient) is so sick, and the nurses are fabulous here. You can talk to them and get nourished too. (58, DNSc, research nurse, oncology)

We all get really frustrated (sometimes) and you think: "Why am I doing this? (nursing)." That's the way it seems in the moment with no support, but I have to say that if I can just give myself some breathing space, I usually can say: "OK, it is just a bad day. Look at the greater good; look at the bigger picture. Just step back and take another look." Usually in the moment I am not thinking about (the importance of nursing). It is not until I can step away from it. (58, PhD, RN, educator, maternal-child)

On days when I am tired and stressed out, I just give myself a mini-break. Sometimes I go to the restroom and kind of talk to myself. I say "OK, you are here to take care of the sick." I pray to God to help me. At that time I will tell myself my first vocation here is to make sure that patients get relief from whatever is happening to them. It helps me a lot. (37, ADN, charge nurse, emergency room)

Sometimes I may have to get a second wind. I may have had a difficult day...I need to get my second wind. I pray for God the Creator to give me strength and knowledge that I have to have in order to work on the patients' behalf....There are sometimes when you are just tired and you know you've "had it," and you just need to draw on the support and resources around you of those other nurses who are supportive. You say, "Look, I need to go and get it together right now," and maybe you take a few minutes or whatever I need to do. And I need the nurses to support me in this because I have to step back for a minute because otherwise I will be emotionally drained. That hasn't happened to me often, but I can say that it has happened at least once that I remember vividly. (43, BSN, head nurse, school health)

When I'm tired, it really cues me that I need to take some time off and rest. I use this as a measure to direct me to take some down time. It does help to think about nursing as a vocation to get me through the days and then I do something to build me up until I get a day off. I use music, a novel, swimming, napping, walking, and seeing nature to build myself back up. (55, MSN, nurse practitioner, mental health)

There may be times you have to pull back...I need to go home. I am not of any help. I would be resentful. I think I love nursing enough that I have to be aware when I am not up to giving and I won't be the best I can be. I feel a little guilty about it. But I know I have to take care of myself in order to come in tomorrow and give it another 8, 10, 12 hours. It is sort of like a tug of war because there is always work to do, and I know that. There is always one more phone call to answer. Families and people who are newly diagnosed want to know what to do. They are always taking from you, which is good. But then you reach a point where "OK, I need to stop, I need to go home, I need to get rid of some stress and get the other part of my life together, and then I can come back." (58, DNSc, research nurse, oncology)

Case Example: Assessing Needs

We had this Asian man in the (intensive care) unit one time, and I'm not sure if it (the family request) was because of their religious belief or their cultural belief but (as he was dying) we had to be sure to put on his pants and slippers on his feet so he could move on to the next life. So in the ICU, with the ventilators and pumps and everything, when it got close to his death, his pants were on the bed and his slippers were on the bed so that we could hurry up and put them on before he died. None of us (staff nurses) were Asian but because the family needed this done, his pants and slippers were there. (45, MSN, team leader, medical-surgical/critical care)

Becoming an Advocate

"To Protect and Defend"

> I will ask the Father and he will give you another Advocate to be
> with you forever.
>
> —John 14:16

The author of a literature review on nursing advocacy observed that while patient advocacy was an appropriate role for the professional nurse, there was a "lack of clarity in operationalizing" the concept (Mallik, 1997, p. 130). Following a concept analysis, Baldwin described advocacy as having "three essential attributes: valuing, appraising, and interceding" (2003, p. 33). Three related core attributes of nursing advocacy, also emerging from a concept analysis, identified by Bu and Jezewski, included: "safeguarding patients' autonomy, acting on behalf of patients, and championing social justice in the provision of health care" (2007, p. 101).

There is a significant body of recent nursing literature describing the importance of nursing advocacy in specific care settings such as mental health services (Ball, 2006), the transcultural care arena (Harrison & Falco, 2005), community health (McElmurry, Gi Park, & Buseh, 2003), and death and dying (Martin, 1998; Ryan, 2007). Nursing leaders, such as case managers, are also identified as "in the ideal position to act as effective advocates" related to their knowledge and skill for working both within and outside the healthcare setting to support patients needs (Hellwig, Yam, & DiGiulio, 2003, p. 53).

The nurse leader, serving as a patient, family, staff member, or student advocate, often has to use creative powers of persuasion in a health care or health education setting to support the needs or concerns of the one for whom the nurse is advocating. A content analysis of the concept of power as reflected in Florence Nightingale's early letters revealed that one of the most prevalent types of power that Nightingale used was persuasion: "Nightingale was very adept at persuasion using facts, statistics, stories, imagery, and tenacity to persuade others" (Whiteside, 2004, p. 1). Writing about the contemporary nurse leader's power, Davidhizar and Shearer observed, "Power is the ability to influence others by persuasion instead of coercion" (2002, p. 33).

In attempting to refine the use of verbal persuasion, a nurse leader should ask him or herself "What do I want (someone) to do as a direct result of what I say to them?" (Milne, 2004, p. 54). Verbal persuasion is also suggested as an appropriate strategy for nurse managers who wish to improve staff practice behaviors (Manojlovich, 2005, p. 271). Nurses may also influence practice through the use of persuasion in areas such as health promotion (Norton, 1998) and general strategies for patient care (Damrosch, Sullivan, & Haldeman, 1987).

Persuasion is a characteristic of advocacy that nurses learn to use early in their profession in terms of working with colleagues, patients and family members. It is well recognized that no one likes to be pushed into any kind of behavior and yet sometimes in advocating for another a nurse must attempt achieve a desired outcome through persuasion. Called to Serve nurse leaders spoke of the importance of patient advocacy in a number of caregiving situations; a subtheme of Becoming an Advocate was that of Protecting and Defending those for whom a leader was responsible.

> I think realizing that patients are more than physical beings you need to let them talk about how they are feeling mentally, emotionally, spiritually. Possibly referring them for medication or to talk to their pastor or priest, their church. You listen for all those kinds of things so that you can try to pull in all their (possible) resources, and become an advocate. (51, BSN, team leader, medical-surgical)

> You really have to become a patient advocate more than anything. Nursing was a vocation, 23 years ago when I started, and it still is a vocation now....I think the more you do it, the more you want to care for the patient because you know their needs, you know what needs to be done. So the wiser you become, it drives you to know what you need to do for the patient. (45, MSN, team leader, medical-surgical/critical care)

> Nursing...is becoming a patient advocate. It is a profession that requires a lot of knowledge and related to that responsibility and accountability in providing nursing care.... In my education, nursing was described as serving others, and providing nursing care, being a patient advocate in nursing. (52, PhD, RN, educator, critical care)

> In education, I was an advocate for the nurse: increasing her understanding and knowledge and awareness of what an integral part they play in patient care. (43, BSN, head nurse, school health)

> As far as my vocation in nursing goes there's a caring aspect. You need to be aware if the patient is coping well or if they

need something and let them know that it's OK to ask, and the family. I might intervene (with family about a patient need) and say, "This is about the patient's care." Sometimes I will leave the (patient's) room and say "Do you want to talk about this?"...I'm a very aggressive nurse...I'll do some kind of advocacy intervention. (49, BSN, charge nurse, burn unit)

I don't like to see people suffer. And if there is something I can do, I will certainly intervene. It distresses me to see patients suffering and whether it is pain medication or anything else I can do to relieve someone's suffering, it comforts me to know that I had a part in easing their suffering....Healing is caring enough to want to improve the quality of their life, to relieve their suffering, make things better for them whatever state they are in. (52, PhD, RN, educator, critical care)

To Protect and Defend

It is the nurse leader's role to protect and defend all those under his or her care. The concept of "protection" is described as a nursing "intervention" by nurse Susan Lorenz who points out, "Nurses protect patients from environmental hazards, themselves, and any perceived threat" (2007, p. 115). She asserts "The concept of protection is inherent in nursing practice" (p. 115). The nurse's role as advocate also includes the obligation to protect a patient from "unethical judgments or behaviors [that] threaten the health and safety" (Fry, 1997, p. 15). The concept of nursing advocacy is noted as critical in terms of care of the mentally ill, prisoners, or any persons who are in a uniquely vulnerable category: "People in vulnerable positions need advocates who will defend and protect their rights" (Rossetti, Fox, & Burns, 2005, p. 1211).

Called to Serve nurse leaders spoke of the importance not only of advocating but of protecting those they served. It was understood that the nurse leader's role vis-à-vis staff, patients, family members, or students was to support, guide, and encourage and also to protect from harm. In some instances it was the leader's advocacy and guidance that both protected and defended those they served:

I can honestly say as a pediatric nurse, in the acute care area, "If you leave your child with me you can be totally confident that I will take care of that child as though that child were my own. I can truly tell you I would give my life for that child." That is how serious I feel about caring for my pediatric patients. That I would love that child and would be there to protect and defend; I would work for and would serve that child. As if it had been an assignment from God. I feel that dramatic about it…. I'm sharing with you how I feel when I take care of a pediatric patient. They are a child, they are at your mercy, and I truly can tell you that I feel compassion, love. I would do anything. I would give my life for that child. (59, PhD, RN, educator, pediatrics)

I think that it is very difficult to see a person suffering, and I think that nursing, as a vocation to serve, gives you the opportunity to protect and defend that patient. But it also gives you the opportunity to say that my job as a nurse is to help this person through and not judge why they are there or the circumstances surrounding (illness). That to me is the vocation….As a vocation, I believe we don't judge a person, we are just there to help them. I think that is an important part of the nursing vocation. (50, ADN, charge nurse, recovery room)

I believe that nursing is a calling, that it is a vocation of service. I think you define vocation in several ways, but in nursing you are acting as an advocate for a person who is someone with a need, whether it be a need in mental or physical well-being. I think the nursing vocation to protect and care for your patients is many things depending on the area of nursing that you work in; then it can have several different meanings in terms of vocation….I think we (nurses) are lucky because there are so many avenues with the profession of nursing to choose from. (53, Diploma RN, head nurse medical-surgical/critical care)

Nursing is such hard work and such long hours. It's emotionally painful; you just don't do it unless you have a need to help people, to protect them when they are sick and in need of caring….We have one patient who is a problem. He is constantly on our doorstep. And being nice to him sometimes takes a conscious effort. I have to remind myself that he is a soul in pain because his personality is not easy to deal with. And sometimes I do have to sit back and remind myself of that. (58, BSN, head nurse, oncology)

The role of the nurse in critical care is a little bit different from other nursing. You play an integral role in protecting the patient and as a human you respect that. So you work hand in hand with whoever the medical director is, the critical care director, or the doctor, and they listen to you during rounds. I have had the opportunity to experience that first hand. It is a time of learning that is taking place, and they (the physicians) want to hear what you have to say. They ask you what is going on with the patient; what does the patient need. I'm responsible from start to finish.... I think in our practice nurses convey spirituality for patients because you are there to protect them through all phases of life. Through the birth of infants and also when they progress to death. Elderly patients and young patients as well, through all the phases of the life process, nurses are there and play an active role in helping patients transcend to where they need to be, and (help) families as well. I definitely see that as an integral part of nursing practice; we look at patients from a holistic perspective. ...No matter what (nursing) arena I'm in I am also an advocate for the nurse, to increase their understanding and knowledge and awareness of what an integral part they play in patients' lives. (43, BSN, head nurse, critical care)

(The vocational aspect of nursing supports care of patients suffering physically, emotionally, or spiritually) because I think they need even more. I think they need the experience of touching more and reassurance more. And it is not just the patients but the families too....I have always felt the vocation of nursing. I can't imagine doing anything else. I'm providing care. I am there for the care of that particular patient...my real role is to be that patient's advocate and protector. (52, BSN, charge nurse, perioperative)

Protecting the patient is a basic nursing principle, whether it be turning a patient, ensuring that IV tubing is changed, that the IV bags are labeled, or being proactive in pain management. For a nurse who really cares, he or she wants to make sure that everything is safe for the patient. That is doing what needs to done to protect and improve the patient's status....You have to care about what you are doing and look at it as more than this is just the essence of a job that I have to get done. It is caring about your patients. (52, PhD, RN, educator, critical care)

I had this woman patient in the ER...on a bedside monitor. She was on a stretcher. She was having a myocardial infarction.

She was in heart block and was very close to dying. I was so frustrated because I knew she needed to be admitted or transferred and kept being strung along. I felt as if I was personally protecting her....We were giving her oxygen, tiny doses of morphine. I had blankets on her; I was talking to her, holding her hand, praying for her....God was keeping her alive until we were able to get her admitted to the hospital....I had to take extra steps of going directly to our medical director of the ER and insist that she either be transferred or admitted....I could have been her daughter, and I thought a woman of this age should not be dying in a hospital where she is not getting the care she needs. (66, MSN, team leader, mental health)

Case Example: Becoming An Advocate

I can give you a perfect example of patient advocacy in pediatrics. A child in a burn unit was going to be bathed after bandage removal so she could be debrided, and the child had had that treatment a couple of times and was obviously terrified because it caused a lot of pain. So, I said "Let's get her medicated before we start"; she only had Tylenol ordered....I said "Let's call the doctor...I won't create that kind of pain in a child." So we called the doctor and...got the appropriate dose (of narcotic)....He ordered morphine, and we gave it, and we waited for it to get to her leg. And then we gave the little girl her doll, and we got her into the bathtub, created the environment to be able to take her dressing off...and she was talking to her doll and playing....It was really a matter for me that I'm here to bring comfort, to be an advocate. I'm here to serve. (59, PhD, RN, educator, pediatrics)

Discerning Decisions

"Staying Focused"

You show me the path of life; in your presence there is fullness of joy.

—Psalm 16:11

In exploring the concept of risk taking by healthcare workers, CCRN Linda Sulzbach-Hoke pointed out that clinical nurse specialists, as nurse leaders, are well positioned to help healthcare workers "make the right decision in risky situations" (1996, p. 30). Making the right end-of-life decisions for a person with a cognitive deficit was discussed by Turnbull (2005); a proposed theory to guide nurses in moral and ethical decision making was addressed by Corley who pointed out that nurses "confront many challenges in making the right decision and taking the right action" (2002, p. 636); and, in an article examining the relationship between decision making and nurse–patient interaction, Millard, Hallett, and Luker suggested the inclusion of patient participation in community nursing decisions (2006).

Nursing leaders from the Called to Serve study observed that the ability to make correct decisions and discern appropriate interventions was an important characteristic of any leader of an organization; for a nursing leader, one who aspires to be a servant leader, it can be critical. In some cases, the nurse leaders pointed out making an incorrect decision may simply inconvenience staff and patients and/or patients' families. In other cases, a wrong decision on the part of a clinical nursing leader, such as a charge nurse or team leader in a critical care unit, could have implications for a patient's future health and well-being. Nurse leaders were very aware, as one put it, that their decisions can make a significant difference in a person's life:

> When it comes to decision making in nursing, I think that discernment is the most important quality that you can have; discerning a decision for a patient or even for a staff member. Discerning the right decision about things like PRN pain meds or treatments or a variety of nursing interventions. The patient's life can depend on a nurse discerning the right decision. (69, PhD, RN, educator, adult)

> I think with maturity I value nursing much more than I did in the beginning. I appreciate things. Well, number one, I was afraid most of the time when I first came to work. There is a fear factor when you are a new nurse that you will make a mistake....I think there should always be a fear factor (to some degree) in the nurse. You can never be overconfident when you walk on that floor to care for someone. You should be confident that you know what to do but not over confident so that if a problem arises you know how to make the right decision....Therefore it makes me secure in my decisions. It makes me confident that I can be a resource for younger nurses,

be a mentor, a (role model).... Carrying out my nursing as a vocation over time has made me more confident that I know what to do...that you know how to make the right decision. It makes me more comfortable in my decisions. I can trust that what I decide is the best thing, the right thing to do. And I'm making the right decisions. I think experience makes a huge difference in that. I'm not saying that I know everything. I have 50 nurses that work for me now, and I turn to their opinion every day. I'll say "What do you think about this or that? How do you feel about this?" (55, MSN, manager, perinatology)

There can be days that are stressing, especially in the management role when you have 50 staff members and 38 patients, plus the doctors, but I always know that in the role, to make the right decision, I can make a difference in someone's life. Many lives. Make a better future for someone, make nursing a better profession, make it easier for someone to do their job. The patients will receive better care, the nurses will be more efficient....So I always know that in the back of my mind, no matter how stressful the day, you prioritize what is important for the future. You set goals for yourself, and you achieve what you can on a daily basis and do the best you can to plan for the future. (55, MSN, manager, perinatology)

You have to figure out sometimes how to bring comfort, decide how you bring comfort....I really feel that as a vocation our job is to bring comfort. You always have to look at the individual patient because there are some patients who just...don't believe what you believe....That is a challenge because obviously I bring my own thoughts and decisions. And it is sometimes not only the patient but the family you have to help. (59, PhD, RN, educator, pediatrics)

Sometimes when there is a problem I run across some nurses who don't (make decisions), and there is a coldness and a nonprobing about what is going on with you (patient). You can't do that....I get so upset. Just reach out and find out what is going on. You might find that you can't fix it, or you might confirm that you really can do something, and this is what the patient needs....You should have compassion. (58, DNSc, research nurse, oncology)

In the DR (delivery room) you have to make the right decision. In the DR it is a little different because some women can
handle pain far better than others. When we do admissions
data we ask for an acceptable pain level by a scale we have, but
it's not written in stone, and I tell them that at any point you
are uncomfortable please let me know. I can look at a patient
(in labor) and tell that she's not coping well. In the DR I keep
asking if people want me to intervene, if I really think they
need something, because some people want to do this naturally. The husbands may say "no" but the patient says "yes."
I will tell the husband politely "Love you dearly, but this is
about the patient. When you are in labor, then we can talk"....
I'm a big pain medication advocate if I think the patient needs
it or is losing control...Labor can be very long and very difficult, so you have to be considerate of how she might feel....
I will stand up for my patient. (49, BSN, charge nurse, labor
and delivery unit)

Staying Focused

To discern appropriate decisions related to patient, family, staff, or student needs and care, nurse leaders admitted needing to stay focused on a
situation as presented. It was also important for nurse leaders to remain
focused on the understanding of their profession as a vocation of service
in making decisions.

Although it is important for nurses working in all specialty areas of
the profession to stay focused on attempting to carry out best practices
in nursing, one healthcare specialty role where continued nursing focus
is critical is that of the certified registered nurse anesthetist (CRNA). A
qualitative study of the occupational stress experienced by practicing
CRNAs, revealed that one of the key coping strategies to combat work-
related stress was identified as "staying focused on the task at hand (i.e.,
patient care)" (Perry, 2002, p. 1).

Called to Serve nurse leaders felt that continuing to embrace their
profession as a vocation of service helped them to stay focused on how
they wanted to practice nursing and the goals they wanted to achieve. It
was the idea of keeping one's eye on the spiritual call to serve that not
only helped nurse leaders to function successfully and make appropriate
decisions in their ministries; this also gave them a significant degree of joy
and satisfaction in the work. In this contemporary era of cost containment
and managed care, nurse leaders admitted that it is easy to lose sight

of the real meaning of nursing, the service component as modeled by Florence Nightingale. If, however, the nurse leaders explained, nursing can remain true to its history and tradition and keep the vocational aspect in mind, nurses will be able to retain their focus on the goal of commitment to caring for the sick that led them to nursing in the first place.

> On those days that I'm stressed and, you know, don't want to be there, it goes back to focusing on why I'm really there. To take care of people and help them cope regardless of what is going on or how crazy life is....you have to stay focused on "I'm here to help...to take care of patients"...even if it's a very basic thing that helps somebody grow that day. Then you've been successful....As crazy as it is...and as stressful as it can be, that just makes it worth it....I'm there to help people... whatever it is they may need...that's what keeps me at work. If I help one child each day then I'm successful. And that's what keeps me focused. (36, BSN, team leader, pediatrics)

> Nursing being a vocation helps you to stay focused. You can understand yourself as being in a vocation versus a job; that is, that you know what you are supposed to be doing, what you are doing. You've got to have the faith that you are given the gifts and the tools to do what you need to do. That is the way I perceive it. It's like having kids. Like the good Lord gave me these children and now will give me the tools to raise them. Well, I know that I need to be a nurse, so I need to be willing and receptive to what I need to do to take care of sick people. (45, MSN, head nurse, school health)

> On days when you are tired and stressed, if you can keep nursing's call to serve in the back of your mind, it always helps you, helps you focus, helps you get back on track. Some days when you are having that kind of a day, you lose sight of the vocation. I believe in the saying that the more stressed you are, the busier your day is, the more time you need to spend on your knees. I believe that 100%, but I'm still not at the point that I can actualize that in my life all the time. (52, PhD, RN, educator, mental health)

> Staying focused on your nursing as a vocation, I think, makes you a better nurse. You are better at what you do, you are happier. If you are just going to work to do a job, you are not going

to be a happy person overall. It is fulfilling to focus on nursing as a vocation. It has meaning, and you are not only offering but are receiving; nursing is a give and take. It the vocational role the makes it a more enjoyable day. It has to be more than just a job—nursing. There are jobs that can just be jobs. But I don't see nursing that way at all. (55, MSN, manager, perinatology)

There was one late evening with a patient…being there at the hospital until 7:30 in the evening, I was annoyed that it was so late…I thought to myself, "Boy, I'm getting too old for this." But then, I focused on this poor patient who was in surgery all day long. I thought, I can be here for an extra 2 hours to get him where he needs to be by 7 o'clock. Do what he needs to make him comfortable and cared for. Then I went home and said "That was really a full day, but that is what my job is in nursing." (53, diploma RN, head nurse, medical-surgical/critical care)

I see God in my patients, and I believe that has grown in a more mature fashion. Over time I have enjoyed the fact that nursing experiences, no matter how much you think you know, can continue to surprise you. In a hospital where joy and respect in caring for the individual is paramount, it helps me to focus on the meaning of a nursing vocation. (54, MSN, head nurse, critical care)

Case Example: Discerning Decisions

There was an elderly man with Alzheimer's who was brought in and had been catheterized in the emergency department, and the family was very concerned that he had it. (His wife) was screaming about the fact that the man had been catheterized (an in-and-out catheterization). I happened to be there, and I made a decision to intervene because I knew that her anger wasn't about the catheterization being done. It was about here is this man who used to be able to get on the Metro, go to the theater, who can't do that any more because he is dependent on the catheter. She didn't say any of those things, but you could tell by the complaints and concern that she was a woman dealing with loss of her husband's functioning. I picked up on what was not said. (49, MSN, supervisor, critical care)

Making a Difference

"Doing Your Best"
"Generating Excitement"
"A Nurturing Environment"

> *And this is my prayer, that your love may overflow more and more*
> *with knowledge and full insight to help you determine what is best,*
> *so that in the day of Christ you may be pure and blameless.*
> —1 Philippians 10

A message from the president of the North Carolina Nurses Association, Dennis Sherrod, included the assertion "Day in and day out, nurses choose to make a difference in people's lives" (2006, p. 3). Nursing education prepares nurses to make a difference in their patients' lives (Kleiman, 2007); student nurses greatly "value projects that enable them to make a difference in the lives of others" (Mansfield & Meyer, 2007, p. 132); and registered nurses' stories continually reveal how their nursing activities lead to "making a difference" in the lives of patients and their families (Donnelly, Leurer, & Domm, 2006).

Other nursing journal articles discussed the various ways in which nurses "make a difference" in the lives of those they care for in such arenas as critical care nursing (Hawley & Jensen, 2007); hospice nursing (Carlin, 1999); infusion nursing (Alexander, 2007); cardiac rehabilitation and intensive care nursing (Premoe, 1995); and older adults in prehospital emergency care (Melby & Ryan, 2005).

One of the servant leadership themes that was very dear to the hearts of the nurse leaders of the Called to Serve study was that of making a difference in someone's life. Nurses experienced satisfaction and a feeling of accomplishment if they felt their nursing leadership had actually made a difference in the life of a person under their care. Sometimes the fact of "making a difference" was obviously related to the outcome of a particular situation; other times it was the personal response of an individual being served who assured a nurse leader that he or she had, in fact, made a difference in the person' s life.

> It's important knowing that I make a difference. And what I contribute, my knowledge, my skills, my touch, just being there makes a difference even when I am tired….I know that providing information to students in a class will have a future impact potentially on hundreds of patients. They (students) can pull on the knowledge that they were told in class; I

should do this, this is my concern. So knowing that is rewarding. (52, PhD, RN, educator, critical care)

I am responsible to have an impact on the staff nurse's lives. Sometimes they will have a bad day, and they will start to question themselves, and every now and again I will say to one of them "You are having a really bad day, but think about some of the patients that you are caring for and the difference that you make in their lives; even a little impact can help. Think about yesterday, what impact you had (on patients) yesterday, and don't let today discourage you because you will have some of those bad days." (49, MSN, supervisor, critical care)

Sometimes you know that you make a difference in people's lives. Somehow God always provides because something will come up that is so phenomenally insignificant to me...for instance an elderly patient that I have gotten medications for from the office that is no big deal for me...and later the daughter will call back and say "Thank you so much, because Mom would not have been able to take her medication without you, and we appreciate it so much." It's those things that I do on a daily basis, say when you are really stressed, and I think that I can't do one more thing, and then you get that phone call to thank you....Somewhere, God sends somebody to you. I can't imagine any other profession. Nursing is so rewarding.... Being a nurse and serving others can make a difference in their lives. Otherwise I would have been out of nursing probably long ago. Without a doubt I would have. I mean think about it. Why would you want to be a nurse? I mean really! If you don't have a calling to serve why would you want to have people throw up on you, be angry when they are not feeling well, scream and holler and tell you "No!" The hours are just fabulous—not! I mean tell me; why would you want to do it? (57, ADN, head nurse, medical-surgical)

Having nursing as a vocation impacts my day-to-day practice in knowing that because of what I do, the patient's day may be better, or their hospital length of stay may be shorted. They may have fewer complications. That they know that someone cares about them as an individual. Nursing is something that I have always loved and wanted to do. And I can't imagine doing anything different....I couldn't picture doing anything else. I love what I do, and it is comforting to know that I have made a difference, and I know there are patients who are alive because of what I've done. They have had improvements in their health because of things that I have done. And truly I couldn't be doing anything else. (52, PhD, RN, educator, critical care)

The people we cared for, we do the exit interview at the very last (prior to discharge), and while doing that interview patients tell us what a difference we have made. One man told us that of all the medical dollars that went into his care for heart disease, it was the cardiac rehab program run by the nurses that was the best; that made the difference. (52, MSN, charge nurse, cardiac rehabilitation)

The nursing vocation helps you make a difference for terminally ill or dying patients. (In regard to care) the family perception is "Well, you are a nurse; you are able to do this better." You know when it's a relative it's a little bit harder, so you can do the simple things to try to make their life more comfortable, their day a little bit brighter. Just simple things like giving a manicure...little simple things that are not monumental but things that could be important to the patient or family.... I think if I didn't see nursing as a vocation I would probably not be in nursing today. I might have chosen something that was easier, that was going to pay more, that the hours would not be so difficult, I wouldn't have to work weekends....So being a nurse is not easy; it's not the easy road. So what am I getting out of it? I'm getting gratification that I'm helping somebody. So, in other words if you're going to take the harder road, there's got to be something that you're getting out of it. I would say that what I'm getting out of it is the feeling that I'm making a difference! I would have a less stressful job, less stressful hours...if I didn't want to serve. (51, BSN, team leader, medical-surgical)

I try to teach and encourage the students, as they care for patients, that these are human beings that need your love and compassion, and if there is anything that you walk away from, from my teaching you clinical, it is to always respect and care for and love a patient as if they were your mother, father, your brother, your sister....You are not just there to pass out meds or give them a shot or take them to X-ray....You still have to deal with them as a person...and hopefully, I made a difference in their lives as future nurses. (50, MSN, manager/educator, quality management)

I can still picture to this day interacting with patients (when I was a student) and that is when I think that it really began to hit me how you could influence patients, that nursing was more than just a job. The effect that a nurse could have on someone's life, providing comfort and encouragement to them. (49, MSN, head nurse, school health)

Doing Your Best

A contemporary expression to reflect doing one's best in a job is to assign the label of "best practice." The "best practice" labeling is beginning to show up in the nursing literature as describing the best way to carry out a variety of specialty care activities, for example

- "Forward: Preparation of a New Intensive Care Unit Nurse: Is There a Best Practice?" (Davidson, 2006, p. 179)
- "Collaboration to Promote Best Practices in Care of Older Adults" (Hertz, Koren, Rossetti, Munroe, Berent, & Plonczynski, 2005, p. 311)
- "The Challenges of Shift Work (Best Practice)" (Blachowicz & Letizia, 2006, p. 274)
- "Development of a Postpartum Depression Best Practice Guideline: A Review of the Systematic Process" (McQueen & Dennis, 2007, p. 199)
- "Best Practice in the Treatment of Patients with Rheumatoid Arthritis" (Oliver, 2007, p. 47)
- "The Quest for Best Practice in Caring for the Home Care Patient with an Indwelling Urinary Catheter: The New Jersey Experience" (Sienkiewicz, Wilkinson, & Emr, 2008, p. 121)
- "Best Practice in Record Keeping" (McGeehan, 2007, p. 51).

Along with supporting the theme of "staying focused" described by the Called to Serve nursing leaders, the continued perception of nursing as a call to serve encouraged the concept of doing one's best at whatever task was at hand. This is also reflected in the nursing vocational attitudinal theme, identified in the previous chapter, labeled the Extra Mile. In many situations the nursing leaders felt that they indeed had to go the extra mile in order to do what they believed to be their "best" for staff, patients, patients' families, and/or students — to make a difference in their lives. It was, however, generally in going that extra mile and attempting to do one's best that the nurses found their greatest sense of accomplishment and peace, that they truly perceived their nursing activities as ministry:

> I think that nursing is a vocation, and no matter what area I work in or whatever situation I'm in, I'm going to fulfill that vocation....When you are in those situations when that patient needs you, and the call light goes on, and you kind of just go "Ahhh!" I think it's a lot like when you have children who call you when you are tired; they need you one more time, and you go "Ahhh!" But still you get up and answer that patient's call, and you are doing your best—do the best you can. You don't give up. You can't. That is your commitment to nursing. (50, ADN, charge nurse, recovery room).

> The concept of service is an essential dimension of my nursing practice. At the end of the day if there is more work to do, you do it. I know that bringing work home, even in your mind, caring for, worrying about, making sure that those who depend on you have gotten their due; that you have done your best to try and help them make another step toward fuller health. (54, MSN, head nurse, critical care)

> I'm committed to my patients, knowing that I've done the best that I can do to make a difference in a patient's outcome. Supporting them through their illness, supporting the family members as they experience critical illness as a family member. Being a cheerleader for patients. Whether it is coughing and deep breathing, or doing cardiac rehab walking the treadmill, being a cheerleader in their support of recovery. (52, PhD, RN, educator, critical care)

> (In a nursing vocation) I think you just do your best job. You want to think about (the fact that) some clients need assistance, information, care and comfort—whatever it happens to be. You just do it, and you don't even think about it. You just do it. It just come naturally....I think (caring) is just something that naturally occurs. That is how I do things. (51, MSN, supervisor, critical care)

> Every day I pray to go out and do a good job and do the best I can to try and be a positive person with my coworkers, with

the people I am caring for. I know in my last clinical position, working as a school nurse with an underserved population, many of the students were uninsured; we really had some difficult situations to deal with. Children not receiving the health care they needed, and…trying to be able to solve the lack of insurance problem. I realized that many things are beyond my control including that. I really felt at that point that I really had to rely on my spiritual side and recognize that I was doing the best job I could and always tried to put others' needs in front of my own as I carried out the job. (49, MSN, head nurse, school health)

I have matured as a nurse…. It took me many years to understand that life is a process; it is not like there is an end point…. God looks at whether we are faithful to the process he has called us to. Not necessarily outcomes. I might have poor outcomes but if I am faithful to what God called me to, that is the most important outcome. I can make a lot more money doing something other than this (nursing), but if I am called to this, I just have to do the best I can and be faithful to what I'm called to. (52, PhD, RN, educator, mental health)

You do the best that you can; you try to understand what a patient needs. You may not be on target exactly, but you have enough insight to realize some of the issues they may be going through. The more you listen to people the more ideas expand out. You still look, and there are just a couple of things that they are dealing with (specifically). What you learn in school is…how to work with people who express things differently…do we talk about this or do we not? Do we bring this up or do we not? How do we say this to him or to her? Because you win some and you lose some. (The patient) is not communicating very openly about how he is doing with this (problem). He is having a hard time. (58, DNSc, research nurse, oncology)

I think you make a commitment to your vocation, and you follow through no matter what the circumstances when you are at work…and if you have chosen nursing as your career you do the best job you can. (50, ADN, charge nurse, recovery room)

Generating Excitement

In the context of doing one's best to make a difference in the lives of those for whom they care, nurse leaders also pointed out the importance of being "excited" about professional practice. A negative relationship between excitement about one's nursing role and the phenomenon of burnout has been identified (Simms, Erbin-Roesemann, Darga, & Coeling, 1990; Sadovich, 2005). Simms et al. describe work excitement as "a prerequisite to effective (nursing) practice and quality care" (1990, p. 177). The authors define work excitement as "Personal enthusiasm and commitment to work evidenced by creativity, receptivity to learning, and ability to see opportunity in everyday situations" (p. 179). Sadovich identified four factors predictive of work excitement: "work arrangements, growth and development opportunities, variable work experience, and (supportive) work environment" (2005, p. 91).

Some ways suggested in the literature in which nurse educators generated excitement for the profession were through providing students with the opportunity to share "ideas related to nursing practice in a specified area with practicing nurses" and inviting them to listen to speakers who could "provide students with a sense of excitement about their chosen career" (Brockopp, Schooler, Welsh, Cassidy, Ryan, Mueggenberg et al., 2003, p. 562). Students were encouraged to consider geriatric nursing, by engaging "faculty, students, and the community in exchange activities that focused on generating excitement for geriatric nursing" (Jeffers & Campbell, 2005, p. 280). Potential nursing students were recruited by creating a summer camp to "stimulate excitement in a nursing career" (Daumer & Britson, 2004, p. 130).

One way of making a difference in working with staff, patients, families, or students, described by the Called to Serve study group of nursing leaders, was that of generating excitement among those with whom they worked in order to help others become excited about the positive benefits of complying with some behavior or activity that the nursing leader was attempting to promote. An individual is much more likely to not only comply with a request but to feel positive about the behavior if he or she can achieve a sense of excitement about an identified aim or expected outcome. This nursing subtheme was particularly reflected in the interview data elicited from the study group nurse educators:

> The excellence in nursing comes just like the excellence in teaching in that relationship with the student. When you can really connect with that person and their needs....I try to be

very open, have good communication processes myself, get students excited, generate excitement...I think I am approachable so a lot of students come to me. I even tell students "What you see me doing with you is what you need to be doing with patients." (52, PhD, RN, educator, mental health)

You catch the excitement generated from the teacher....You know, seriously I can honestly say that every instructor, every professor, that I had, they were proud to be a nurse. And they will promote nursing till the day that they die. The really will! (26, BSN, charge nurse, pediatric clinic)

I have always been happy to be a nurse, and I am very happy now to be able to teach inexperienced or new nurses, because I think that if they don't catch the excitement you try to generate, the inspiration, if they don't get the feeling that this is more than a job, that this is a vocation, that their work with people is so important, then they don't get turned on; they don't get persuaded of the value of nursing. They don't get what they should be getting out of their education. (66, MSN, team leader, mental health)

I think when I was young and first starting out I was all caught up in trying to do a good job from a clinical standpoint...It was almost a matter of just survival in my first jobs working in understaffed areas. But as I have grown older and matured, I think each year I recognize more and more of the excitement of nursing being a calling. And I speak to people who are new in the profession or thinking about entering nursing about that... do they have that dimension (of calling) that they will need to be a successful nurse.... For me the excitement generated was a kind of "click," having watched some of my instructors in action and they way they care for patients and interact with them. It really made a profound impression on me. As a nurse educator, I really hope that I can have that impact on someone one day, on students. (49, MSN, head nurse, school health)

Probably a number of things first attracted me to a call to serve the sick...actually a combination of things, like seeing a movie (about nursing) and thinking it was exciting or the nuns coming to visit us, who were nurses, or going to the clinic where the Sisters of Charity of St. Vincent de Paul worked, when I was little to get vaccinations. Just really loving the sisters and the work they did...it was obvious that there was something in the profession that I was attracted to, that I found exciting. (59, PhD, RN, educator, pediatrics)

I'm excited because my family, they are excited about it (nursing). Even my son who was only about 4 years old when I graduated from nursing. He told me "Oh, Mommy is a nurse, and I'm proud of you." My family, especially back home, viewed nursing as rewarding, and it is also symbolic when you're a nurse. It means something. Not only you're doing patient care; it's a big deal serving others. My family verbalized to me that they are very proud of me. (36, MSN, charge nurse, medical-surgical)

One of my close friends had decided to go into nursing, and she said, "You like helping people, this might be a route for you to go...why don't you start in it, and you can quit if you don't like it?"...And in that prenursing year, the second semester, we had a chance to do therapeutic communication with people in assisted living. And I was so excited; I loved it!...So, I was like "This is for me!"...Just having a bond with this nice little old lady and helping her. It was great! I was so glad I did it. (38, MSN, charge nurse, maternal-child)

A Nurturing Environment

The Called to Serve nurse leaders spoke about the importance of nurturing and having a nurturing environment in which professional practice is carried out. A nurturing environment has been found to be critically important for both faculty and students in a school of nursing (Melland & Volden, 2001; Riffel, Peterson, & Insley, 2004), and for patients and their families in a variety of healthcare settings, especially those where life-and-death decisions are sometimes made, such as the neonatal unit (Brockopp et al., 2001) and the intensive care unit (Rashid, 2007).

A nurturing work environment is also important for staff nurses in contemporary healthcare settings, especially those working in hospitals, medical centers, and clinics. In promoting a "nurturing work environment," Mills and Pennoni emphasize the fact that "open nurturing communication (among nursing leaders and nurses) is...basic to job satisfaction and professional growth" (1986, p. 117). "Nurse manager support of staff nurses" is described as "an essential component of a productive, healthy work environment" (Kramer, Maguire, Schmalenberg, et al., 2007, p. 325).

Three other key factors that contribute to a nurturing healthcare work environment are:

1. An environment of compassionate caring (Turkel & Ray, 2004)
2. "supportive communication that creates trust and expresses appreciation" by organizational leaders (Apker, Zabava-Ford, & Fox, 2003, p. 226)
3. "a shared decision-making structure that promotes an empowering work environment in which professional fulfillment and personal satisfaction can flourish" (Moore & Hutchison, 2007, p. 564).

To nurture the healthcare work environment, nursing leaders from the Called to Serve study reported attempting to create and maintain a positive attitude among staff members at all levels and also in relation to nurse–patient and nurse–family interactions. While the staff's primary role was to nurture the patients and families for whom they cared, the managers and supervisors felt a responsibility to nurture the overall healthcare environment. Nurse leaders spoke about having worked in "nurturing" and "nurtured" environments, where the majority of the staff were "like-minded" and supported similar ends and goals for the practice of nursing. Providing for the equal sharing of work responsibilities among staff was also a key to nurturing the work environment:

> I was working in a hospital of young people with cancer who were terminally ill. We were a regional referral center for the whole West Coast and the whole Pacific. And that was very challenging for me as a young nurse working with many patients who were my own age that were terminally ill. But I found myself working with a community of nurses who were like-minded…, and we also had the support of our administration of the hospital to really make it a nurturing environment, (a place) where people truly felt cared for. I think this not only helped the patients but also helped me. (49, MSN, head nurse, school health)

> In a nurtured and nurturing environment the nurses are, in a way, giving spiritual care to their patients because of their presence there. It is the time you spend with the patients that demonstrates your concern. Even a simple touch on the hand

or on the arm to show the patient that this is a caring nurse: "She is very concerned for me. I know she can't do everything for me because they are short staffed, but at least I have a feeling of trust, a feeling of presence of her being here for me." (54, MSN, supervisor, medical outpatient clinic)

Working in an environment where they recognized nursing as a vocation, the environment was more nurturing, this was a calling as opposed to just coming to work and going home.... This would be the environment I want to work in. (50, ADN, charge nurse, recovery room)

Where you work and how people in the environment see the work that they do has a huge influence on how the nurses perceive their own personal practice. Where I work now and where I worked before have similar cultures. The culture is one where you care about and support your patients and you support each other. You are allowed to spend some time thinking beyond the day to day about what it is you are doing and why. I think that makes a difference....It has been very good for the nurses to actually spend some time thinking about "How do I make an impact everyday, what do I leave behind?" I think once nurses really started to think about how they practice, they become better. (49, MSN, supervisor, critical care)

I certainly think that environment impacts your practice. When you are in an environment in which nursing is seen as a ministry, because of the way the system is set up and because of the people who are practicing in it, more people reflect that attitude of caring ministry. And the further you get away from an environment where you have a vocational or religious philosophy and involvement of other practitioners, I think nursing becomes just a job. People don't have the same seriousness about compassion and maintaining a caring environment....I think if you work in a (religiously affiliated) hospital...nurses are offered a much greater opportunity to work with the calling to serve....To connect with that vocational component is an intrinsic component or dimension, I would say, because it is really not just a piece of (nursing); it cut through your whole practice. And there are so many issues in day-to-day practice—understaffing, the critical nature of our work, the clinical component, the technology...then it is easy to forget unless there is something in the environment supporting the (vocation to serve) and supporting the nurse in keeping that in the forefront of your thought. If that environment is not there, it is real easy to get away from it, just to forget what it is you are here to do. (59, PhD, RN, educator, pediatrics)

If you are not nurtured and nurturing, which to me is nursing, I don't know how you can do it. Because you can't start just being professional, especially when people are terminal or long-term care, because they know it, and it has got to be pretty scary and upsetting. I still cry, and when I stop crying, I will stop being a nurse. That's when you look at nursing as a vocation and not just a profession. I think when you go home at night and turn everything off, I guess that's what a professional can do; I cannot. (57, ADN, head nurse, medical-surgical)

I have been in clinical with students who are so scared they are actually shaking. I always tell them I am here to teach you. I don't expect you to know everything. I'm not looking to see how your going to make a mistake or what you don't know. Quite the contrary, it's my job to teach you, to nurture you; that's what I do, and so I want to do it with compassion, I want to do it with love. And it is truly that feeling that makes us a community of nurses, that permeates teaching as a vocation. I have a tremendous amount of reward when I can help someone else be a nurse. Then also help teach them how they can be compassionate.... and trying to understand what love means....We love another person when we desire to help them and help us together as a team....We are doing something together; we are sharing our lives together. (59, PhD, RN, educator, pediatrics)

Nursing to me is nurturing all the way around the body, soul, and physical components, the emotional components also. When I take care of a patient, I think I am helping their mental psyche as far as just talking to them and trying to find out what they need. (Nursing) is to me a definite calling of helping someone else in need. (57, ADN, head nurse, medical-surgical)

The calling to serve influences practice because in the old days a patient stayed in the hospital for 14 days. Where now you don't get a whole lot of time to know about the patient because they are in and out in one or two days. But you still have to, while they are in… get to know the patient and the whole person. It's not just the heart or the stomach, it's the whole entire person and everything that is involved whether it is their home life, the stress of their job, or whatever the case may be….I look to see that the physical needs as well as the nurturing environment of care and other needs of the patient and family are met. (45, MSN, team leader, medical-surgical/critical care)

Case Example: Making A Difference

We had this patient come in to the rheumatology clinic…he comes and asks me where his shot is (but he was from another clinic) so…I ask him who he is and what clinic he's in…and "Since you were in the lab did you have lunch?" The patient says, "No, I'm not hungry. I just wanted to get my shot." I said "Let me do you a favor while we are trying to figure this out. Let me try to get you a bag lunch."….I gave him a bag lunch while I looked at this chart….It took us maybe an hour to get it resolved, and he finally got his shot, and we took him to the lobby to catch a cab. I stayed there with him, and he said "You know, I really appreciate all that you did for me, all the attention." I said, "I just wanted to make sure you are okay." He said…"I never realized anybody would go to all this extent, someone who doesn't know me from the clinic but who is willing to help me"….This is the real focus of our nursing practice, to be responsible for our patients, to make a difference. It is our patient. If you have to stop at the moment to do something extra, then you do it….This is an example of what a nurse is. (54, MSN, supervisor, medical outpatient clinic)

Being There to Serve

"Beyond the Ordinary"

> *Serve one another with whatever gifts each of you has received.*
> —1 Peter 4:10

The concept of service within the nursing profession is so widespread that it would be impossible to cite all of the extant literature references to the term in this chapter. One important reflection of the concept of service in nursing education that might be noted is that of "service learning" undertaken by most contemporary schools of nursing. In service learning projects, the students are engaged in some community nursing activities in which they have a learning experience and at the same time are providing nursing care for an underserved population. Service learning projects are often carried out in urban inner-city facilities or in impoverished rural areas. Two examples of service learning experiences are a service-learning project in maternal-infant health that was designed to "enhance services to teen-age mothers" (Bentley & Ellison, 2005, p. 287) and student-supported mobile wellness services provided to rural older adults (Neill, Hayward, & Peterson, 2007).

As discussed in the previous chapter, the study nurse leaders were very open and comfortable in describing their understanding of their nursing vocation as a call to serve others. The idea of servanthood or being of service to the sick was not in any way perceived as placing the nurse in a lower position. It was in fact considered a privilege to serve the sick. For a number of the nurses, most of whom were Christian, the positive attribution placed on the concept of service was derived from the Christian scripture; that is from the example of Jesus, who as "the Son of Man came not to be served but to serve" (Matthew 10:45). (This is discussed in Chapter 4 under "A Christian Mandate").

> What I do is help the patient understand that, one, I am there to serve them; they don't have to apologize for whatever their problem is. You have patients that say "I'm such a bother." I say, "This is what I do. I love doing this. The reason I am a nurse is to help you feel better. Whether that means moving you again, repositioning you, changing the dressing, reevaluating the IV, or getting you your pain medication." (59, PhD, RN, educator, pediatrics)

> Nursing is very much the type of caring profession where the nurses are always there to serve the patient. The nurse is always there consulting with the patient, listening, giving education, giving some guidance about the infrastructure of the hospital. I think it is the nurse who is always there at the battle line more so than any other type of profession....The people who go into nursing basically because it's a job, just a job, won't last long. They will find another easier job. There is a separation between what is your vocation of service versus a job. And if you are a nurse, it's the vocation, the call to serve first...you have to love your vocation. (54, MSN, supervisor, outpatient medical clinic)

My real role is to be the patient's advocate; to be there to serve them. (52, BSN, charge nurse, perioperative)

Sometimes I find out that a family member has a concern. My immediate response upon seeing that person approaching is to greet them and offer assistance....I just see it as that is what I am there to do. I'm there to serve people usually in the worst times of their life. They are usually not happy. They usually have a concern because they are seeing their mother, father, or husband—whoever—had been discharged, and nobody had told them anything, and they haven't made arrangements....I feel like you do nursing with people probably in the worst time of their life. And it is still your job to put a good face on it and energy on it and to serve. (59, PhD, RN, educator, pediatrics)

I just believe that nurses are there to serve people. Often I don't take any kind of break. I get very concerned about these elderly folks who have a fall risk, and they don't have a sitter, and they put them down the hall away from the nurse's station and hope that the bed alarm works. I would much rather prevent a fall than have the patient hurt. (58, ADN, charge nurse, chemotherapy treatment)

If I didn't see nursing as a vocation to serve I wouldn't be here. I would be like some nurses I run across. I think not everybody is called to do this, and they figure it out; hopefully, they figure it out sooner than later. They always feel underpaid, underprivileged, and they come to work angry. They don't want to be there, and they are not there for the clients they serve; they're not there for the families. They are just there for the paycheck. It's reflected in the job they do....It's reflected in the care they give and in the patient's responses....they respond to you when they know something is for their well-being. They respond to you differently. (43, BSN, head nurse, school health)

For people who want to be nurses....there's technology and all these things that can get you sort of interested in nursing. And there's so much that nursing offers in terms of so many different things in nursing that you can do, but if we could market just one, it's that feeling that you get from helping someone. You can't bottle that....If you could put that on a poster you'd have a lot of people signing up. But I think that's where the challenge is (in nursing): people have to feel the call to serve — to be serving others. Those are the people you want to be nurses. (51, BSN, team leader, medical-surgical)

The concept of serving is essential to nursing because any time you're a nurse you're always caring for people. That's considered a service that you do for patients regardless of what kind of nursing you do. (51, BSN, team leader, medical-surgical)

Service is what your practice is. You are serving, you are caring for, helping whether it be bathing a patient...or giving medication, it is all part of the service for the patient who can't do it for themselves....Just serving someone who needs your help and your professional knowledge to help them recover...or to come in the next day for a procedure....It is just serving and helping them to do something that they otherwise would not be able to do on their own. (53, Diploma RN, head nurse, medical-surgical/critical care)

I was attracted by a call to serve the sick in a sense (because) I know in life I have been very blessed to have what I have. You know we all have good days and bad days when we feel sorry for ourselves, but there are people out there who really, really, really need help. And if you, you know, if God gave me my health and my mind as a way to help others than that is what I need to do. I feel as though nursing, you can look at two ways. You can look at it as very task focused...we are taught to draw blood, we are taught to give meds...we are taught to do (physical) assessment, but there is also nursing that is almost a way of life and a personality — an ultimate frame of mind of serving. (26, BSN, charge nurse, pediatric clinic)

When I went back to school to do my bachelor's, that's when my professors really pointed me in the right direction (about nursing as a vocation); that you are called to serve, and your nursing career is a gateway to serve others. Nursing is not just a job, it's a service to serve others....Most of my patients are underprivileged or underserved, and when I talk to them or go visit them at home, I see myself as being of service...being a servant and then pointing them in the right direction. (40, MSN, manager, public health)

Beyond the Ordinary

In a study entitled "Take Patient Care Beyond the Ordinary," qualitative interviews were carried out with a sample group of 24 hospital clinicians in order to identify caring and compassionate behaviors that went beyond ordinary patient care. Analysis of the interview data led to the development of a "model of affective clinician/patient interactions" (Graber & Mitcham, 2004, p. 87). It was also reported that the clinicians involved "did not appear to sacrifice objectivity in practicing compassionate care" (p. 87).

Many contemporary nurses carry out caring activities beyond the ordinary in the course of their nursing practice. Two examples cited in recent literature include: "Out of the Ordinary," which describes the ministry of a psych-mental health nurse who ministers "wherever the patient needs him" (Price, 2003, p. 60); and "Julie's Bath," a brief article that asserts that "performed with a dose of kindness, a humble nursing task becomes something out of the ordinary" (Jaramillo, 2004, p. 61).

The theme Beyond the Ordinary describes the dimension of nursing practice reported by Called to Serve study leaders that encompassed a variety of caring activities the nurses carried out above and beyond their usual role responsibilities. These actions were often done without charting, without reporting, sometimes without anyone other than a patient or family member, the nurse, and God even knowing of the act. Repeatedly in nurse leader–staff, nurse–patient, and nurse educator–student interactions reported by nursing leaders, caring ministries of serving were identified and described that touch the heart and the spirit with their mercy and compassion. These activities, while not specifically part of a nursing role, were like the poetic "random acts of kindness" that generous individuals do for others simply because a need for such generosity is recognized.

Beyond the Ordinary

> If we could continue to nurture people's spiritual reasons for going into nursing then we could really elevate the profession. I think nursing has always had a lot of respect because nurses were nurtured into that sort of spiritual role as nurses. But I hear some horror stories about nurses who are just not caring about their patients; they can have really bad attitudes. I think it is because they have not stopped to take inventory and try to figure out where they are spiritually in nursing. I think it is

nurses' responsibility to help each other with that, and I think if we could do that then it would be really positive in nurses facing their awareness of why they go into nursing. I know that people are not doing it for the money because nursing is not always pretty; it is not a pretty job when you are dealing with some serious illnesses. It is really easy to become disillusioned. I think the reason that some nurses become disillusioned is because they don't recognize that there is something there that needs to move them beyond the ordinary patient care. You don't do nursing for the paycheck. You really need that spiritual force inside you that moves you beyond ordinary patient care, beyond death. I think otherwise you can't do nursing. I know that if I didn't have that spiritual calling; this idea of calling to serve I wouldn't have been in the hospital 29 years. But I think I could do another 29 years because I have that (spiritual calling) within me; because of how I see nursing. (49, MSN, supervisor, critical care)

If I didn't see nursing as a vocational calling to serve, then I would just think of it as another job. Another day, another dollar. Not as a profession where I am giving something in which I don't expect anything in return. I think the more you get into nursing and you see it as something where you care, where you go beyond the ordinary care and not as just a job, it tends to make your days go better. (40, MSN, manager, public health)

I see nursing as a spiritual calling beyond just the day-to-day ordinary patient care. I think it is sad when I see a nurse and she is doing nursing and it is not her calling. I feel she can't enjoy it. He or she can't enjoy nursing and be as enriched from the profession as I have been…they don't reap the same rewards from serving as I do. (52, PhD, RN, educator, mental health)

I always try to tell a student that in that moment when they are upset about a patient or family situation (they have encountered), that is what excellence in nursing is. It is going beyond doing just what you have to do, but it is really caring for that person. The excellence in nursing comes, just like the excellence in teaching, in that relationship. When you can really connect with the person and their needs. Especially when you are connecting on a spiritual level, and patients are willing to share with you their concerns and you are willing to hear that and connect. (52, PhD, RN, educator, mental health)

I had to care for patients whose babies had died. And it was very difficult. It was probably the hardest thing I did because most of the time my job was happy (with new moms). But those were really hard times. I think you grieve with the family. I was like a grief counselor for those patients....And a lot of times if the mother didn't want to be with the baby (at the end), I would sit with the baby under the warmer until they breathed their last breath. I brought myself and my own spirituality into that nursing, not only in labor and delivery but in working with other patients and staff. I think patients can sense when you feel like you are doing something that's more than what's ordinarily expected; it's giving yourself, but it's bigger than yourself. I think you bring aspects of your own spirituality into your nursing every day. (51, BSN, team leader, medical-surgical)

Nurses go way beyond the ordinary role responsibilities when they see nursing as a vocation, as a calling to serve others. We had this one case, a gentleman who was here from the South for a job for a short time and ended up in a terrible industrial accident; he was burned pretty badly...he was so bad, we could not do too much for him. But a small core of us (nurses) became like his family. We got money together to get his family from Kentucky to come up. They lived here almost three months, and we all took turns helping them, and it was amazing to see the nurturing and the love; the family still write and keep in touch. (57, ADN, head nurse, medical-surgical)

Case Example: Being There to Serve

Seeing nursing as a vocation made joy and respect in caring for the individual paramount. It helped to bring to the front of my mind how indeed the power of using myself in serving others, in being there to serve, made the work that I do not only better but more joyful. In working with other human beings and seeing their worthiness, and literally seeing God in them, you can't help but expect from yourself the best job you could possibly do....A patient care interaction comes to mind, one where I was working with a student. The woman was unable to speak, and the student had turned on a radio station that frankly would not have been appropriate for the woman...So, I asked if I could help, and I took over the bath. I spoke to this woman each time I started washing a new part of her body. I talked to her, I rubbed her back, I used myself in many different ways....After we finished...the student...said to me "She can't hear you, you know." And I asked her "Are you sure?"...I said to the student that I would much rather err and have this patient not hear a word I said...than to ever find out a week later, or later on in my career, that that individual patient felt demeaned by the way I treated her by not ever really speaking or comforting her or allowing her to know that I was attending her while I bathed her. I like to think that the student learned from this experience. That she understood that you are always there for that patient, that respecting them for the many experiences that make up the human person. Even though you cannot share with them (verbally) at the time, you are, in a way, giving of yourself and making sure that no matter what, even if it was simply the sense of touch, that the way you touched them meant a great deal. (54, MSN, head nurse, critical care)

Embracing a Higher Purpose

"A Caring Vocation"

> *I lift my eyes to the hills; from where will my help come? My help comes from the Lord who made heaven and earth.*
>
> —Psalm 121:1–2

M. Patricia Donahue, in discussing the fact that nursing is both an art and a science, described the central core of nursing as "not merely a technique but a process that incorporates the elements of soul, mind, and imagination. It's very essence lies in the creative imagination, the sensitive spirit and the intelligent understanding that provide the very foundation for effective nursing care" (1996, p. ix).

The description of the servant leadership theme of Embracing a Higher Purpose suggests that servant leaders perceive something greater and more important and spiritual in the inherent nature of their profession. Nurses in practice, nurses in education, and nurses conducting research consistently embrace this higher purpose in order to develop and enhance the profession of nursing.

The understanding of nursing's higher purpose has been identified in the literature by describing nursing as "more than just a job" (Penney, 2000; Kiger, 1993, p. 309). This higher purpose is also explained in a 2006 editorial in the *Vermont Nurse Connection* entitled "Nurses as Advocates: A Higher Calling" (p. 3). Articles and books abound describing nursing as a spiritual vocation of service, a call to a higher ministry of service; many of these are cited in Chapter 1, "Called to Serve: The Nurse's Vocation of Caring." Nursing has been identified in one recent book, *A Sacred Covenant: The Spiritual Ministry of Nursing*, as encompassing a holy and blessed covenant in the bonding commonly known as the nurse–patient relationship (O'Brien, 2008b).

Many of the nursing leaders interviewed for the Called to Serve study perceived the overall profession of nursing as a spiritual calling to serve the sick and, from that posture, were able to envision unique and beneficial ways of carrying out a caring ministry to the ill. Nurses spoke about how their understanding of the nursing profession led them to view their ministry as having a "higher purpose," that is a spiritual calling to service. For some nurses the spiritual calling related to religious beliefs, such as those derived from the Judeo-Christian perspective; for others, the spiritual purpose was humanitarian based in one's belief in the equality of all members of the human family and the right of all to care and compassion when ill or infirm.

> I think (nursing) is a higher calling. I knew very early on what I wanted to do. I think you can do a whole lot of things in life where you never get that tingle or that satisfaction or that fulfillment. The higher purpose is ordained. It is something that you are called to do, and you know it when you are there; you embrace that higher purpose. I know because no matter how tired I get I am always refueled. When I'm there in the (hospital) setting, serving the patient, I am there for them more than 100%....I have to have down time when I go home. Then I say (to myself) "Did I do the best that I could do today?" (43, BSN, head nurse, school health)

> I have a certain pride in the fact that I do something (in nursing) that stands above what other people do. I could be working in a nursing home, working in the community, working anywhere, doing any kind of nursing, and I still think the

profession, the vocation, is elevated above other professions. I think, in a lot of ways, it is because people hold nurses to a higher standard, a higher purpose, that might be higher that what other roles demand of people. So you need to be a role model as a nurse. (49, MSN, supervisor, critical care)

Where you work and how people see the work that they do has a huge influence on how the nurses perceive their own personal practice. Where I work now....the culture is one where you support patients and you support one another. You are allowed to spend some time thinking beyond the day to day about what it is you are doing and why. I think that makes a difference. I think... you have time to reflect on your calling—a higher calling. I think reflection is an important piece of the whole process....why you do what you do, what it is that you do, how does your practice reflect who you are, those kinds of things. It is very good for nurses to actually think, spend some time thinking about "How do I make an effect every day? What do I leave behind?" (49, MSN, supervisor, critical care)

(Understanding nursing as a calling to serve) it forces me to be less abrupt, more gentle. When you have doctors shouting a million orders at you and patients calling, and you are hungry and you are thirsty and you are going on no sleep. From a physical sense, you know, remembering how that patient is suffering, you can fly into that room to do what you need to do. (You can stay with the patient) or you can fly out of there as fast as you can. But you know what the difference is between a nurse who is nurse who is just there to do a job and a nurse who truly believes in what she does, who sees nursing as a higher vocation. (26, BSN, charge nurse, pediatric clinic)

Nursing definitely is a spiritual vocation for me; we are called to a higher standard of caring, and I think it's been that way from the beginning when followers of Jesus cared for the sick in their communities. Then we think of Florence Nightingale and how she saw nursing as a calling to serve sick brothers and sisters, especially during her ministry in the Crimea. (69, PhD, RN, educator, adult health)

When I try to describe what comes to mind when thinking of nursing as a vocation or calling to serve the sick, what really comes to mind is the higher expectations. First of all, the fact that you are working with people, that every individual is unique and every (nursing) situation is just a little bit different, or perhaps very different from the one before. A profession as a vocation calls for caring, ingenuity, flexibility; words that I don't necessarily think can define a job…. I do believe that nursing goes beyond simply doing what is necessary to a higher level of doing what is necessary in a right manner, in a correct manner, and having it done well to the satisfaction of the patient with whom you are working. (54, MSN, head nurse, critical care)

I don't think people go into nursing for the money because they are not going to get rich or make a lot of money (in nursing). I think people do it for a higher reason. You know, to help people or to change people's perspectives about their illness or generally to have a positive impact on people who are sick. (51, BSN, team leader, medical-surgical)

I've worked as a nurse for 29 years in a variety of settings. I've been in many situations that I found personally to be somewhat difficult, frustrating, challenging, due to either the work situation or the challenges of the patients who I am caring for. I think by being able to look at nursing as a higher calling to serve, at times when I felt like I was hitting my head against a brick wall or really dealing with a frustrating situation, I feel that I was able to look beyond the problems and recognize that I needed to be patient. I needed to remain kind, to truly show the patients that I cared for them. (49, MSN, head nurse, school health)

I was planted where they grew nurses who were really about the ministry. And they did encourage that idea. In my role as a nursing administrator what we did during Nurse's Week, we did a blessing of the nurse's hands. It was really important; we ritualized it and the nurses came. Many nurses came. I thought it was important for nurses to see the spiritual side, the higher purpose of the work they do. For them to really feel like they were a part of the community of nurses who saw their role as ministry. One of the things I learned from the woman who was our vice president for mission effectiveness was that we need to ritualize some of the things we do in order for nurses to see our work in that sort of higher realm. It's more than that paycheck that I get at the end of the day....And nurses are realizing that they can have an impact on people's lives. (49, MSN, supervisor, critical care)

A Caring Vocation

In Chapter 1, "Called to Serve: The Nurse's Vocation of Caring," contemporary professional nursing is described as a caring vocation. While the perception of nursing as a "vocation" or "calling to serve" was somewhat downplayed in the scholarly literature of the 1960s, 1970s, and 1980s, which saw a heightened emphasis on nursing as a profession, the vocational aspect of nursing is currently being resurrected in a number of quarters. This is evidenced by the emergence of recent nursing literature exploring the understanding and operationalization of a nurse's vocation to serve, as identified in Chapter 1.

Nursing leaders in the Called to Serve study spoke eloquently of the importance of their profession of nursing as being a caring vocation of service:

It's the caring vocation part of nursing that makes nursing so special; so different from any other kind of work. It's not just a job that you do for money. Nursing is something you are called to do deep in your heart—to care for those who are weak and fragile and sick. It's not what you do; it's who you are. Nursing is a privilege and a blessing. The caring vocation is a privilege and a blessing. The vocation is a gift to all of us who are nurses. (69, PhD, RN, educator, adult health)

Viewing nursing, which is my career, as a caring vocation impacts my day-to-day practice whether I am on a nursing unit, role modeling for my students, or in the classroom trying to help them understand...they have a bigger impact on patients than just here and now....A nurse who cares can impact a group, a patient, or family member in such a way that experiences can stay with that person, that family unit, that group of individuals in the community for years to come....We needn't be limited by space and time but... when we care enough to really treat individuals with respect then it can make a great deal of difference in their lives...I try to help (students) see, in day-to-day practice, that they can be a special nurse for every single patient they care for....This is more than just a job....The (vocational) frame of reference shows a person utilizing themselves to honestly meet the needs of another in a loving and caring manner. (54, MSN, head nurse, critical care)

I think of the nursing vocation of caring in terms of the whole idea of selflessness and helping someone out. And it is for me this idea or this notion that I'm helping a patient and I am doing good for someone, and the benefit of doing those things is that there is good for me....And I think one of the things that keeps me in nursing is that I know I can make a differ- ence, and I learned...years ago...that no patient interaction is ever neutral. And although now I am not at the bedside (as an administrator) I know what I do has an impact on people's lives....Even if I didn't get paid for it, I would still want to do (nursing), just because I think it is more about my soul than it is about my body or making money. (49, MSN, supervisor, critical care)

Viewing nursing as a caring vocation is definitely a motiva- tion to keep going, not throw my hands up and walk out. It (nursing) is definitely trying at times, but the vocation is the motivating factor. It helps me deal with some of the harder things. I think it helps me be supportive and be aware of what patients' needs are. I feel like it is my job if they are in pain, address that pain immediately, make that my first priority.... That is just how I operate, but I think that subconsciously I am motivated by seeing nursing as a service calling. (33, BSN, team leader, medical-surgical)

You learn pretty fast how to be a devoted nurse and set your priorities. You always have to remember that it is the patient's presence...that is your immediate concern, and even if you are rushed to do many things, it is the suffering patient out there who really needs to be looked after. As a vocation it can be a test for each nurse to see if you could hang in there during your first few years....If you didn't have that caring vocation to serve, you wouldn't stick to that type of environment at all. (54, MSN, supervisor, medical outpatient clinic)

Seeing nursing as a vocation of caring supports my practice because it's not just a job. I mean if it was just a joyful job all the time, it would be easy to do, but there are a lot of times when I have had really difficult days, and I thought, "Why am I doing this again?" And I think that is because at the end of the day you know that you did something positive for somebody, that you had an impact, even if the patient had a negative outcome. You know that you made their last hour or two comfortable. So I think even when faced with difficult patient situations or staffing crises, that was what kept me in nursing — the good that I was able to do. Most of the time you don't get direct patient feedback, but it's the gratification that you get personally from what you are doing. It's really not for thanks that you are getting...it's gratification from doing something that you think is good and positive and caring for others. (51, BSN, team leader, medical-surgical)

I've always viewed nursing as a calling. I read nursing articles and nursing books. I like to read about history (of nursing) and lives of other nurses like Florence Nightingale who have made big contributions to nursing or medical fields to keep me in touch with the meaning of nursing as a caring vocation. I don't think that will change....I think nursing should always be a calling. It should be a profession where you care for people, but you don't only consider their medical needs, but also their spiritual and emotional needs. I believe that nursing always needs (to include) caring. (36, BSN, charge nurse, medical-surgical)

I know a lot of nurses that treat nursing as a vocation. For some newer nurses coming in I don't always see that calling, that service piece, and it could just be that they are new, and they are trying to get into the role, and when you are stressed and things are new, it's really hard to relax and see your true calling....I hope the calling doesn't ever die out when older nurses leave or retire. Hopefully, when they mentor some of the younger nurses, the baby nurses that we have, they can pass that on and lead by example. Then these younger nurses will develop their nursing role into a caring vocation-oriented professional. Hopefully. (45, MSN, team leader, medical-surgical/critical care)

I think with maturity, the longer I am in nursing, I value things more…I have so much more confidence in my abilities, obviously, and my judgment. Therefore it makes me secure in my decisions. It makes me confident that I can be a resource for younger nurses, be a mentor, a (role model)….Nursing is more than just a job, it is more than just a profession, you are dealing with people's lives. It is an emotional, caring field. (55, MSN, management, perinatology)

I never feel like nursing is a job that you can go to and come home and you are done. I remember people saying to me, who worked in the business field, "You go to work, you do your job, and you come home." I never felt like I left my work at work, and I still don't. I don't feel you ever just shut the door and go home….I don't think you forget about (patients) when you leave. I think you are touched by the people you deal with on a daily basis….I always think too, when you talk about a priest (or minister) having a calling to serve, I think nursing has the same calling. And I don't feel like it is a job…. I think you get some idea…that the calling you have…is not unlike being a religious person. (47, BSN, head nurse, obstetrics and gynecology)

Case Example: Embracing a Higher Purpose

I realize that seeing nursing as having a higher purpose can make a difference in patients' lives. One of the first areas I worked in, in nursing, was labor and delivery. And I realized not only did I help the women get through labor, but I also helped them with their parenting skills, how to bond with their babies, how to take care of their babies. This helped their self-esteem. It not only affected the woman, it affected the family unit. It affected the relationship with the child, so eventually it affected the entire family. So, I see that as very gratifying that I can have—that one person can have—that kind of impact on a family….to have a positive impact on the lives of others, that what you do every day can affect positive change in people or make their lives better.... Seeing your chosen career as a vocation with a higher purpose impacts practice because it's more than just the tasks you do; it is the value of actually caring for the person, to be there with them. Like for instance during a patient's labor, that's such a personal experience, and I tell the nurses to (be there) and..."Check, check, check" (on the mom). And actually take time to have empathy, you know, to really try to make the (laboring mom) comfortable or explain things to her family—to actually feel like you're part of the birth experience. You are not just an employee, you are part of the birth experience, and they (patient and family) welcome you, and it impacts the kind of care you deliver because you put in your own emotion. I think you have to care; it's caring. I can't imagine being a nurse and not being a caring person and really caring about your patients. I think it comes through if that's how you feel about nursing having a higher purpose; that's why you became a nurse. (51, BSN, team leader, obstetrics)

A MODEL OF SERVANT LEADERSHIP FOR NURSING

Following analyses of the phase 1 and phase 2 Called to Serve study data, a model of servant leadership for nursing was created. From initial analysis of the phase 1 study data five attitudinal themes emerged representing the nursing leaders' perceptions of and experiences in the lived experience of a nursing vocation of caring for the sick. These themes are:

1. A Blessed Calling, which describes the nurse leaders' understanding of their vocation as a spiritual calling to serve
2. Passionate Caring, a theme identifying the depth of feeling that nurse leaders possessed for their ministry to the sick
3. Ingrained in the Spirit, which demonstrated the nurse leaders' innate self-identification with professional nursing
4. The Extra Mile, an expression used by the study group of nurse leaders to describe their perceived degree of commitment to their vocation
5. A Privilege, which was a theme representative of the nurse leaders' appreciation of, and gratitude for, their vocation as nurses.

A subtheme that emerged from data analysis related to A Blessed Calling was that of A Christian Mandate. As the majority of nurse leader study participants were Christian, many described their calling as related to Christ's mandate to care for the sick; some nurses quoted scripture, especially Matthew 25:36, as the guiding principle for their nursing practice (details of the themes and subtheme are presented in Chapter 4).

The five key nursing vocation attitudinal themes are related as they describe five major facets of a professional nurse's practice:

1. The nurse's calling or attraction to the work (A Blessed Calling)
2. The nurse's emotional investment in the ministry of caregiving (Passionate Caring)
3. The nurse's personal sense of appropriateness of his or her vocational choice (Ingrained in the Spirit)
4. The nurse's depth of commitment to the work (The Extra Mile)
5. The nurse's gratitude for the vocation of nursing (A Privilege)

To summarize, during the initial data analysis, from which the above themes emerged, it was recognized that the nurse leaders almost universally, at some point during an interview, spoke of nursing as being a "service," a role in which the goal was "to serve" others and to embrace the concept of "servanthood." This emphasis on service directed the investigation to an exploration of the concept of "servant leadership" in nursing, the living out of which might, of course, be mediated by the nurse leaders' specific leadership role in an institution and by his or her length of time in nursing.

To describe the "lived experience" of servant leadership in nursing, a secondary analysis of the phase 1 study data and analysis of the phase 2 study data were carried out. The 9 key nursing servant leadership themes and 16 subthemes, which emerged from the secondary analysis, were found to be supported by contemporary servant leadership literature as discussed earlier in this chapter.

The 9 themes and 16 subthemes related to servant leadership identified from content analysis of data elicited from the study group of 75 nursing leaders included:

1. Listening with the Heart—The Sounds of Silence, the Mystery Behind the Visit
2. Giving of Yourself—Crossing Over, Compassionate Care
3. Doing Ministry—Making Connections, A Wounded Healer, A Sacred Trust
4. Assessing Needs—Being Grounded, Taking Time Out
5. Becoming an Advocate—To Protect and Defend
6. Discerning Decisions—Staying Focused

7. Making a Difference—Doing Your Best, Generating Excitement, A Nurturing Environment
8. Being There to Serve—Beyond the Ordinary
9. Embracing a Higher Purpose—A Caring Vocation

As with the 5 nursing vocation attitudinal themes, the 9 nursing servant leadership themes and 16 subthemes are related in that considered together they reflect a beautiful tapestry of nursing practice as carried out by one who is a true servant leader in the profession. Nurse servant leaders listen with their hearts both to the words and to the silence of those for whom they care. Nurse servant leaders attempt to cross over to truly understand the problems and concerns of their staff, patients, family members, or students. Nurse servant leaders give of themselves consistently in their compassionate caring for those they serve. Nurse servant leaders work to remain grounded so they can continually assess the needs of those for whom they care. Nurse servant leaders advocate for all those under their care. Nurse servant leaders perceive nursing as having a higher purpose and conceptualize how best that can be achieved in day-to-day practice. Nurse servant leaders remain alert to discern right decisions for those they serve. Nurse servant leaders accept the responsibility of serving those entrusted to their care. Nurse servant leaders continually strive to make a difference and to achieve positive outcomes for those under their care. Nurse servant leaders attempt to use their leadership positions to nurture the environment wherein they practice.

As Figure 5-1 demonstrates, a description of servant leadership in nursing involves a vocational perception of the profession as encompassing a strongly positive attitude toward one's calling, a passion for the ministry, a feeling of belonging in nursing, a desire to do more than required, and a deep gratitude for nursing as a personal life vocation. These attitudes direct the nurse to become a servant leader, a ministry which might, of course, be somewhat mediated by the nurse's leadership role and length of time in nursing. And, flowing from the attitudinal perception of nursing as a calling to serve, are the servant leadership characteristics, operationalized for nurses in terms of 9 nurse servant leadership themes and 16 subthemes reflecting heartfelt caring, understanding of others' problems and needs, giving of oneself in nursing ministry, accepting responsibility for the good of those under one's care, being a servant of others, and doing one's best to achieve a positive outcome for all of those for whom the nurse servant leader is responsible.

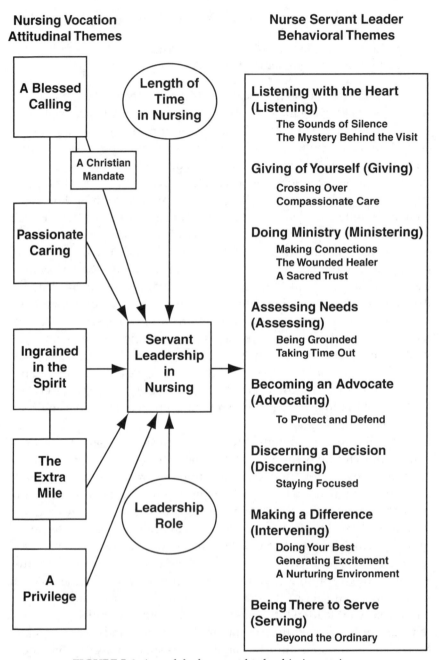

FIGURE 5-1 A model of servant leadership in nursing.

REFERENCES

Alexander, M. (2007). Infusion nurses: Making a difference. *Journal of Infusion Nursing, 30*(2), 73–74.

Alligood, M. R. (1992). Empathy: The importance of recognizing two types. *Journal of Psychosocial Nursing and Mental Health Services, 30*(3), 14, 33–34.

Apker, J., Zabava-Ford, W. S., & Fox, D. H. (2003). Predicting nurses' organizational and professional identification. *Nursing Economic$, 21*(5), 226–232.

Arif, Z. (2006). Who has time for a break? *Nursing Standard, 21*(2), 26–27.

Baillie, L. (1995). Empathy in the nurse-patient relationship. *Nursing Standard, 9*(20), 29–32.

Baldwin, M. A. (2003). Patient advocacy: A concept analysis. *Nursing Standard, 17*(21), 33–39.

Ball, S. C. (2006). Nurse-patient advocacy and the right to die. *Journal of Psychosocial Nursing and Mental Health Services, 44*(12), 36–42.

Barrere, C. C. (2007). Discourse analysis of nurse-patient communication in a hospital setting: Implications for staff development. *Journal for Nurses in Staff Development, 23*(3), 114–122.

Bentley, R., & Ellison, K. J. (2005). Impact of a service-learning project on nursing students. *Nursing Education Perspectives, 26*(5), 287–290.

Biley, F. C. and Chiocchi, N. M. (2007). Nursing: A sacred healing dance. *Reflections On Nursing Leadership, 33*(3), 2–6.

Blachowicz, E., & Letizia, M. (2006). The challenges of shift work (Best Practice). *MEDSURG Nursing, 15*(5), 274–280.

Britto, M. T., Kotagal, U. R., & Boat, T. M. (2005). Listening to families: First steps toward improved hospital care. *Archives of Pediatric and Adolescent Medicine, 15*(2), 187–188.

Brockopp, E., Schooler, M., Welsh, D., Cassidy, K., Ryan, P., Mueggenberg, K., et al. (2003). Sponsored professional seminars: Enhancing professionalism among baccalaureate nursing students. *Journal of Nursing Education, 42*(12), 562–564.

Bu, X., & Jezewski, M. A. (2007). Developing a mid-range theory of patient advocacy through concept analysis. *Journal of Advanced Nursing, 57*(1), 101–110.

Bulley, M. (2001). Listen, share then lead. *Nursing Standard, 15*(39), 24.

Campinha-Bacote, J., Yahle, T., & Langenkamp, M. (1996). The challenge of cultural diversity for nurse educators. *Journal of Continuing Education in Nursing, 27*(2), 59–64.

Carlin, C. (1999). Hospice nursing: More than a job. *Caring, 18*(1), 8–9.

Carson, V. B. (1989). Spirituality and the nursing process. In V. B. Carson (Ed.), *Spiritual dimensions of nursing practice* (pp. 150–179). Philadelphia: W.B. Saunders.

Caserta, J. E. (1989). Listening to families. *Home Healthcare Nurse, 7*(6), 3.

Chang, P., Chou, Y., & Cheng, F. (2006). Designing career development programs through understanding of nurses' career needs. *Journal for Nurses in Staff Development, 22*(5), 246–253.

Claflin, N. (2005). Continuing education needs assessment of acute care and long-term care nurses in a Veterans Affairs Medical Center. *Journal of Continuing Education in Nursing, 36*(6), 263–270.

Corley, M. C. (2002). Nurse moral distress: A proposed theory and research agenda. *Nursing Ethics, 9*(6), 636–650.

Cowling, W. R. (2006). Healing as appreciating wholeness. In W. K. Cody (Ed.), *Philosophical and Theoretical Perspectives for Advanced Nursing Practice* (pp. 155–169). Sudbury, MA: Jones & Bartlett.

Dagenais, F., & Meleis, A. I. (1982). Professionalism, work ethic and empathy in nursing: The nurse self-description form. *Western Journal of Nursing Research, 4*(4), 407–422.

Damrosch, S. P., Sullivan, P. A., & Haldeman, L. L. (1987). How nurses get their way: Power strategies in nursing. *Journal of Professional Nursing, 3*(5), 284–290.

Daumer, R. D., & Britson, V. (2004). Wired for success: Stimulating excitement in nursing through a summer camp. *Journal of Nursing Education, 43*(3), 130–133.

Davidhizar, R., & Giger, J. N. (1994). When your patient is silent. *Journal of Advanced Nursing, 20*(1), 703–706.

Davidhizar, R., & Shearer, R. (2002). Taking charge by 'letting go'. *Health Care Manager, 20*(3), 33–38.

Davidson, J. E. (2006). Foreward: Preparation of a new intensive care unit nurse: Is there a best practice? *Critical Care Nursing Quarterly, 29*(3), 179–181.

Davis, C. M. (2003). Empathy and transcendence. *Topics in Geriatric Rehabilitation, 19*(4), 265–274.

Decker, S. A., & Blecke, J. (1999). Environmental complexity and aesthetics: Developing integrated awareness in nursing students. *Complexity and Chaos in Nursing, 4*(1), 27–34.

Donahue, M. P. (1996). *Nursing, the finest art* (2nd ed.). St. Louis, MO: Mosby.

Donnelly, G., Leurer, M. D., & Domm, L. (2006). Making a difference: A story from the research revealing the voices of experience: Insights from registered nurses. *SRNA News Bulletin, 8*(4), 4.

Downey, M. (1993). Compassion. In M. Downey (Ed.), *The new dictionary of Catholic spirituality*. Collegeville, MN: Liturgical Press.

Duffin, C. (2007). Pick your own path. *Nursing Standard, 21*(22), 22–23.

Edwards, C. (2002). A proposal that patients be considered honorary members of the healthcare team. *Journal of Clinical Nursing, 11*(3), 340–348.

Felgen, J. (2004). A caring and healing environment. *Nursing Administration Quarterly, 28*(4), 288–301.

Fry, S. T. (1997). Protecting patients from incompetent or unethical colleagues: An important dimension of the nurse's advocacy role. *Journal of Nursing Law,* 4(4), 15–22.

Gerber, L. (2007). The sacred path. *Nursing 2007, 37*(5), 43.

Graber, D. R., & Mitcham, M. D. (2004). Compassionate clinicians: Take patient care beyond the ordinary. *Holistic Nursing Practice: The Science of Health and Healing, 18*(2), 87–94.

Gray, A. (2002). Taking time out. *Nursing Standard, 16*(34), 14–15.

Gray, A. (2005). A private matter. *Nursing Standard, 19*(39), 31.

Greiner, P. A. (1989). The idea of empathy in nursing: A conceptual analysis. Unpublished doctoral dissertation. University of Pennsylvania School of Nursing.

Haggard, A. (2007). Administration. *Journal for Nurses in Staff Development, 23*(4), 193–194.

Hagerty, B. M., & Patusky, K. L. (2003). Reconceptualizing the nurse-patient relationship. *Journal of Nursing Scholarship, 35*(2), 145–150.

Hall, J. (1996). Challenges to caring: Nurses as wounded healers....part A. *Australian Journal of Holistic Nursing, 3*(2), 12–18.

Harrison, E., & Falco, S. M. (2005). Health disparity and the nurse advocate: Reaching out to alleviate suffering. *Advances in Nursing Science, 28*(3), 252–264.

Hawley, M. P., & Jensen, L. (2007). Making a difference in critical care nursing practice. *Qualitative Health Research, 17*(5), 663–674.

Hellwig, S. D., Yam, M., & DiGiulio, M. (2003). Nurse case managers' perceptions of advocacy: A phenomenological analysis. *Lippincott's Case Management: Managing the Process of Patient Care, 8*(2), 53–63.

Hemsley, M., & Glass, N. (2006). Sacred journeys of nurse healers. *Journal of Holistic Nursing, 24*(4), 256–268.

Hertz, J. E., Koren, M. E., Rossetti, J., Munroe, D. J., Berent, G., & Plonczynski, D. J. (2005). Collaboration to promote best practices in the care of older adults. *MEDSURG Nursing, 14*(5), 311–315.

Hostutler, J. J., Taft, S. H., & Snyder, C. (1999). Patient needs in the emergency department: Nurses and patients perceptions. *Journal of Nursing Administration, 29*(1), 43–50.

Hunt, B. (2007). Managing equality and cultural diversity in the health workforce. *Journal of Clinical Nursing, 12*(12), 2252–2259.

Irvine, K. N. (2004). *Work breaks and well-being: The effect of nature on hospital nurses.* PhD dissertation, University of Michigan.

Jackson, C. B. (2003). *Medical-surgical nurses self-perceptions as healers.* Unpublished doctoral dissertation, Union Institute and University, Cincinnati, OH.

Jaramillo, D. M. (2004). Julie's bath. *Nursing 2004, 34*(10), 61.

Jeffers, B. R., & Campbell, S. L. (2005). Preparing to care for older adults: Engaging college constituents. *Journal of Nursing Education, 44*(6), 280–282.

Jensen, L. E. (2004). Mental health care experiences: Listening to families. *Journal of the American Psychiatric Nurses Association, 10*(1), 33–41.

Kiger, A. M. (1993). Accord and discord in students images of nursing. *Journal of Nursing Education, 32*(7), 309–317.

Kleiman, S. (2007). Revitalizing the humanistic imperative in nursing education. *Nursing Education Perspectives, 28*(4), 209–213.

Kramer, M., Maguire, P., Schmalenberg, C., Brewer, B., Burke, R., Chmielewski, L., et al. (2007). Nurse manager support: What is it? Structures and practices that promote it. *Nursing Administration Quarterly, 31*(4), 325–340.

Laskowski, C., & Pellicore, K. (2002). The wounded healer archetype: Applications to palliative care. *American Journal of Hospice and Palliative Care, 19*(6), 403–407.

Legge, L. (1995). Renaissance nurse: Naida Colby suggests return to natural, spiritual healing. *Minnesota Nursing Accent, 67*(4), 3–4.

Lomax, B. (1997). Learning to understand a patient's silence. *Nursing Times, 93*(17), 48–49.

Lorenz, S. G. (2007). Protection: Clarifying the concept for use in nursing practice. *Holistic Nursing Practice: The Science of Health and Healing, 21*(3), 115–123.

Mallik, M. (1997). Advocacy in nursing-a review of the literature. *Journal of Advanced Nursing, 25*(1), 130–138.

Manojlovich, M. (2005). Promoting nurses' self-efficacy: A leadership strategy to improve practice. *Journal of Nursing Administration, 35*(5), 271–278.

Mansfield, R., & Meyer, C. L. (2007). Educational Innovation. Making a difference with combined community assessment and change projects. *Journal of Nursing Education, 46*(3), 132–134.

Marelli, T. (2006). Nursing in flux: Are you ready to meet the challenge of the future? *American Journal of Nursing, 106*(Suppl. 1), 19–25.

Martin, G. (1998). Ritual action and its effect on the role of the nurse as advocate. *Journal of Advanced Nursing, 27*(1), 189–194.

Mathias, J. M. (2004). Listening to staff key for hospitals on Fortune's top list of employers. *Operating Room Manager, 20*(3), 1, 10–11.

MacDonald, J. (2007). Reflections of a nurse healer (Foreword). In J. E. Koerner. *Healing presence: The essence of nursing* (pp. xvii–xix). New York: Springer.

McElmurry, B. J., Gi Park, C., & Buseh, A. G. (2003). The nurse-community health advocate team for urban immigrant primary health care. *Journal of Nursing Scholarship, 35*(3), 275–281.

McGeehan, R. (2007). Best practice in record-keeping. *Nursing Standard, 21*(17), 51–55.

McGilton, K., Robinson, H. I., & Boscart, V. (2006). Communication enhancement: Nurse and patient satisfaction outcomes in a complex continuing care facility. *Journal of Advanced Nursing, 54*(1), 35–44.

McGonigle, T. D. (1993). Ministry, ministerial spirituality. In M. Downey (Ed.), *The new dictionary of Catholic spirituality* (pp. 658–659). Collegeville, MN: Liturgical Press.

McQueen, K., & Dennis, C. L. (2007). Development of a postpartum depression best practice guideline: A review of the systematic process. *Journal of Nursing Care Quality, 22*(3), 199–204.

Melby, V., & Ryan, A. (2005). Caring for older people in prehospital emergency care: Can nurses make a difference? *Journal of Clinical Nursing, 14*(9), 1141–1150.

Melland, H. I., & Volden, C. M. (2001). A nurturing learning environment: On or off-line. *Nursing Forum, 36*(2), 23–28.

Millard, L., Hallett, C., & Luker, K. (2006). Nurse-patient interaction and decision-making in care: Patient involvement in community nursing. *Journal of Advanced Nursing, 55*(2), 142–150.

Mills, D. S., & Pennoni, M. (1986). A nurturing work environment: in philosophy and practice. *Cancer Nursing, 9*(3), 117–123.

Milne, D. (2004). The power of persuasion. *Professional Nurse, 20*(2), 54–55.

Moore, S. C., & Hutchison, S. A. (2007). Developing leaders at every level: Accountability and empowerment actualized through shared governance. *Journal of Nursing Administration, 37*(12), 564–568.

Neill, M., Hayward, K. S., & Peterson, T. (2007). Students' perceptions of the interprofessional team in practice through the application of servant leadership principles. *Journal of Interprofessional Care, 21*(4), 425–432.

Norton, L. (1998). Health promotion and health education: What role should the nurse adopt in practice? *Journal of Advanced Nursing, 28*(6), 1269–1275.

Nouwen, H. J. M. (1979). *The wounded healer: Ministry in contemporary society.* Garden City, NY: Image Books.

Nurses as advocates: A higher calling. (2006). *Vermont Nurse Connection, 9*(1), 3.

Nursing is the most emotionally rewarding career. (2005). *Nursing Standard, 19*(30), 22–28.

Nussbaum, G. (2003). Spirituality in critical care: Patient comfort and satisfaction. *Critical Care Nursing Quarterly, 26*(3), 214–220.

O'Brien, M. E. (2001). *The nurse's calling: A Christian spirituality of caring for the sick.* Mahwah, NJ: Paulist Press.

O'Brien, M. E. (2003). Navy nurse: A call to lay down my life. *Journal of Christian Nursing, 20*(4), 32–33.

O'Brien, M. E. (2008a). *Spirituality in nursing: Standing on holy ground.* Sudbury, MA: Jones and Bartlett.

O'Brien, M. E. (2008b). *A sacred covenant: The spiritual ministry of nursing*. Sudbury, MA: Jones and Bartlett.

Oliver, S. (2007). Best practice in the treatment of patients with rheumatoid arthritis. *Nursing Standard, 121*(42), 47–56.

O'Meara, T. F. (1990). Ministry. In J. A. Komonchak, M. Collins, & D. A. Lane (Eds.), *The new dictionary of theology* (pp. 657–661). Collegeville, MN: Liturgical Press.

Parachin, V. M. (2003). The power of compassionate touch. *Journal of Christian Nursing, 20*(2), 8–9.

Pask, E. J. (2005). Self-sacrifice, self-transcendence and nurses' professional self. *Nursing Philosophy, 6*(4), 247–254.

Penney, W. (2000). The story of fable: Connecting with the real world of being a registered nurse. *Australian Journal of Holistic Nursing, 7*(2), 12–19.

Perry, T. R. (2002). *The certified registered nurse anesthetist: Occupational responsibilities, perceived stressors, coping strategies and work relationships.* Unpublished doctoral dissertation. Virginia Polytechnic Institute and State University.

Premoe, M. L. (1995). Nurses make a difference! Two patients: two stories… caring nurses make the difference. *Michigan Nurse, 68*(8), 4.

Price, D. H. (2003). Out of the ordinary. *Nursing Standard, 17*(32), 60.

Ramos, M. C. N. (1990). *Empathy within the nurse-patient relationship.* Unpublished doctoral dissertation. University of Virginia.

Rankin, W. W. (1988). Listening with the heart. *Journal of Pediatric Nursing, 3*(2), 127–129.

Rashid, M. (2007). Developing scales to evaluate staff perception of the effects of physical environment on patient comfort, patient safety, patient privacy, family integration with patient care, and staff working conditions in adult intensive care units: A pilot study. *Critical Care Nursing Quarterly, 30*(3), 271–283.

Reid, K. (2006). Sacred moments: The human-to-human encounter between palliative care nurses and people who are dying. *International Journal of Human Caring, 10*(2), 55.

Rew, L., Becker, H., Cookston, J., Khosropour, S., & Martinez, S. (2003). Measuring cultural awareness in nursing students. *Journal of Nursing Education, 42*(6), 249–257.

Riffel, K., Peterson, J. A., & Insley, C. (2004). Nurturing the nursing spirit. *Journal of Christian Nursing, 21*(3), 39–41.

Rigolosi, E. L. (2005). *Management and leadership in nursing and health care: An experimental approach* (2nd ed.). New York: Springer.

Rossetti, J., Fox, P. J., & Burns, K. (2005). Advocating for the rights of the mentally ill: A global issue. *International Journal of Psychiatric Nursing Research, 11*(1), 1211–1217.

Russell, R. F., & Stone, A. G. (2002). A review of servant leadership attributes: Development of a practical model. *Leadership and Organization Development Journal, 23*(3), 145–157.

Ryan, K. (2007). The role of the nurse as advocate in ethically difficult care situations with dying patients. *Nevada RNformation, February/March,* 22.

Sadovich, J. M. (2005). Work excitement in nursing: An examination of the relationship between work excitement and burnout. *Nursing Economics, 23*(2), 91–96.

Sanghavi, D. M. (2006). What makes for a compassionate patient-caregiver relationship? *Joint Commission Journal on Quality and Patient Safety, 32*(5), 283–292.

Schantz, M. L. (2007). Compassion: A concept analysis. *Nursing Forum, 42*(2), 48–55.

Schreiter, R. J. (1993). Trust. In M. Downey (Ed.), *The new dictionary of Catholic spirituality* (pp. 982–983). Collegeville, MN: Liturgical Press.

Sherrod, D. (2006). Accept the challenge: Focus on Nursing. *Tar Heel Nurse, 68*(1), 3.

Sienkiewicz, J., Wilkinson, G., & Emr, K. D. (2008). The quest for best practice in caring for the home care patient with an indwelling urinary catheter: The New Jersey experience. *Home Healthcare Nurse: The Journal for the Home Care and Hospice Professional, 26*(2), 121–128.

Simms, L. M., Erbin-Roesemann, M., Darga, A., & Coeling, H. (1990). Breaking the burnout barrier: Resurrecting work excitement in nursing…practice excitement project (PEP). *Nursing Economics, 8*(3), 177–187.

Smith-Stoner, M. (2004). Home care nurses' perceptions of agency and supervisory characteristics: Working in the rain. *Home Healthcare Nurse: The Journal for the Home Care and Hospice Professional, 22*(8), 536–546.

Spears, L. C. (2004). Prescription for organizational health: Servant leadership. *Reflections on Nursing Leadership, 30*(4), 24–26.

Sulzbach-Hoke, L. (1996). Risk taking by health care workers. *Clinical Nurse Specialist: A Journal for Advanced Nursing Practice, 10*(1), 30–37.

Sutherland, J. A. (1993). The nature and evolution of phenomenological empathy in nursing: An historical treatment. *Archives of Psychiatric Nursing, 7*(6), 369–376.

Thornby, D. (2006). Beginning the journey to skilled communication. *AACN Advanced Critical Care, 17*(3), 266–271.

Thornton, L. (2005). The model of whole-person caring: Creating and sustaining a healing environment. *Holistic Nursing Practice, The Science of Health and Healing, 19*(3), 106–115.

Trimm, D. (2003). A listening heart. *Journal of Christian Nursing, 20*(4), 18–19.

Tripp-Reimer, T. (1994). Crossing over the boundaries. *Critical Care Nurse, 14*(3), 134–141.

Turkel, M. C., & Ray, M. A. (2004). Creating a caring practice environment through self-renewal. *Nursing Administration Quarterly, 28*(4), 249–254.

Turnbull, H. R. (2005). What should we do for Jay? The edges of life and cognitive disability. *Journal of Religion, Disability and Health, 9*(2), 1–25.

Watson, J. (2000). Leading via caring-healing: The fourfold way toward transformative leadership. *Nursing Administration Quarterly, 25*(1), 1–6.

Watts, S. (2007). Taking a break. *Practice Nurse, 34*(3), 34, 36–37.

Webb, C., & Hope, K. (1995). What kind of nurses do patients want? *Journal of Clinical Nursing, 4*(2), 101–108.

Whiteside, C. L. (2004). *The sources and forms of power used by Florence Nightingale as depicted in her letters written July 1, 1853 to August 7, 1856.* Unpublished doctoral dissertation, Gonzaga University, Spokane, WA.

Widerquist, J., & Davidhizar, R. (1994). The ministry of nursing. *Journal of Advanced Nursing, 19*(4), 647–652.

Wilson, E. M. (1996). The mobile emergency department: One nurse's foresight into the future. *Journal of Emergency Nursing, 22*(2), 138–139.

Wolf, Z. R. (1986). Nurses' work: The sacred and the profane. *Holistic Nursing Practice, 1*(1), 29–35.

Wright, S. G. (1995). The competence to touch: Helping and healing in nursing practice. *Complimentary Therapies in Medicine, 3*(1), 49–52.

Yegdich, T. (1999). On the phenomenology of empathy in nursing: Empathy or sympathy? *Journal of Advanced Nursing, 30*(1), 83–93.

Youll, J. W. (1989). The bridge beyond: Strengthening nursing practice in attitudes towards death, dying and the terminally ill, and helping spouses of critically ill patients. *Intensive Care Nursing. 5*(2), 88–94.

6 Servant Leadership in Contemporary Nursing

Serve the Lord with all your heart.

—1 Samuel 12:20

In my role as a nursing leader it is vital to support an environment of serving and healing...I have to give of myself, creating an environment of healing, just like listening and having empathy – all this promotes healing. It is vital that everyone who walks into my office or walks into this hospital sees that here is an atmosphere of serving, of caring, of healing....You cannot be aloof of your surroundings or what is going on. You have to be in tune with needs of the contemporary environment...you have to make yourself available. Nursing is caring with my whole heart and putting my best into it....It could be in terms of defending others, protecting others, serving others. It is the role of a nurse to serve those who cannot take care of themselves.

—Cindy, nurse administrator critical care units

When I first encountered the concept of servant leadership some years ago, I was immediately struck by its appropriateness for nursing leaders. Robert Greenleaf's (1977) understanding of the fact that in order to be a good leader one must first be a servant of those he or she seeks to lead supports the heart of leadership in nursing. As reflected in Chapter 2 of this book, "The Spiritual Heritage of Servant Leadership in Nursing," nurses have a long and honored tradition of service for the patients, family members, and staff with whose care they have been charged. From their initial vocational inspiration to minister to the sick or the disabled, to the most fragile members of our society, nurses are directed to become the servants of those for whom they care. Just as Jesus taught that he had come "not to be served but to serve," so nurses are called not to be served but to serve others—those to whom they have dedicated their lives and their ministry of caring.

219

Before exploring the unique servant leadership roles of a variety of levels of nursing leadership, it is appropriate to identify who exactly might be considered a "nursing leader" in contemporary society. Nursing leadership is described as referring to "the ability to guide, motivate, and inspire, and to instill vision and purpose" (Ellis & Hartley, 2008, p. 471). "To provide leadership," Ellis and Hartley add, one must "be able to influence beliefs, opinions, or behaviors of others and to persuade others to follow your direction" (p. 471). Nursing claims many distinguished leaders according to Valiga and Grossman (2007, p. 7). Some of the most famous include Florence Nightingale; Lillian Wald; nurse theorists Dorothea Orem, Imogene King, and Martha Rogers; and a variety of other well-known scholars in nursing education, practice, and research (pp. 7–8). Each nurse, however, has the potential to be a leader if he or she has a "vision," is "passionate about realizing it," and "invests energy" to accomplish the vision (Valiga & Grossman, 2007, p. 8).

Based on the above criteria, nurses ministering in a variety of healthcare settings can be considered nursing leaders. Although their names may be recognized only by a relatively small cadre of individuals whom they serve directly, their nursing is conducted with vision, passion, and energy, and with the ability to influence the beliefs and behaviors of others. In accessing participants for the Called to Serve nursing study of servant leadership introduced in Chapters 4 and 5, nurse leaders were found in such settings as hospitals, clinics, long-term care facilities, home health agencies, parishes, schools, colleges, and universities. The nursing servant leaders in the study carried the titles of nurse administrator, nurse manager, nursing supervisor, nurse clinician (head nurse, charge nurse, team leader), advanced practice nurse (clinical specialist, nurse–midwife, nurse practitioner, and nurse anesthetist), parish nurse, nurse educator, and nurse researcher.

THE NURSE ADMINISTRATOR AS SERVANT LEADER

Nursing administrators may be found in myriad contemporary healthcare and health education settings. Some administrative roles of today's nursing leaders include CEOs (chief executive officers) and COOs (chief operating officers) in hospitals and long-term care facilities, clinic administrators, directors of home health agencies, and deans or vice-presidents of nursing in colleges and universities. Obviously, the scope of responsibilities that a nurse administrator is called upon to assume varies depending upon the organizational goals, operating structure, and size of a healthcare or health education facility. Nevertheless, the philosophy and behavioral character-istics of servant leadership are both appropriate and desirable and may be found operative in many nursing administrators.

One overall approach for nurse administrators to promote staff morale is use of concepts from the Bowen's Family Systems Theory; especially useful is the concept of differentiation of self, which may help individual staff members to establish their place in the setting and thus reduce anxiety (Glasscock & Hales, 1998, pp. 37–38). This is congruent with the behavioral characteristics of servant leadership that reflect the leader's commitment to the well-being of those under his or her care.

Also noted as critical elements of administrative leadership are the establishment of trust: "The nurse administrator who earns the trust of the staff can create the high-performance synergy required for excel-lence in today's healthcare setting" (Newhouse & Mills, 2002, p. 67). Job satisfaction among staff can be achieved by "a structure that meets the needs for professional practice" (Cumbey & Alexander, 1998, p. 45). These concepts are also consistent with the nursing servant leadership characteristics of Listening with the Heart as well as Advocating for and Nurturing those one serves.

The comments of nurse administrators who participated in the Called to Serve study reflected a variety of nursing servant leadership themes such as Being There to Serve, Listening with the Heart (the Mystery Behind the Visit), Assessing Needs, Becoming an Advocate, Generating Excitement, Staying Focused, and perceiving nursing as A Caring Vocation.

Megan, a 50-year-old master's-prepared, vice-president for nursing, shared the following comments:

> I've always thought of the role of service, or the role of servant leader, as one where my responsibility really lies in supporting those people (staff) who support the patients. As a chief nurs-ing officer I am really cognizant of what I do every day to sup-port patient care. Whether it is budgeting, fighting for an issue of human resources, working on overtime so that each of the units has a supportive nursing director....I learned to listen to people and what their concerns were; that was early on in my role as chief nursing officer....One of my very first experiences was to really listen and hear what was going on with staff. The other part of my role was to try and identify whether or not a person who was in a role was happy, confident that they could do the job and whether they would be successful if I kept them on as a nursing director....I think I needed to read between the

lines....As a servant leader you learn lessons. You try and want to support people, you want to be empathic, and you need to do it in a way that does not negatively impact others.

Megan added:

Being committed to your staff is primary, because if you don't come to work energized and happy then it creates difficulty for many people. It has a ripple effect. You really want to try as a nursing leader to do what you can to put patients first and then nurses....We as servant leaders can make sure that the middle management group are well cared for, that we are not pulling them in a lot of different directions.

Megan concluded:

The nursing management job is one of the most difficult jobs in the organization. Being committed to your employees is treating them fairly, making sure they are not overworked...to find ways to give them time to renew themselves. It is important for me to give them time off when they went above and beyond.

Joanne, a 51-year-old master's-prepared nursing director in a large healthcare system, related her perception of nursing as A Caring Vocation of service and advocacy:

I became a nurse because I felt I had an inner need to help people. I felt that I not only wanted to serve patients but my colleagues and the community at large. I got my master's degree and proceeded up the corporate ladder, so to speak, and felt that I acted not only as a liaison for management but also as a leader, as an advocate, for my employees. I took the information I learned as a staff nurse and kind of superimposed the leadership responsibilities on top of that....I think that is how I came to my leadership style.

Joanne also spoke of the importance of Listening with the Heart "to what people are saying but also what they are not saying":

One of the things I was taught as a nurse practitioner was that being able to listen and hear what the person is saying is probably more important than any kind of clinical skills you can obtain.... There can be issues with patients and with staff; sometimes the important thing is just to listen. People just want to be heard, to have you listen to them and to try to understand what they are going through....I have gotten letters of praise from patients, not so much for what I did, because sometimes there was very little I could do for them, but just for listening and caring.

Joanne explained her manner of Being There to Serve her staff:

When I need somebody to do something, it is really never an issue because I'm always willing to do it myself, and they know that. I am not concerned about getting my hands dirty or doing something below my level. If files need to be refiled, I file them; I do Xeroxing.

Joanne also spoke of nursing as A Caring Vocation:

I can't imagine how someone can do nursing and not care. If you don't care for people how can you possible clean them up? How can you deal with some of the things we have to do as nurses?...From a leadership point of view, if you don't care for the people who work for you, you probably need to be in another job. Leaders need to be committed to their staff. They need to trust them, listen to them, and need to help them be the best they can be. I really think that caring is the core to everything we do (in nursing) today.

Sue, a 36-year-old, baccalaureate-prepared assistant department head in a hospital setting, spoke of the importance of commitment and providing Compassionate Care for patients and staff:

As a nurse, my passion for everything I do for my patients, my staff, and my (patients') families is out of compassion for taking care of others....A good nursing leader looks out for him or herself and staff members — commitment to make things better in the community and the (healthcare) facility, in the nursing unit, and with your staff. I think that is important, because if you have commitment to and from your staff members it is going to show in patient care. The patients are going to know that your staff are committed to taking care of them and giving them the best healthcare possible.

And Cindy, a 39-year-old, baccalaureate-prepared administrator of the a hospital's critical care units, spoke of how listening to staff and patients can support the development of a Nurturing Environment in the healthcare facility:

> To be a nurse in a leadership role, it is imperative that you are a good listener.….listening to what is being said and…to what is not being said. I find that as a good nursing leader you have to have that skill. People can tell whether you are listening or not. The way you respond to what was said or not said will tell how much of what was said you heard. So to be a nurse leader you have to listen. You cannot get away from it!

Finally, Caitlin, a 48-year-old director of a hospital-based palliative care unit, described the Ministry of a nurse servant leader:

> I think that a core component of nursing is truly be a servant, being for the other and truly having a disposition of heart that avails oneself to care for the other in the manner that you would want to be cared for. The image that I think of, I have also pondered in my role as a nurse is that of Jesus washing the feet of the disciples. It is a posture that is one of being there present, accompanying, caring, and attentive to the needs of the patient and or their families. Often in caring for the dying I have truly said in my own prayer in asking God to give me the strength to continue to be his instrument. I ask God to help me to strive to understand versus being understood. I think that is what a servant does. A servant in the strength of that role is not a demeaning role but a very active, engaged, truly powerful posture. I think it is really primary to every thing that we do as a nurse and everything that we are as nurse.

Caitlin next explained the importance of Listening with the Heart:

> I go back to the work or the ministry that I have been privileged to be a part of as far as accompanying those at the end of life and often newly diagnosed with advanced illness. Listening is, on any given day, sometimes 95% of what I do. I've learned over the years that listening, if passive, really I'm not listening, but an active listening…is really hard work. It calls forth from me a disposition or a posture of truly trying to hear at times what is not being said. For example, I remember caring for a patient who truly was demonstrating signs of actively dying. When I went in to visit with her, I said to

her "Are you in pain?" She said, "No." I said, "You appear uncomfortable." She said, "I am." I said, "What is the source of your greatest pain or greatest discomfort?" I thought at that point because she had cancer with bone metastasis, that she was going to say something about her back pain or something physiologically, instead she said, "My son is (far away), and I really don't think I am going to get to see him before I die." I was really struck by that response, because number one, it called forth from a need to deepen the conversation with this patient, but also to be sensitive to the fact that pain is often not simply physical, it can be emotional, mental, spiritual, sometimes far more difficult for a patient. But also perhaps if I hadn't been listening inventively, I wouldn't have pursued asking or reflecting back to her what I was seeing. The fact that I perceived that she was uncomfortable, and then I rephrased the question, caused her to be able to respond in truth to what she was going through. The other thing that I think about in nursing with listening is sometimes in our present healthcare system, we seem, myself included, to be so caught up with tasks that we lose sight of really being present. I think when we are present with another person that is when the greatest active listening takes place.

The nursing servant leadership theme of Crossing Over to try and understand a patient's suffering was also highlighted in Caitlin's perception of nursing leadership:

I try as best as I can to walk in the other's shoes. Enter into their space, their world, their mind as an invited guest; to enter as best as I possibly can to try to imagine what their life at that point in time must be like. I think certain rephrasing has helped me as a nurse when sitting at the bedside of someone who has an advanced illness when empathy I think has become the most well demonstrated. I can say back to the patient, "Help me to understand, help to know, what matters most to you, what are you most afraid of." To ask questions that draw them, to share with me what they are experiencing. When I am able to hear that, then I can more readily enter into a sacred space and hopefully actively empathize with them. Not feeling sorry for them but calling forth in them what is good and holy and true.

Caitlin also described the importance of the ministry theme the Wounded Healer, as well as that of providing Compassionate Care:

There was a book years ago, *The Wounded Healer*. I very much have appreciated that concept of healer because I think to the degree that we are able to recognize our own woundedness, it is then that we are able to actively engage in the work and ministry of healing. I think the same way with compassion. The degree that I believe we have suffered and have entered into our own suffering is the degree that we can empathize, be sensitive to, and actively accompany another and bring forth and call forth healing.

Caitlin related an anecdote that well reflects the nursing servant leadership theme of going Beyond the Ordinary in providing care to a patient:

I have had the privilege of dreaming with patients that are dying of the most common simple wish. A man who truly longed to be able to get back into his red pickup truck and listen to country music. For him that was his dream, his longing before he died. Although we couldn't get his pickup truck from (his home in) Florida, we were able to get a red pickup truck from one of the car dealerships and CDs of his favorite country singers and played it. We got him out to the pickup truck in the hospital parking lot. It was truly leaving life with no regrets and marking his memories in a powerful and profound way. I think with patients as well as for us as nurses, when we stop dreaming, or stop daring to say what if, why not. Look outside the box, I think we tend to limit what God is really calling for us and what we are really about and the privilege we have to serve.

THE NURSE MANAGER AS SERVANT LEADER

A distinction is sometimes made in the literature between leadership and management; however, the difference is not always clear cut. It has been suggested that there is sometimes a lack of agreement about the definitions of the two positions: "Often leadership is conceptualized as the broader of the two concepts, with managing including such tasks as controlling resources, budgeting and staffing...nurses in leadership roles are responsible for such activities, but their most important role involves the development of mission and goals for their areas of responsibility that support those of the organization" (Garrison, Morgan, & Johnson, 2007, p. 15). There can also be some confusion between understandings of the roles of management and administration. Administrators, however, are generally considered to be those individuals who assume a higher or broader level of leadership within a particular organization. For example, a hospital administrator oversees the operation of the entire healthcare facility, while a middle manager may assume a supervisory leadership role over a particular area, such as an intensive care wing, within the larger institution.

Nursing managers may hold such titles as manager of surgical services, manager of critical care areas, division officer, organ donation manager, outpatient clinic manager, or emergency services manager. Those with management responsibilities may also have the title "supervisor": house (hospital) supervisor, shift (7-3, 3-11, 11-7) supervisor, or area (medical-surgical units) supervisor. It is generally difficult to distinguish differences in role responsibilities between nurses with the title "manager" and those whom a healthcare facility designates as "supervisor." For the study participants discussed in this book, the assigned titles, either manager or supervisor, are those reported by the nurses themselves when asked to identify their leadership role.

As with nurse administrators, the nurse manager/supervisor may be expected to assume a variety of responsibilities depending upon the organizational goals, operational structure, and size of the area or department that he or she supervises.

Some roles and competencies of nurse managers identified in the literature include: "(personal) self-management, collaborator, networking; (client) advocate, provider of care, coordinator of care; and (organizational) member of the profession and communicator" (Garrison, Morgan, & Johnson, 2007, p. 26). Some related activities identified by Garrison, Morgan, and Johnson include:

- Values clarification
- Lifestyle management
- Goal setting
- Nurtures relationships with organizational leadership
- Liaisons with healthcare leaders in the community
- Recognizes needs of clients
- Maintains evidence-based practice
- Supports "interdisciplinary team care"
- Represents the organization to the community

- Mentors new nurses
- Facilitates communication (2007, p. 26).

These roles, competencies, and related activities described for nursing managers are especially consistent with the servant leadership characteristics of listening, assessing, discerning, and nurturing.

The concepts of trust, empowerment, and respect, both toward and from staff and clients, are important for nurse managers to cultivate and can be helpful in addressing the current shortage of staff that exists in many healthcare facilities (Laschinger & Finegan, 2005, p. 6). Trust between the nurse manager and his or her staff is especially relevant in today's culture of "unprecedented challenges and uncertainties" related to such issues as the pressure to "downsize services, reorganize patient care delivery systems, and provide adequate staffing at a time when the profession is facing one of its most severe nursing shortages" (Rogers, 2005, p. 421). Also critical during this time of nursing shortage is promotion of the element of job satisfaction and its related concept of nurse retention (Andrews & Dziegielewski, 2005, p. 286). Supporting a nurse manager is identified as one dimension of improving staff nurse retention (Pinkerton, 2003, p. 45) and "building high reliability organizations in health care" (Kerfoot, 2006, p. 274).

The attributes of trust, empowerment, and respect are appropriately derived from the nursing servant leadership characteristics of giving of oneself, assessing needs, and being there to serve.

Pat, a 47-year-old, baccalaureate-prepared nurse manager of a critical care area spoke of making sure that her staff were Doing Their Best in providing patient care, as well as the importance of Listening with the Heart and Becoming an Advocate for both staff and patients:

> My...number one priority is to my patients on my unit, and in order to better take care of my patients on my unit I have to make sure I have staff that are competent to take care of those patients. To do that I have to make sure I hire the best staff. I educate them appropriately. I also help educate physicians, any auxiliary staff..., and the ancillary personnel that may come in to meet the needs of the patients, keeping within what the hospital wants us to do. My number one priority is the patient all the time, and to get that I have to ensure that I have all of the support staff that meet with that patient up and functioning and understanding what their role is and how they should interact with the patient.

Pat added:

We managers always have to listen to both the hierarchy and what they are mandating downward, and we have to listen at the level in which we manage and also down to the patient. We are in the middle, listening on both sides and trying to help the communication go upwards and downwards. We can meet an awful lot of barriers a lot of time. Another thing that comes into play with listening effectively is time and interruptions and the length to which somebody does or doesn't explain whatever is going on, to get the full story. Sometimes information from higher up may come down, and you will take the time to explain it to staff or coworkers, and it may be misinterpreted as people start to talk about it so then you have to reexplain for clarification to make sure everybody is listening.

Pat explained that advocacy for both patients and staff was also a critical characteristic of the leader in a managerial role:

It's (advocacy) important for helping to heal the patient. As managers we want to ensure that the patient understands what is going on with them, answering their questions, at the bedside when I have to or either to guide the less experienced nurse, maybe to reassure the patient, reassure the family member…talking to family members about processes or talking to physicians on behalf of patients a lot of times. Be their advocate because they are scared; the physicians are going in and out and not spending enough time, explaining processes. Ensuring that nurses, especially the less experienced, understand the importance of communication to relieve some of the anxiety that patients have. We have to be thinking about from the time the patient is admitted to the time of discharge; what needs to be put in place so that patients can reach the best outcome for that patient.

Pat continued:

You have to advocate for patients and staff. Again going back to the patients being cared for, do I have the coverage if it is really busy? The staff is out there, and I can see that they are overwhelmed, and I'm out there at maybe 9 or 10 o'clock at night, but I am still out there because that is where the need is. My first priority all the time is the organization. It sometime can be a detriment to me. But again it is for the patient with the reputation of the organization and for the staff because I can emphasize with them 100% when it gets to be busy like that. What keeps people here is not just a paycheck, it is the environment in which they work.

Pat recounted a detailed anecdote about an elderly patient admitted from the ER with cardiac problems for whom protective services was needed; this was related to perceived abuse by a mentally challenged son. The staff initiated a complex intervention strategy and ultimately concluded that it had to be done:

So that we could ensure the person's safety as well as the safety of the greater good out there because if this patient's son had gotten off meds and was just going wild, could he go and hurt someone else? We had to look into all the resources for that. And talk to the physician about what was going on, as well as setting up plans for case coordination to follow-up and deal with adult protective services. And explaining to the staff that the patient had the right to refuse to press charges, but they could not refuse to file a report because that was the law. That was just that one; then we got a second one back to back on that. This had to do with a son abusing his mother and how to handle that and how to document in the charts to support and again be the advocate for the patient. So even if the clock says it is time to go home, but you have less resources available, you need to make sure again the patient or whoever is related to the patient is taken care of.

Advocacy for staff was also noted:

The reason I came in here was to help develop the new individual and less experienced practitioner. Even in my 5 years in this role, we have instituted a really good working relationship with physicians. We helped educate the physicians that they are going to be seeing a turnover of new grads, and they can be part of the process or they can interfere with the process. So we have them be part of the process, and as a result they do monthly in-service to the staff. We set up educational opportunities with sister departments, like the cath lab; we have set up education series with critical care educators, but we are also orienting and teaching people to identify an area that needs more development. We will set up one-on-one teaching. For example, if you needed more IV access or phlebotomy or even just doing an EKG, or on this floor if you are not really good with identifying arrhythmias because we have a lot of nurses that are senior nurses that may come from other institutions so they are not as proficient in reading arrhythmias or EKG, we will set up sessions so they can have that one on one. So there is not this sense of institutionalized phobias or being blamed because you don't know how to do something. They can become better at their skills.

Pat concluded her comments with her personal perception of the overall leadership role in nursing; this included both the nursing servant leadership themes of Compassionate Care and Giving of Yourself:

I think the role as a leader has a lot of responsibility, a lot of hidden responsibilities that people don't realize. I think people look at you, and you have to set the example, you have to be compassionate, and you have to be willing to give a lot of yourself to do a good job. It is not a 9-to-5 job, and you have to be willing to be there. It is always a challenge, and you are learning something every day.

Christine, a 43-year-old, baccalaureate-prepared nurse manager of surgical services first described her perception of the meaning of service as a nursing leader:

The idea of service is providing either care or some kind of function to another person. Whether it be a patient, a family member, another staff member, a surgeon, a coworker, anything like that, in my leadership my service is to everyone that reports to me or that I come in contact with.

Christine linked Listening with the Heart to service:

I think the most important part (of serving) is with the listening; that is, you have to hear, and when you really listen you really hear what others are trying to say.... You have to respond using...the verbal or nonverbal cues that you got to provide the best answer or direction for patients or staff. You have to be understanding to what people are saying, to issues they may have, to realize that that is what they are feeling and that is just what they are complaining about and not to put your ideas on to them. I think this has a lot to do with your creditability.

Christine gave an example:

A staff member came up to me and was very upset over the current way preadmission department was being run. I understood what she was saying and her frustration level; lots of patients do not get enough time. We don't have anything… to help us out, but we are currently in the process of…doing process changes and making it more efficient. I asked her if she was frustrated. She is on this committee with me to help me make these process changes. Things are not happening fast enough, and I think being understanding with her, saying "I understand what you are saying. You are really frustrated right now, but we are doing a lot of good things. It is coming together," (helped). I think she believed me that things were going to happen.

Christine noted the importance of assessing both her own needs and those of staff, especially related to the concept of Taking Time Out:

A common thing for nursing is that you take care of every-body but yourself. I think we tend to spend all kinds of time doing for others because others need us, but then we need to stop and think about how do we get our bucket filled with the things that we need so we can continue to give to others. It is one of those things I think nursing in general has to reflect on because that is what we do. We do it for 8 hours a day, 5 days a week, or 12 hours a day for 3 days a week. Sometimes we are just too wiped out to do anything else. I think we have to remain grounded and stay focused.

Lastly, Christine spoke of the importance of Generating Excitement about nursing among the members of her staff through education:

My biggest commitment, and I say this until I'm blue in the face, is continuing education. I say it to my staff thousands of times. I think the nurse's professional accountability is raised to a higher level when you have that commitment to continuing education, whether it be a certification in your specialty, or fur-thering your degree, or a skill. Always keep that commitment to the nursing profession and be willing to review the latest literature and keep up on your latest journals. I think that just grows the nursing profession in itself, and overall you are just giving better patient care.

Maria, a 53-year-old master's-prepared nurse manager of a surgical/gastrointestinal service, described the meaning of nursing as a caring profession of service:

Our leadership role in nursing is to be a generous role model to others. To make sure the kind of care I used to give at the bedside is given by the nurses under my leadership — the same kind of care. I believe in role modeling.

Maria linked this idea to the importance of Listening with the Heart to her staff and also her patients:

A good example of listening to my patients and to my nurses relates to what happens in the relationship to nurse and patient. Many, many times I have realized sitting with patients and listening carefully to them was important. By my listening to (the nurse and the patient) and understanding where they were both coming from I was able to help the patient understand where the nurse was coming from.

Maria added:

I believe that as leaders we take not only responsibility for the physical body but also the spirit. Personally I have a mission for my life on planet Earth, and I take that to work with me. I try to communicate this to my staff. Why am I getting up everyday and going to work? What is the mission of my life? I encourage them, by helping them to have a dream, to have a mission, to have hope, because this is the force behind their daily nursing activities. I am open to sharing my own philosophy of life with my staff. I need to help my staff find their nursing mission by sharing my own mission. I try to be a mentor to help them see beyond the daily mundane tasks. Nursing is a true sacred profession, by serving patients. I try to help the staff to understand how much they give to patients and thus how much peace and satisfaction they can take home at the end of the day.

Maria concluded:

> As a committed servant leader in nursing I take ownership for this department, this group of nurses that have to work with me to achieve the goal of patient safety and patient healing. My commitment is not only to my patients but to my staff. So that my staff know what they need, they know what their job description is and why they are working in my department. I do this by working side by side with them, making them aware of the profession, making them aware of the purpose of the work...why they are here and how they can be their best selves — to call the best out of them. We all have the potential (for leadership), but it's like a mirror; show it to them. This is who you are; this is what you do.

Anna, a 40-year-old, baccalaureate-prepared manager of medical-surgical services in a medical center, spoke of the relationship between Listening with the Heart and Compassionate Care:

> In listening to staff, you have to have compassion. I can think of a particular example when I was a manager of an ambulatory care clinic. I had a young (staff member) who was newly married with three children, and she had this issue of not showing up on time to work. She was getting a lot of flack from other people in that department. After sitting down and talking with her I realized that not only was she married with three children but she didn't have a drivers license, and her husband wasn't willing to get up and take her early in the morning. So instead of taking the approach of just saying you need to be at work on time, we looked at different solutions for her. One of the solutions that we came up with was riding with someone who lived near her, including myself. So we partnered up so that would relieve part of the stress and some of the issues she was having with coming to work on time.

Anna also gave a patient example:

> (At the time) I worked in the recovery room. I came across this military member who was active duty army, and he had lost both legs. He was recently married and had a child and had a lot of anxiety about going home without his limbs. (He was) very angry. His issues were basically that his body was

disfigured and that his family and wife would not love him any more. Showing empathy in taking care of him and showing him kindness and compassion were instrumental in helping with the healing process with him. Being that we were both from the same hometown helped him. Just talking about what positive things to come from this as far as he may not have his limbs but he has his life. With rehabilitation, he would be able to work and be able to take care of his family.

Margaret, a 45-year-old, baccalaureate-prepared supervisor of critical care areas, described her perception of nursing's call to serve:

I feel like it (nursing) is not an obligation, it is something that I want to do, that I care about people. I want to show that I care about people while I'm doing my job. It is a service, it is not an obligation in the fact that I care and want to take care of people. Most nurses go into nursing because they care about people and want to do better for people and provide better care. Overall I think that good nurses do have those characteristics.

Margaret linked caring service to Listening with the Heart:

I think listening is very important because you have to take care of the (whole) person. Sometimes there is a lot more involved than just what you see. There are family issues, and if you send someone home they have to be cared for properly. You need to know all about it. I think nonverbal communication is important especially because there are some that don't like to always talk so sometimes you have to "hear" the nonverbal. A lot of times people can't communicate, and you have to look at nonverbal.

Assessing patients' needs was also described as important for a nursing leader:

You have to assess and respect the cultural differences and the care that you give patients. You might have to provide a little different care. You have to respect each individual and their beliefs. You try to provide them the knowledge. If there is a cultural problem, then of course you respect that by maybe changing nurses. Some cultures don't let women take care of men. You would provide what the patient needs as far as the care. If it is somebody doing something I don't believe in, you still have to understand they are human, and you have to take care of them whether you believe what they do is right or wrong. You provide them the knowledge of how to do better. They are human, and everyone makes mistakes. As you grow in the nursing field, you become much more aware. I think that comes with experience. The more different types of people you take care of, the more that you are able to assess much more. I think that grows as you grow as a nurse.

Margaret spoke about nursing leaders' patient advocacy in terms of Protecting and Defending those for whom they care:

I think of when I was young and working in a nursing home, and those elderly people who you needed to take care of if they were not able to mentally protect themselves. Every day we take care of patients who are unable, because of medical reasons, to protect themselves. You have to do the best for them and care for them. You also see kids who come in abused who you have to report to social services and things like that. So every day nurses should be looking at opportunities for their patients and determining if there is something they can do to provide for them or protect them. Just in your daily nursing care you are protecting patients from harm every day. I try to go a step beyond all the time.

Several other nursing leaders serving in the manager/supervisor role also identified specific themes or subthemes relating to nursing servant leadership.

The Mystery Behind the Visit

I think sometimes patients cry out spiritually. People who are dying cry out spiritually, and it is not understood as that, that they want to talk about something. I think nurses, sometimes in their haste, overlook that. I try to get nurses to understand and pay attention to what people are trying to say but what they (nurses) are not hearing. This may be the end of a patient's life…so I encourage nurses to get families to connect with the patient somehow. (Talking about death) is not something we should not talk about. It is not something we should shy away from, it is not something we need to avoid, and yet I find a lot of people avoiding that very important topic in the family member who is dying. (49, MSN, supervisor, critical care)

Embracing a Higher Purpose

I believe that spirituality is a very healing thing not only for the patient but also for nurses. It is a reflection of who you are as a person....You have to have some kind of belief in yourself and in a higher being in a meaningful, purposeful way to give of yourself....You've got to have the spiritual aspect in your life to survive. (54, MSN, supervisor, medical-surgical outpatient clinic)

Giving of Yourself

(Part of giving yourself in a vocation of service) part of that is your spirituality and what that means in your life. Some people, it doesn't mean anything to. They take it for granted. But in the nursing vocation or profession, I think you have a unique position to experience spirituality at a different level. I was raised in a religious family...therefore religion and spirituality played a role in my ability to what I believe is my service to humanity. (64, PhD RN, educator)

THE NURSE CLINICIAN AS SERVANT LEADER

There are currently a variety of labels applied to the role of an expert nurse clinician identified as a nursing leader. One of the most recent is that of the clinical nurse leader (CNL) a title identified by the American Association of Colleges of Nursing (AACN) to describe nursing graduates who are "prepared for clinical leadership in all healthcare settings; are prepared to implement outcomes-based practice and quality improvement strategies; will remain in and contribute to the profession, practicing at their full scope of education and ability; and will create and manage microsystems of care that will be responsive to the healthcare needs of clients and families" (Grindel, 2005, p. 209). The goal of the clinical nurse leader is to improve patient care and assist in implementing new models of patient care delivery (Smith & Dabbs, 2007, p. 157). The CNL role also supports "provision of continuity of care to a complex aging patient population" (Tachibana & Nelson-Peterson, 2007,

p. 477). Nurses "in this new role will be prepared at the master's level and will act as the lateral integrators of care, patient advocates over the many components of the care continuum, and information managers to the multiple disciplines involved in care delivery" (Wiggens, 2006, p. 341). "Ultimately," it is admitted, "the CNL, just like every nurse, works for the benefit of the patient" (Hartranft & Garcia, 2007, p. 263).

Also identified by the AACN as a new nursing role, which might fill a gap in the nursing care delivery system, is that of the doctorate in nursing practice (DNP). The DNP-prepared nurse is envisioned as one who has earned a practice-focused doctorate (in distinction to a research-focused PhD) in nursing. The DNP-credentialed nurse is also an expert nurse clinician whose role centers on initiating and implementing new and creative strategies for the delivery of patient care.

For the present discussion of nurse clinicians as servant leaders, however, the more traditional roles of head nurse (HN), charge nurse (CN), and team leader (TL) are addressed.

The Head Nurse

Many healthcare facilities, especially hospital based inpatient units and outpatient clinics, continue to use the title "head nurse" (HN) for the nursing leader who has overall administration and management of a particular nursing area. Most intensive care units (ICUs) have their own head nurses, as do general medical-surgical units, specialty care areas such as neurosurgery, EENT (eye, ear, nose and throat) units, perioperative suites, emergency departments, pain clinics, diabetic clinics, and so forth. As with administrators and managers, the head nurses' roles may vary to some degree depending upon the healthcare focus and the structure and size of the unit or clinic. A few large areas have assistant head nurses, but that is not usual in average size institutions, especially those in which team nursing is implemented.

In a study to determine the essence of what head nurses actually do, researchers observed the work behaviors of 48 head nurses using a "semistructured observation technique for 6 hours each" (Drach-Zahavy & Dragan, 2002, p. 19). The study results showed that head nurses spent a great deal of time in "clinical practice," "coordinating care," "operating the unit functions," and "leading staff" (p. 19). The study concluded that "head nurses exhibited a management style oriented to maintenance rather than creation, focusing more on the 'doing' and the 'here and now' aspects of the job" (p. 19). A study of work empowerment among head nurses, however, concluded that head nurses experienced "quite strong verbal and behavioral empowerment," verbal empowerment relating to the ability "to state one's opinions and debate views" and behavioral empowerment in "the ability to work in groups to solve problems" (Suominen, Savikko, Puukka, Doran, and Leino-Kilpi, 2005, pp. 147–150). And, results of a study of gender-related characteristics between male and female head nurses revealed differences in "men's direct and women's roundabout ways of communicating"; men's orientation "toward technical matters and women's toward relationships," and men's perceptions of needing to "show what they can do to a greater extent than women" (Nilsson & Larsson, 2005, p. 179).

The three research studies cited above point out the importance of the head nurse's role in coordinating care, communicating with and leading staff, as well as being able to work in groups to solve problems. The nurse servant leadership behavioral characteristics of assessing needs, becoming an advocate, and making a difference would seem to be highlighted in the role of the head nurse as servant leader.

Tim, a 33-year-old, baccalaureate-prepared head nurse of a medical-surgical unit, spoke of leaders' need to provide Compassionate Care to both staff and patients:

> When I think of service, this is an interesting concept. A service you are not only providing to your patients who need your care and compassion but you also provide services, not so overtly but it can be, to your staff who also depend on your leadership role. You provide a service to them as well by keeping them abreast of new changes in technology, giving them the benefit of your experience and passing that down. So you are also servicing not only your patients but people you work with and work for. That is what I think of as service. You are treating your patients, and you are also treating the people you work with, and that occurs on many planes.

Tim also noted the importance of Listening with the Heart in providing care:

> Listening kind of helps you break down barriers, the perception of the patient's trust; they start trusting the provider, in this case the nurse, that they actually care about the situation. Staff also feel like they need to talk to you about something; they feel like you are actually hearing them, that you are actually taking the information from what they are saying and

possibly doing something with it that is very key. It was most apparent when I started my nursing career, and I worked on an oncology, hematology floor. Listening was pretty much the staple of what we did. The cancer patients I was treating, you would see some of the more chronic patients who came in for treatment, and you develop a relation with them. I had noticed that some of my coworkers who hadn't developed great listening skills, had harder times communicating with the particular patients that were coming on a regular basis. I myself really try to focus on listening. I felt like I made a difference. I felt like patients could trust me and speak to me on many issues. Many times I was requested to be the nurse for a certain patient. One of the reasons was that I was a good listener and communicator. So that is key in displaying that to other people who see that listening is a pretty important skill. And with your core staff and colleagues, the people you work with, listening is essential. Open lines of communication, this kind of goes down the list of things to do. Listening is key, listening with your heart of course, I think people can sense sincerity in your voice and posture and your mood and being receptive and open to listening. So listening is very key to know as a nursing leader or any role where you are having to constantly communicate with people.

Tim also described the value of Compassionate Care as a nursing leader:

As long as I can remember, compassion has been pretty much ingrained in my role as a nursing leader and is exemplified in the way I interact with my patients: being kind and compassionate to others. It kind of creates a bond when I'm with the patients.

In discussing compassion, Tim also identified the nursing servant leadership characteristic of Giving of Yourself:

Whether it be a physical treating of a medical ailment that is bothering a patient or treating them on an emotional, spiritual level, healing can occur on many levels. It is basically giving of yourself that is key. People can kind of sense that you care about their situation. An example of this occurring in my work place: About 8 years ago when I was working on oncology, hematology, one of my patient was chronically ill, and had a relapse to her primary cancer. Going and talking to her and treating her, no matter how much I explained her situation as far as she was getting a lot of pain from her cancer and treating her pain physically with all medication, didn't seem like it was making a lot of difference, so talking to her and obviously developing a relationship with the patient helped me to understand that she was hurting from more of a spiritual standpoint and emotional standpoint. She was concerned about her daughters and their welfare, the constant going into the hospital; she was more worried about how that was kind of weighing on her kids. So me being there and trying to treat her on a more of a spiritual, emotional level was probably better time spent than actually treating her physical pain with just the medication alone....As a servant leader with patients, colleagues, and staff, you have to be in tune with what is going on. Assessing patient needs is a big role for a servant leader.

Tim spoke about assessing staff needs and then Generating Excitement among the staff:

One situation in particular is when I worked in oncology, hematology, in which we had to combine with (another unit), which was the cardiac step-down unit due to space renovations on their floor. Once hearing this message, our staff became very disheartened by that only because the thought was they would have more work, and there would be confusion, training new people to come; they wouldn't know where all the resources were. Many people saw it as a big, big task that would take a lot of their time and effort. So communicating to them was essential, explaining to them that this was a great beneficial move for everybody involved and kind of helping them to see the long-term benefits from this. Let them see it through a different perspective; we are going to make the best of it. The excitement in my tone, my voice, my overview on it probably helped a lot. The respect that the staff showed with me, at least showed that my excitement probably would be key to this being a successful situation.

Finally Tim spoke of Becoming an Advocate for his patients and staff and of providing a nurturing environment:

My advocacy for patients that I serve also goes with the colleagues that I work with. My commitment is to make sure that their welfare is taken care of. It goes throughout the normal day of working. Being able to be that person that people can rely on because advocacy is a concept that is highly respected. Take care of the environment that you are in, the people that you work with and work for. Make sure that is a nurturing place where people can work with each other for a common goal, common good.

Rosemary, a 54-year-old, diploma RN and head nurse of a PACU (postanesthesia care unit), explained the value of a nursing leader Listening with the Heart:

To be a good nurse you definitely need to listen with your heart because how are you going to know what is wrong with the patient or what they need? You can think you know what they need, but you might be way off the mark too. You have to talk to them and listen to them and find out really what is going on because you don't know this person. If you don't you might think they are in pain, but maybe they are just having a bad day or maybe they aren't. (Like) if you have an older person, and they are not showing an outward sign of pain but they are laying there in agony. I think when I was precepting nurses, I think now especially younger nurses need to slow down and listen to the patient. It is hard at first. You have to actually sit down and have a little conversation with them.

Rosemary also reflected on the nursing servant leadership theme of Staying Focused:

In trauma, you could be taking care of the person who shot the person in the next bed. Or the alcoholic who crashed his car. You do have to focus—you are taking care of a patient, a person who needs you. You do have to put a lot aside. It is a hard thing to do here unless you are focused on that person. You can't narrow it down to just taking care of a body, but you take care of that person. That person needs you now. It is not your place to judge. It is a big part of nursing. If it was you in that bed, you would want someone to care for you. A lot of times they start demanding stuff, but you have to care for them.

Because of working in a trauma unit, Rosemary recognized the need for occasionally Taking Time Out:

As a nurse if you get too burned out, then you lose it. So you do have to take the time away and make sure you take care of yourself. Like there are two of us here today, and we have had 2 really, really hard days. You have to start fresh every morning. Heal yourself emotionally. This place is kind of hard, so you do have to get away.

Rosemary described the importance of Assessing Needs of patients:

You kind of have to get a feel for your patient as to whether they are going to clean up. Like here, they are still kind of groggy, so we do have to have a lot of assessing. Like how are they going to be, how are they going to turn out. You just get a gut feeling about someone. We actually hung on to two patients yesterday because we didn't want them to go to a lesser care floor. You just kind of feel for what's going on with them. You will know something is wrong with them before their lab shows, or X-ray shows. You gain that as you are working a little longer. Probably the older experienced nurses have better assessment skills.

Lastly, Becoming an Advocate was important for Rosemary. She also mentioned the nursing servant leadership concept of Making a Difference in her comments:

That (advocacy) is a little bit of why we became a nurse. You do that in many ways. Like in your own life, you do that. Especially here because we have some patients that we have taken care of for over a year. You run into them outside, there is fine line, you can e-mail people or follow up on them and given them a little bit of encouragement outside when they leave here. Check up on them when they go to rehab places. We are lucky because we see them come back and we can help them out that way. Like the older lady we were trying to help, encouraging her family to come in and have a discussion about her. She is not aware of what is going on; we are trying to protect her. She has a living will, and we are trying to protect what she has written. Nurses make a difference in lives of others, but letting them know that someone genuinely cares for and is taking care of you and your interest. Trying to make their lives better.

Rosemary concluded:

Two days in a row we haven't had lunch, we haven't really gone to the bathroom, and we are back here for a third day. It is making a difference for patients. And its self-fulfilling. You feel good about yourself when you leave.

Maureen, a 63-year-old, diploma RN and head nurse of a medical-surgical unit, described her philosophy of being a nursing servant leader:

> Service, to me, is giving unselfish caring, caring for others and not thinking about what my own personal gain would be. In the end, feeling self-satisfaction that you have helped mankind. I mean like putting in many hours, not looking to be reimbursed. I think the current day nursing leadership, looks at it as our job. I see it in myself 10–12 or more hours a day, and I help other units if need be or wherever else is needed in the hospital. I try to be a role model for new staff coming aboard.

From this philosophy of nursing leadership flowed the theme of Listening with the Heart:

> Listening, to me, is active, not interrupting the other person, not interjecting what I feel at the time. Not interrupting them, giving them your complete time and giving feedback at the end. Be nonjudgmental, and listen to whatever the issue is at hand and seek to solve it. This applies to patients, staff, or anyone, including families.

Two other head nurses identified nursing servant leadership themes or subthemes in their discussions.

Being Grounded

> My nursing vocation supports situations like when a baby is born with disabilities, you think, you were there to get them through the pregnancy, and now you have to take them beyond to help them deal with whatever it is to come. At whatever point they find out that there is something not right with the baby, the vocational aspect of your nursing takes over. You are not just dealing with the baby now, you have to be ready to be dealing with the mother, the father, the siblings, the grandparents who now have this devastating news. It is not a wonderful thing anymore. You hope that your vocation to serve, your vocational aspect, will help you deal with the patient (and family) in a way that they can cope. I lot of times

they can't understand...but the process is helping them get to the point where life becomes normal, whatever normal is after that. I think you have to trust, you have to believe even though this is a tragic situation, that there is going to be some acceptance of this down the road a bit. (47, BSN, head nurse, obstetrics and gynecology)

A Caring Vocation

Often I have worked in areas where patients can't do for themselves so we need to do for them, or you're helping them with something they will benefit from. There may be aspects that are not very appealing. I had a patient who after surgery and anesthesia was very nauseated. He was sick, and you clean him up and you think you are done, and then it happens all over again. Then he was so apologetic. I just said "It's OK. Do you feel better now?" and he said "Oh, yes I do!" I can think of many examples whether it's holding a patient's hand or having them ask questions that you can either answer or get them the information for and the fact that they just appreciate that. This is the caring aspect of nursing. (53, diploma RN, head nurse, medical-surgical)

The Charge Nurse

As with the head nurse role, most hospital units and clinics have nursing staff members who are assigned the role, either consistently or periodically, of charge nurse (CN). The charge nurse role differs from that of the head nurse in that the charge nurse does not have oversight of the broader administration of an area in terms of such responsibilities as planning the staffing schedule; dealing with persistent staff problems; updating equipment and supplies; submitting weekly or monthly reports on admissions, transfers, and deaths as required by a healthcare facility; or communicating with the higher administration of the institution. The charge nurse may on occasion assume one or more of the above duties, if mandated by the head nurse. Generally, however, the charge nurse's responsibilities revolve around maintaining order on a unit or in a clinic, supervising staff and patient care activities during a particular shift, and preparing and communicating the end-of-shift report to the oncoming staff. Charge nurses may help with certain patient care activities, such as administering medications, if an area is short-staffed, but ordinarily the role activity tends to be more that of a supervisory nature.

A list of charge nurse competencies identified by Mary O'Keefe include such activities as:

- Identify patient acuities
- 24-hour report
- Update (patient) census
- Assist staff
- Act as a clinical resource
- Delegate workload
- Handle unit emergencies
- Provide direct patient care as needed, balancing patient care with charge nurse duties
- Provide for patient safety (2007, p. 81).

In some instances the charge nurse is able to acquire unique clinical education to position him or her for service in a particular care area. One example is the Geriatric Training Academy, at Texas Tech University Health Sciences Center, which has developed a program to prepare individuals for charge nurse responsibilities in long-term care facilities (Cherry et al., 2007, p. 37).

The importance of the charge nurse role is emphasized in an article in *Nursing Economics* entitled "Don't Forget Our Charge Nurses." The title of the paper was derived from "a clear message communicated during... research interviews by the author with nurse managers" (Sherman, 2005, p. 125). "During the interviews, nursing managers expressed concern that their charge nurses were key leadership staff on their units yet most had received no leadership training" (p. 125).

From the lists of competencies expected of charge nurses it would seem that the corresponding servant leadership characteristics of listening, giving, assessing, ministering, and discerning are most desirable in this population of nursing leaders.

Sally, a 35-year-old charge nurse working in an inner-city trauma unit, spoke of nurses not only Listening with the Heart but going Beyond the Ordinary in caring for adolescent trauma victims:

> Part of our assessment is listening because you learn a lot just from talking to patients. Sometimes you have to read between the lines. You get a lot from hearing them, listening for their concerns. A lot of times here at the trauma center, it is not just about the patient, you have to listen to the family. So if you have a minor that has been beat up and you are not sure who by, then the mom starts to (admit to the problems at home). Our unit is a

short stay unit. Some young patients come here and literally in 40 minutes they are ready to go back. But others, they are very upset, they might have lost a friend and they don't even know that they lost a friend yet. Later on that day they are going to have 20 teenage visitors. Sometimes we go above and beyond, try to hook them up with music or something just to let them pass the time and get their mind off of things. I think that is important. It is the little things. You just do the extra stuff. Whether it is calling the peds unit to see if they have an extra Nintendo for a 12-year-old or something like that. Breaking the visitation rules. It means a lot to the patients.

Sarah, a 28-year-old charge nurse on a medical-surgical unit, emphasized the importance of Listening with the Heart to patients:

I think listening is huge with nurses. We are pretty much the voice of our patients a lot of time because we spend the entire day with them, the entire shift with them. We hear the happy things they are feeling, when they are upset, when they are in pain, or feel like they are out of the loop. I definitely think we are the voice more than other disciplines, like doctors, physical therapy, or nutrition. Like when it comes to meals, just their complaints of what meals they want, what they do like. I think that is huge in what we do. That is one of our main things in nursing.

Sarah explained how Listening with the Heart can help a charge nurse to cross over and empathize with a patient:

I had a patient that came in with a GI bleed. Here at this hospital we have to ask these patients what does very good care mean to you, and just asking her that question and then asking her how do you feel right now, how are you feeling. She said she didn't know, like how would you feel if you were me. So I had to think about that and I realized it is kind of easier to understand what they are going through and maybe what I would have done for myself, if I kind of put myself in their shoes. When you do that it kind of helps the whole empathy aspect of that.

Sarah spoke of being a patient advocate as well as identifying the nursing servant leadership theme of Embracing a Higher Purpose:

I really love nursing. It is my Cinderella shoe that fits. I really like being part of the healthcare team. I love the part that I play in nursing. I think things are going well; I am a good advocate for my patient. Advocacy is another thing that is huge in the nursing field; being the patient's advocate. Just making sure things are being done for the patient. Just addressing issues, such as pain meds. Maybe a physician or somebody is not trying to order something, but you see with your own eyes that something isn't right. Just follow your heart, keep pushing for it.

Sarah added:

I want to be part of that role that is a leadership role where you are kind of in control or in tune to have more of a say in the type of care patients get, more of a voice. I think that is my higher purpose, or my higher level of nursing.

Paula, a 25-year-old, baccalaureate-prepared charge nurse on a medical-surgical unit, shared her understanding of leadership and service:

I definitely believe that leadership is all about service and serving others. Although you are in a position of power, your place of power is to serve and represent the people who are supporting you. I think leadership in general is about service and leadership in nursing is more specific to serving others.

Serving, for Paula, included Becoming an Advocate and providing Compassionate Care:

I think when you are a charge nurse on the floor lots of time your job is to put out fires of the patients who are emotionally distressed. A lot of time it takes a lot of compassion to understand why they are angry, why are they upset, and to figure out the reason of why they are having these emotional upheavals. Maybe they are just sick and they got really bad prognosis from the doctor, and so they are taking it out on the nurses, then you have to basically create boundaries for them. Or maybe their needs are not being met and they are trying to communicate it, but it is not being actually supported by this faculty because they either had been not understood or they were not heard.

Paula also mentioned the need for charge nurses Taking Time Out:

I think actually one of the biggest problems amongst nurses in general is the fact that they don't take enough time to care for themselves. They give so much of themselves to their patients that they have nothing left to give, and lots of times they end up being burnt out because they haven't taken the time to take care of themselves. Sometimes nurses give all of themselves to their patients and when they get home they give all of themselves to their children with nothing left for them. There are very few examples of nurses actually making time to care for themselves. Nurses need to allow themselves time out to take a break.

The nursing servant leadership themes of Being Grounded and Discerning Decisions also emerged in the interview with Paula:

I think some of the best leaders and best managers that I ever worked with are the one that are so grounded and self-aware. That they are able to put their ego aside and actually make a fair and observant decision. When I was unit council chair I created a petition to stop the management from making the staff nurses float instead of the travel nurses. I dealt with a lot of managers who were not self-aware. One was so empowered; she was taking the power from others to build her own talent. It is those kinds of situations that make things very difficult. I think for me is it always a constant challenge to be in a leadership position and not let the power consume you and be aware of your ego getting in the way because ultimately you are going to observe other people and depend on other people. Actually make a fair decision in the interest of everyone. I think probably it is something that has remained very challenging that unless the vision is also shared from within the other person, it is very difficult. The vision you are proposing is actually the one that everyone should embrace. Everyone has an idea. I think the best way to handle things is usually to get everyone at the table and everyone to say their opinion and actually to go with something that is a good compromise for everyone.

Paula added:

It is very important as a leader that you try and actually find common ground with other leaders in the hospital. Because without that it is really impossible to conceptualize any kind of vision unless there is some kind of teamwork.

Lastly, Becoming an Advocate for staff, was identified as an important leadership quality by Paula:

I really think that…my role is to defend the nurses on my unit, defending the new grads, defending the nurses on the floor. It is really a conscious decision. Not to mention a reflection of the communication between the unit nurses and management. I think advocacy is really important. You have to be willing to take the heat that will be focused on you and be able to manage that well while not having a tough exterior and not let people get to you.

Alice, a 27-year-old, baccalaureate-prepared medical-surgical charge nurse, began her comments by explaining her perception of the importance of Listening for a leader:

When I think of listening, what I understand from listening as my role is pretty much always knowing, and I think that not just listening with your ears but just listening with all your senses. I think a lot of time, listening in the sense of being a leader or as a role model, means not just listening to what the person is verbally telling you, but also listening to the person as a whole. Given the holistic approach to listening which is knowing that that person is obviously not telling you something for whatever reason. You know that the way your body language or gestures mean something completely different. It is definitely something that in that role of leader you want to say, "Okay, obviously you are telling me yes, but if you can't, it is okay." Allowing yourself to look beyond your personal objective or your personal goal of having enough staff. Allowing yourself to listen to what the person is truly saying. That also helps you a lot. Listening not just with your ears but also looking at the person and trying to listen to what their heart is telling you. It is definitely a very deep commitment because it is almost looking beyond your needs. It is looking into the other person's needs and knowing what they really want to tell you.

Alice also perceived Listening with the Heart as allowing a leader to Cross Over and empathize with patients and staff:

I think understanding in my role as a nursing leader means that you are trying to put yourself in the other person's shoes without any limitations. Maybe as I have experienced it in my nursing leader role would be putting myself in the other person's shoes with no limitations in regards to feeling for that person or how they would feel if I was in that position without thinking about my status or my experience or my title. As an experienced nurse, a lot of time experienced nurses tend to forget how it is as a new graduate nurse. When you first get out there and you start taking your first load of patients, there is anxiousness and the feeling of hopelessness at a time when you can't help a patient out for whatever reason. I always remember when I first became a nurse, and I remember leaving late and being anxious and not being confident yet about having it together and knowing what I was supposed to do....I think when I have new graduates or when I'm training or being somebody's preceptor I really try to empathize with them and remember what it meant when I first got on the floor. It is hard to do that when you're not a good nursing leader. In the sense of being in a charge role, a leadership role, I think you really have to be able to know what it means—the complete experience of putting yourself in somebody's else shoes, looking at it from their perspective and feeling it from their perspective. That goes also with patients. Knowing or trying to understand what it means to be in a bed sick with cancer, after surgery, not knowing what is going on. Or a patient's family, really thinking that could be your mother, your aunt, or your father. All those feelings that you have when you are in the hospital. Really connecting with that person through that. Empathy allows connections; it builds a relationship. I think that even more so than just understanding them, it allows you to really captivate and understand and feel what they are going through and know.

Alice described both Generating Excitement among staff and providing a Nurturing Environment as part of her leadership role:

Generating excitement, as nursing leader, means trying to help others understand that we are a team and that we try to get the team to work together, and when we do that it is very easy to convince others and do something that benefits the whole group.

That always works better than just saying I need to do this, or I need you to follow these rules. I am helping them understand and explaining the meaning behind the protocol, not just doing it because you have to do it, but doing it because we are helping each other out, and it makes a better environment. Knowing and letting other staff or coworkers know that you are part of the team, that whatever needs to be done, it's because it is for the common good. It is not just one task that needs to be completed. Getting others excited about that and getting others to understand the purpose of team work; you don't want to sound just like you are dictating. You want to make them part of your decision. Being a good nursing leader you transmit that to your staff and patients.

Six other charge nurses reported the presence of the following nursing servant leader characteristics as important to their practice.

Assessing Needs

When it comes to spiritual matters, I try to find out whatever it is a patient can relate to. If they are Jewish, find a rabbi; if they are Christian, find a minister or a priest. Or if Moslem, an imam. Find their leaders or their churches to help them through (an illness); first determine their belief systems. And in terms of emotional problems...I would have to appeal to a psychologist or psychiatrist to help me understand what the patient's needs are, what they are undergoing and to help them cope. Essentially the need is for them to learn to cope. And that is what a nurse's job is: to determine what a patient's needs are, what are their priorities and to address them. (50, BSN, charge nurse, medical-surgical)

Being There to Serve

I shifted in the DR (delivery room) for 12 hours so you could have a patient all the way through. One woman wrote a letter that basically addressed my professionalism, caring, and kindness. Those are the words she used. She said: "(she) was my nurse through my entire labor and before I could ask for anything or any need she had it covered. She knew what I needed before I said it. She was there. She was more instrumental than the doctor could ever have been in my care. She is an outstanding nurse. She was caring to my family"....She (the patient) also said, "She was everything a nurse should be, and it was effortless for her. I felt that she was sincerely caring." What an incredible experience I had; that was the most beautiful letter anyone had ever written (for me). (49, BSN, charge nurse, obstetrics)

Compassionate Care

With all the suffering that we see in the units and in patients' homes, how else can nurses understand if we didn't see it with the eyes of the Divine? There is an invitation to be more compassionate, to be merciful and to be more connected to humanity, to our patients, and perhaps to be able to see from God's point of view. How he would view our patients if he were standing right there with me...in front of both of us — the patient and myself, in the way I am treating the patient....I think we are invited to become nurses, and I think that's the real clincher, to be invited to become more in the eyes of God. (50, BSN, charge nurse, critical care)

Becoming an Advocate (To Protect and Defend)

You have to plan down the road with terminally ill patients. Dying is part of the life cycle. Some of us will be lucky enough to know when we are going to do it and be able to do so in a peaceful way surrounded by our friends and families. For others of us, it is not going to be like that. As far as critically ill and dying patients are concerned, you have to plan. They want comfort, they want information, they want to trust in having alleviation of pain, they want to die with the best sense of dignity they can, and that is something that I feel that nurses can facilitate. (26, BSN, charge nurse, pediatric clinic)

Staying Focused

(Viewing nursing as a calling) impacts my practice. I think it is enthusiasm. When I am in a setting that I feel is my heart, I ask God to lighten the path so that I don't trip and fall. So I really feel like I'm where he wants me to be at that time....I have confidence that I'm where I'm supposed to grow, and the workplace feeds into that....Many times...I see the younger nurses getting angry.... I'm not doing that. By being able to see nursing as a calling to serve, this is where I'm supposed to be, maybe I'm supposed to learn something from it, I see this as a kind of release to go forward, to be consistent, to keep going on, and to see what else is there. (52, MSN, charge nurse, cardiac rehabilitation)

Doing Your Best

I can call to mind for instance, being a cardiac nurse, a patient coming in, a woman with terrible chest pain and she had a stress test. The stress test is negative, and she is beside herself because she is having terrible, terrible chest pain. And she is in tears because she is afraid we are going to miss something, and she is going to drop dead. As I started talking to her, getting her ready for discharge, I find that her husband is out of work and her mother just moved in with her and her one child is flunking out of school. All of a sudden you recognize that the good news is that her heart is safe at the moment, but if you don't do anything, she may have serious problems down the road....Because she is not fine, and she will be back, and she will have problems if we don't do something. So, you pull up all kinds of stuff about stress from the computer, and you sit down and talk with her. A lot of times it's that little band-aid that the patient needs to know that "Okay, stress can cause this (chest pain). My heart's okay, I'm not crazy, and it's okay to feel this way" (52, MSN, charge nurse, cardiac rehabilitation).

The Team Leader

Depending upon the size and organizational structure of a nursing unit or clinic, patient care may be organized into several teams designated according to such characteristics as patient location or acuity of illness. The members of a nursing team may consist of an experienced registered nurse (RN) team leader, several RN staff members, one or more licensed practical nurses (LPNs) and, in some cases, one or more certified nursing assistants (CNAs) or technicians depending upon the needs of the specialty area.

"Effective team leaders" are described as being able to understand "the concepts and theories that explain how teams function so they can meet the challenges inherent in this complex leadership role" (Seavor, 2007, p. 195). The team leader's role is to make sure that all members of the team are functioning to their greatest potential to achieve the goal of the team, which is excellent patient care. The team leader may assist with direct patient care, assist other team members with their care activities as needed, and communicate directly with the head nurse or charge nurse.

Some particular skills identified for a team leader include defining the teams' goal and explaining how individual tasks will "contribute to the accomplishment of the goal," explaining the nature and importance of "difficult tasks" to the team, and valuing and trusting the other team members (Seavor, 2007, p. 196). Seavor suggests that "in most circumstances, team leaders should expect, acknowledge, and reward collaboration over competition" (p. 196).

In examining the impact of leadership by a nursing team leader in an acute medical nursing development unit (NDU), it was found that the outcome of skilled and insightful leadership was well-planned patient-centered care (Graham, 2003, p. 213). An exploration of team leadership in a mental health setting revealed that patients' satisfaction and quality of life were positively associated with transformational team leadership styles and inversely associated with a *laissez-faire* type of leadership approach (Corrigan, Lickey, Campion, & Rashid, 2000, p. 781).

In an article entitled "Follow the Team Leader," Marjorie Barter asserts that "Successful team leaders exude certain competencies that enhance patient care, including the ability to teach, coach, and foster effective delegation strategies" (2002, p. 54). The latter competency may perhaps be the most critical asset for a team leader; in order for a team to function effectively and with a high level of efficiency, the leader must not be shy in delegating appropriate responsibilities to other members of the team. "An effective team leader," Barter notes, realizes that the roles and responsibilities assigned to other team members "must be congruent with the team member's expectations to prevent role conflict. An ability to consciously adjust leadership style according to the environment's demands and the work's nature is a hallmark of an effective leader" (p. 55).

For the team leaders, as for the charge nurse, the servant leadership attributes of listening, assessing, serving, discerning, caring, and perceiving a higher purpose in nursing are critical to the achievement of the team's goals in relation to patient-centered care.

Lynn, a 51-year-old, baccalaureate-prepared team leader on a medical-surgical unit, described how nursing involved Embracing a Higher Purpose in her life:

> I remember always hearing about nursing as a helping profession. That's basically what attracted me to it; it was that I knew, by being a nurse, I would not just be serving myself, I would be serving others, helping others, you know. It's kind of something higher than yourself, doing something that will

have an impact on people. And you may affect their lives; temporarily you may have a great impact on them. I don't think many people go into nursing because they think they are going to get rich. I think people do it for a higher, a bigger reason, to have a positive impact on others.

And Elizabeth, a 53-year-old baccalaureate-prepared team leader in a critical care unit, spoke about the characteristics of Listening, Assessing, and Nurturing as a nursing leader:

Nursing is basically nurturing—everything. If a Mom is sick, I have to support her. Her husband can cooperate. We have to support her and what she needs. I think nursing is responsibility for caring for my patient and being involved with all the patient's lifestyle. In order to care for my patients I have to worry about them.

Elizabeth added:

When you are taking care of patients the first thing is you have to assess the patient. When you are assessing the patient, you are not just assessing the patient's eyes and heart and bowel sounds, skin. When you are talking to patients; what is your patient saying to you? Sometimes the patient is nonverbal, or a patient is really tired. You should initiate talking. "Can I help you? Can I do anything for you?" When taking care of my patient or some other patient, we have to have a patient–nurse relationship. That is the first thing—trust. If we don't have a good relationship, it is very hard to do my job.

Nursing is nurturing a person especially if the person is sick and needs help. Without nurturing, I don't know how you can treat your patients. When you talk to patients, you have to listen. You cannot put in your judgment and tell your opinion. I am trying to listen what patients say to me. Whenever I am taking care of a patient, we all came from different families, different cultures, and different beliefs and values. You have to listen patiently and nurture the patient.

Kelly, a 23-year-old baccalaureate-prepared team leader in critical care, shared an altruistic view of service in nursing; her thoughts included the concept of Assessing, Crossing Over, and Staying Focused:

Service in general and especially nursing, for me, certainly means putting your patient above yourself and sacrificing things for the betterment of others, whether that means their health, mentally, physically, for recovery purposes or for whatever reason. Putting yourself aside and taking yourself out of it and focusing on what that person needs. The important concept is that we want to heal people in one way or another. Being able to interpret what your patient needs whether they are able to tell you, or you are able to listen in other ways. Whether it is recognizing their physical cues or their emotional cues or even just looking at their vital signs if they are completely unable to communicate with you. Just sort of putting yourself in that place or even your family or knowing what that means to understand how they are feeling. So you can better treat them and better help them as well as just be open to everything around them. Being aware of all that is going on with your patient, with the physicians, anyone you have to interact with, their families.

To assess and cross over to understand a patient's needs, Kelly also highlighted the importance of Listening with the Heart:

As I mentioned, it is very important to be totally aware and to be exactly listening for what is actually not being said — to hear what a patient is saying. If the patient says "I'm fine," but you see they are showing a lot of emotion or tears are welling up in their eyes, you have to pay attention to that even if they say they are fine. That goes a long way with the people you work with as well. Sometimes we are just tired. Just knowing your patient and staff, getting intimately involved with that patient from the moment you meet them, to get down to their bare bones of understanding how they feel.

Kelly also admitted that as a nursing team leader, sometimes she and her staff needed to Take a Time Out:

When the unit is stressful we can help each other. Being aware of each other and our own weaknesses. Sort of knowing, especially when it gets busy, I need to stop for 5 seconds, sit down, and have a drink of water. All of a sudden it is 6 p.m., and I haven't eaten all day. There was a nurse who had a couple of patients and someone else coming into the OR, and she said, "If my patient comes out, could you please set him up for me?" I said, "Sure, but would you rather me transport?" She said, "No, I just need to leave for 5 minutes. I'm overwhelmed, and I just need to take a breather. The patient will be fine if you can set him up on the monitors and make sure everything is okay with him." That was a good thing for her, just to know she needed a breather, she was going to explode.

Kelly identified the theme of Generating Excitement with patients, if that could help their recovery:

It's knowing which patients, it is very important from the get go when we tell them you need to do this or you are not going to get better. Some people you joke around with, and they are…okay, and then they are happier about it, and they will do it. Just making them excited about it, saying "Listen, we've got this incentive spirometer, and it is kind of like a game: we need you to take a deep breath and watch this go up." Just to make them feel good about it, as dumb as it might seem for an 85-year-old man, do whatever we can to make them excited. We will clap and cheer and do whatever we can to make a patient excited about a therapy.

Kelly related her perception of Doing Ministry:

Sometimes you just have that connection with someone, you share the same faith and you can pray with them or talk with them. Sometimes it is totally different: I've had families ask me to step away from the bedside, because they wanted to pray. They didn't ask "Would you like to pray with us?" which some of us will, and I said "Okay, that is fine." I do feel like it is a calling to do this.

Finally, Kelly gave an example of the nursing servant leadership characteristic of going Beyond the Ordinary nursing practice activities:

I had a patient, and she got discharged home, and we could not find her Bible and her purse. I gave her a call the next day and said "Did you ever find those? If not we will get you something, a voucher or something." Something as small as just calling her the next day. She talked to me for about 10 minutes on the phone about how she was feeling and thanked us so much for everything we did. It was just little thing, I didn't necessarily have to do it. I wouldn't have felt good about not calling her back, but it wasn't necessarily required. Other people have done that many times. Just give the patient a call, it is not part of our job but just for them to be able to say, "You know, I am actually feeling better today and doing well and thanks so much," means the world to them. That helps them too with their healing.

Luke, a 26-year-old baccalaureate-prepared team leader in a critical care unit, explained his concept of being a nursing servant leader:

I think that if you are going to be a nurse you have to have a sense of service. You have to be humble enough to know that you are a servant, not only to your patients but to your fellow nurses as well. You have to be willing to bend over backwards for your patients and the people you work with to help them out and help your patients get better because that is your job.

Luke spoke about Listening with the Heart:

You have to listen to your patients, you have to understand where they are coming from. You need to try to understand what the patient is feeling. A lot of patients don't want sympathy from you; they want empathy. They don't want you to feel sorry for them; they want you to understand what they are going through. I think if you can do that you can better help them. Listening with the heart—that is what we do everyday. That is just our job—second nature. You have to listen and become intimately involved with what is going on with the patient; otherwise, you are not going to be able to care for him or her the way you need to. Listening to what is not said—you have to look at nonverbal cues; you need to look at their body language and see what they are communicating other than what they are saying.

Luke added:

You have to be able to put yourself in the patient's shoes. You have to imagine going through what the patient is going through and try to consider what your needs would be if you were in that situation and care for the patient accordingly.

Luke gave examples of empathy and Crossing Over, as well as the themes of Taking Time Out and being a Wounded Healer:

We have patients in this hospital all the time, and they are coming back from overseas and are wounded. Having been overseas myself, although I wasn't wounded, I can put myself in the position they are in, having been there, knowing that things are going to be much more difficult coming back: having to deal with the injuries and long recovery, just trying to help them recover one day at a time. Not trying to push them too hard, but setting small achievable goals for them. Just helping them along. Healing is your job as a nurse. You help heal patients. They say it is *nursing* back to health not *doctoring* back to health.

In addition to healing your patient you have to remember to take care of yourself, and I think that is something a lot of nurses neglect; they forget they have to take care of themselves before they can take care of their patients. You've got to take a little time out for yourself every now and then. But always remembering that you are a "wounded healer" as well. There is always going to be something going on in your mind; you are always going to be dealing with something if you are in fact being empathic to your patient and being a caring nurse where you are getting involved with what is going on with the patient. A lot of time you have to push through that and do you best to take care of them.

Luke also spoke of Giving of Yourself:

I think if you are not going to come to work with a smile and if you are not going to come to work giving 100% you shouldn't come to work. Especially as a nurse because that bad energy that you bring to work is going to rub off on your colleagues and patients, and it is not going to help anything. We have to try, myself especially, to remember to try motivate without talking down to people. I think that is where nurses eat their young, to use the popular phrase, because I think a lot of the young nurses get burned out and don't stay in because it can be very fast paced, and they don't get the support they need from their seniors."

And, of seeing a Higher Purpose, including Advocacy, in his vocation:

Every nurse when they are taking care of their patients sees some higher purpose to their job. Myself as a Catholic, I see it as a corporal work of mercy to take care of people in their need. I don't do nursing for the sake of doing nursing, I do it because

I do believe it is my vocation, and I sincerely believe in taking care of people. We are all stewards; we are all in charge of our patients care, and that is synonymous with being the servant for your patient. The word *stewardship*, I think I would replace with *advocacy*. That is what nurses are: we are advocates for our patients. We have to be there for them, we have to defend them, we have to protect them…from themselves, their families, an order that we don't think is appropriate, care that we don't think is appropriate. That goes back to ethical and humanitarian treatment. You have to have a higher belief, something driving you to want to do good for these people. If you see that I think advocacy for your patient comes naturally after that.

Finally Luke described the importance of Staying Focused, Going the Extra Mile, and going Beyond the Ordinary as well as providing Compassionate Care and a Nurturing Environment for patients and staff:

You have to be committed to this job. It is a very strong sense of community in the nursing profession. Like I say, before you have to look out for each other and your patients become part of your community. Commitment is a challenge sometimes. Staying focused and going beyond the routine. It is easy to just come to work and do an assessment and pass meds and call it a day. It is important to take the extra minute and sit down with your patient and just simply chat with them sometimes. A lot of times you will find out more from your patient just from casually talking to them than talking about their disease process. It has been an issue as long as I've known about nursing, is that nurses don't have enough time to sit and talk to their patients and do that casual chat every now and then. I think it is important that we really try to go that extra mile and prevent the job from becoming routine.

When you are taking care of your patient, even though you may have three, four, or five other patients to take care of, you have to make that patient feel like he is the only patient you have. You can't let them think that you are rushed, that you are just trying to make them swallow their pills, and you are on your way to do the rest of your work with the other patient. You have to sit and take time. You need to facilitate that patient getting better. You can't expect him to be relaxed and put his best foot forward and give 110% if you are not willing to do that for him. On the same token, if you really do feel like that is happening, you have to tap your resources and get help from your fellow nurses or anyone you can to make sure the patient gets what he needs. In doing that I think we can provide a better recovering environment for our patients.

Emily, a 40-year-old Diploma RN working as team leader in a clinic setting, also spoke of the value of viewing her profession as having a Higher Purpose:

(After a stressful period) it helps to take just a second to recoup; recouping may give you another way of thinking about the situation, another way of handling the situation. Seeing a higher purpose: I think if you see your job as a profession in terms of a higher purpose, meaning I am trying to help this person be the best person they can be, it can give you some pep in your step. It helps keep me motivated and optimistic that I am doing some good.

Emily added:

Commitment at the end of the day is what makes you stay on the path of service. It will help you treat your job as more than a job. Serving people who came to you with their need. It is about what is going to make you do the best that you can for this person. It is what is going to make you at the end of the day feel good about what you have provided.

And Cathy, a 39-year-old master's-prepared team leader in critical care, echoed the thoughts of Emily in terms of helping others as a nursing leader:

Nursing is… just something that comes from my heart. I started nursing school years…years ago because I really loved nursing. I saw nursing as something that I can do to help my patients, and at the end of the day I can be satisfied with myself. At the end of the day I feel like I have helped somebody.

Three other team leaders also spoke about nursing servant leadership characteristics and themes:

The Sounds of Silence

Sometimes you don't get people to talk to you about what's going on. I had a specific interaction with a client's parent the other day. She did not want to talk, did not want any help at all. But it sort of made me think, "Oh well, maybe there is something I can do for this family anyway." It was bringing this thought out in me because I was the one caring for the family so much. So I thought maybe I can reach out to this family more, and in doing so I can build a relationship slowly (even if they are not talking about what's going on). It's these more difficult interactions that sort of solidify that I'm doing the right thing (in nursing), that this is my calling. (35, BSN, team leader, medical-surgical)

Beyond the Ordinary

Seeing nursing as a vocation informs and inspires nurses to go an extra measure with people: to think of things other people maybe hadn't thought of, to show empathy, or think of more creative solutions for patient problems. You have several different ways you can handle any situation with a patient. You can do just what is written down on a piece of paper and go out the door. Or you can spend extra time and try to figure out if there is some alternative; is there some reason why this woman is not taking her medication? Spend some time trying to figure out what the barriers are. (66, MSN, team leader, mental health)

Discerning a Decision

We've sent dying children home on palliative care, and that is very challenging, knowing that you're stopping all your care and sending them home. But it may be best for their future illness trajectory. I think that at times like this, viewing nursing as a vocation, we had to put our own emotions aside and help the family make the best decision. When you think about the needs of the child and the family, that's important to do. I think your personal faith comes in a lot in that situation.... I think that if you view nursing as a vocation, you're able to have more open conversations with the family, about what all this means, and help them make the decisions they need make. (34, BSN, team leader, pediatrics)

THE ADVANCED PRACTICE NURSE AS SERVANT LEADER

Among the titles included for advanced practice registered nurses, those commonly identified are the clinical nurse specialist (CNS), the certified nurse–midwife (CNM), the nurse practitioner (NP), and the certified registered nurse anesthetist (CRNA). One of the earliest of these advanced nursing roles, and sometimes one of the most ambiguous, is that of the clinical nurse specialist.

The Clinical Nurse Specialist

A clinical nurse specialist (CNS) is defined by the American Nurses Association as an "expert clinician and client advocate in a particular specialty or subspecialty of nursing practice" (ANA, 1996, p. 3). The clinical nurse specialist is an advanced practice nurse with graduate education, usually a master's degree, whose primary role may include that of consultant, patient educator, specialty healthcare provider, or case manager in a variety of healthcare settings. The CNS can work with individuals, groups, or families to improve care and enhance quality of life in situations of illness or injury.

Because CNSs work in so many different venues and carry myriad titles within the healthcare system, the role is often misunderstood. Clinical nurse specialists "account for the second largest group of advance practice nurses in the United States" (Henderson, 2004, p. 38); however, the role "elicits… confusion both inside and outside of the nursing profession" (p. 38). This role disconnection was also acknowledged in a 1997 article entitled, "Clinical Nurse Specialist Role Confusion: The Need for Identity" (Redekopp, 1997). Monica Redekopp admitted that "role confusion" for a clinical nurse specialist "may lead to frustration, hamper collaboration, contribute to conflict, prevent the CNS from optimizing knowledge and skills, and even result in deletion of the position" (p. 87). Redekopp points out that "clarification of the role requires identification of and insight into the specialty setting and the needs to be addressed" (p. 87). The bottom line is that CNSs must be able to articulate and defend their role and role responsibilities to others in the healthcare system in order to be effective.

The clinical nurse specialist role competencies are vast and varied depending upon the setting and specialty within which he or she functions. In 1998 the National Association of Clinical Nurse Specialists (NACNS) identified three broad domains of CNS core competencies; these focused on "patient/client, nurses and nursing personnel, and organization/system. These three competency domains were named the CNS spheres of influence...(and) became the organizing framework to describe CNS practice" (Baldwin, Lyon, Clark, Fulton, Davidson, & Dayhoff, 2007, p. 299).

Despite the issue of role confusion, many practicing clinical nurse specialists are well accepted and respected by the healthcare systems within which they function. The CNS can be "considered an important member of the healthcare team with an important contribution to make in improving the health of the general public and the quality of nursing care provided" (Henderson, 2004, p. 40).

For the clinical nurse specialist it would seem that the servant leadership characteristics of listening, assessing, and discerning might be his or her greatest gifts to the healthcare community.

The Nurse–Midwife

The certified nurse–midwife (CNM) is a title assigned to a registered nurse with a degree in midwifery who is trained to care for women during pregnancy, childbirth, and the postpartum period. The CNM is certified by an examination reviewed by a National Board of the American College of Nurse–Midwives. These nurses practice in hospitals, clinics, and physician's offices in both rural and urban areas of the country.

The Nurse Practitioner

The nurse practitioner (NP) is an advanced practice RN with a graduate degree in one or more specialty healthcare areas in which he or she is credentialed to practice.

The NP role is a very popular career choice among younger graduate nurses today. Nurse practitioners practice in myriad settings including hospitals, clinics, schools and, especially, in physician's offices where many NPs carry their own group of individual patients within a practice. Nurse practitioners specialize in such areas as adult health, family health, pediatrics, geriatrics, cardiovascular disease and community health. Nurse practitioners sit for credentialing exams in their field of study. The appropriately credentialed nurse practitioner has the authority to "diagnose and treat diseases and to prescribe" (Griffiths, 2006, p. 13). Thus, the nurse practitioners now undertake some of the "tasks and assume responsibilities traditionally associated with medicine" (Wilson & Bunnell, 2007, p. 35).

Some tasks of the nurse practitioner include those of "teacher, researcher, consultant, mentor and coach, leader, and ethical decision maker....The care the NP provides includes information on health maintenance and disease prevention, counseling, and patient education" (Rhoads, Ferguson, & Langford, 2006, p. 32). In some settings the NP role is "characterized by extended practice (including) prescribing of medications, requests for diagnostic investigations, referral to medical specialists, and admitting clients to inpatient facilities" (Allen & Fabri, 2005, p. 1202). It is also noted that "The nurse practitioner is in an ideal position to develop a therapeutic relationship with the patient and loved ones through use of clinical expertise, interpersonal skills, and presence" (Anderson, 2007, p. 14). NPs who are in private practice can avail themselves of the plethora of contemporary nursing research reports in order to "more effectively assist patients with healthcare decision making" (Kania-Lachance, Best, McDonah, & Ghosh, 2006, p. 46).

The servant leadership characteristics of listening, crossing over, advocating, discerning, and making a difference are especially appropriate for the daily practice of the nurse practitioner.

The Nurse Anesthetist

The certified registered nurse anesthetist (CRNA) is an advance practice nurse who has participated in a graduate education program of nurse anesthesia leading to a master's degree. The curriculum is overseen by the American Association of Nurse Anesthetists (AANA), Council on Accreditation of Nurse Anesthesia Education Programs. CRNAs are licensed to administer anesthesia to patients in multiple settings. The CRNA is certified by sitting for a national certification examination administered by the Council on Certification of Nurse Anesthetists.

All of the nursing servant leadership characteristics may be found in the population of advanced practice nurses; significant are those of Listening, Advocating, Discerning, and Nurturing.

Mark, a 30-year-old master's-prepared clinical specialist in pain management, and working in a critical care area, described his view of a good nursing leader:

> There are certain qualities in nurse leaders. Probably the first thing is that a good nursing leader definitely has a good, well-rounded bedside nursing experience. They can say they know what nurses go through day in and out. It can be a relatively challenging profession to be in because of the unpredictability and increase amounts of workload that are placed on nursing and increasing responsibilities that nurses have to take on during day-to-day activities. A nursing leader that understands that definitely shows far more superior characteristics in nursing leadership than someone who was never oriented to be a bedside nurse.

Mark spoke about Listening as a leadership quality:

Listening is a very important characteristic. We, here at the university, have an outstanding CNL, chief nursing officer. I've had conversations with her a few times, and every time I have spoken with her, she has always taken upon actually listening to what I have to say or what other people have to say. She definitely takes the time to stop whatever she is doing to listen to whatever someone has to say. It really trickles down the line as far as directors and patient care services. A lot of them also display a lot of the same characteristics. They are genuinely interested in what the frontline clinical nurses have to say and what their input is. They are valued and want to know what it is that is on the minds of the clinical nurses. I definitely think listening is a very important part of being a leader. You want to get the input of your staff because they are more of your eyes and ears in making an organization more successful. You want to know what their concerns are and be able to act on those concerns.

Mark added:

A good leader understands what the concerns are among their staff and is able to act on them and use their own opinions in order to make a decision that will positively affect nursing staff. Listening to someone, it could be "How can I help you?", going the extra mile, and trying to look at someone else's life. Healing doesn't always have to be some sort of pharmacological or technical intervention. It can be as simple as something like "How can I help you? Can I get something for you in order to correct the problem?" I think in nursing leadership it goes right up the line as far as from the bedside nurse all the way up to the highest nurse. They need to promote healing and a nurturing environment.

Being Grounded and self-aware were also considered important leadership characteristics by Mark:

One needs to identify what strengths and weaknesses they have. One, to focus on the weaknesses in order to make them stronger in that area. And to continue in those areas where one is strong. A nurse needs also to identify, especially in the leadership role, their weaknesses so they can find potentially the resources they need in order to facilitate healing. One needs to identify weaknesses in themselves. They can't set a good example as other nurses as far as helping them identify weaknesses. Because as humans we are all going to have weaknesses, and we need to identify them and be able to provide adequate resources to the patients and staff to facilitate success."

Mark embraced the nursing servant leadership role of Advocacy:

The middle management is in between their own staff and also in between more senior management, in advocating for their staff. Do they need more staffing? Do they need more resources? And what do they need to help facilitate a more efficient environment to work? The same holds true for upper management. Persuading the president or vice-president, "Hey, we need to make a change," "We need to give our nurses a raise," or "We need to provide better benefits for the nurses." If there is a need for a certain area of nursing in order to recruit, as far as offering a certain specialty of nursing, a different incentive, a different package in order to help build a unit. Even though health care is about health care, but health care is also a business. A lot of time in a nursing role a lot of nursing leaders are forced to make business decisions. Thus, the importance of advocacy for staff and patients.

Mark added:

Advocacy in the nursing leadership role becomes very effective as far as serving the needs of others. Looking out for what is needed for a nursing unit, looking out for what is needed for patient care technicians and nursing systems. A lot of times unfortunately they are overlooked. They are usually a very hard working corps of individuals that go unrecognized. So being able to advocate for these individuals and nurses is very important as far as the whole structure of healthcare leadership: in order to be able to speak out to their needs to others as far as providing better hours, better tools in order to facilitate better patient outcomes. It is very important in making a difference in their lives but also in the lives of the patients because they would be able to provide better patient care.

Mark believes that most nurses serve Beyond the Ordinary nursing role responsibilities assigned:

> There are a few nurses out there that come in do what they have to do and go home. There are a lot of nurses who come in, besides doing all their patient care, they also serve on committees, they also serve on groups and are looking for ways to improve efficiency in the unit and efficiency in patient care. Process improvement, quality assurance, all these factors, going above and beyond the call of duty, looking at "What are we doing now?" "What can we be doing better in order to facilitate optimal patient care?"
>
> I think this comes from the top down. A lot of times as a nursing leader they see nursing leader hop in and help out. That really sets a good example of true team work. Rather than the nursing leader that goes in her office, stays in her office all day and the unit is crazy busy and not even going to come out and help. It really makes a difference when they see their manager or nurse leader out there with them in the fire, in the trenches, helping out when there is a need. They really foster an environment that portrays team work. Teamwork in nursing is critical in providing optimal patient care, which then also usually leads to providing a nurturing environment. Nurses who feel like they are wanted on the unit are definitely going to provide more nurturing care to other patients but also to other staff.

Judy, a 58-year-old doctorally prepared nurse and nurse–midwife spoke about the importance of Making Connections:

> I am a nurse–midwife…and I had a young woman who had a miscarriage, actually had two, and we just connected for whatever reason. I see a lot of women who have miscarriages, but we connected! What is that that connects you to some people?…We connected very well, and I feel like I really helped her, but it may have been just my presence of being there. I certainly couldn't fix things for her, but I could be present.

Joan, a 48-year-old family nurse practitioner in a medical-surgical area, described nursing service as a religiously oriented Ministry:

> When I think of service, I always think about Jesus when he, I think just before his Last Supper and they were going to the

upper room and all of the disciples walked into the room, no one was given the job to wash feet. Jesus realized they had placed themselves too importantly. So he got up from the table and he washed their feet. Not to humiliate them, but to make them realize that even if you are in a position of authority, the most important call is to care for others. So when I think of service, I try to remember Jesus wrapped in a towel kneeling at his disciple's feet. It was the lowest task that he could possibly do. So when I think of servant leadership, no matter what city I've been in, in the hospital, I always try to communicate to people under me that I'm not too important to kneel down and wash their feet. I am never above doing one of the dirty tasks that you might do at bedside nursing. I just always try to remember humility. To be a good example like Jesus was for his disciples.

In speaking about the importance of Listening, Joan took up the problem of language incongruencies that can occur in today's urban hospitals:

It is hard right now to listen in the OB/GYN clinic because of the foreign languages. I try to communicate without words using touch, looking at someone if they are speaking to me, trying to help them understand that whatever they are saying is important to me. In community health I am seeing a whole lot of patients. People have called me a listener. When we are together I really try to hear what people are saying and to get at the heart of it. Not just listen to the words but find out what is behind the words. I can't think of a specific example, but I just end up finding myself helping to explain what is happening to them.

Joan added that in nursing there is definitely a Giving of Yourself:

You have to empty yourself in order to listen to what is going on with the other person. In order to be present and to be aware of their needs, you have to…empty yourself. I think self-awareness is really important. You always have to be aware of your framework—where you are coming from—because it colors how you hear what the other person is saying. When I forget that, then I have trouble. One time as a school nurse, I was back from Germany, I had been living as an American in Germany. I came back to serve in a school where it was mostly Americans. I don't know whether it was just a change from cultures, from Europe to America, or I was encountering a difference in cultures. I would be surprised with a parent who would be unhappy with my communication on the phone. I had to think more like the person I was talking to. I have to know more about their life, so I tried to find out more. That is one of the areas where I have a need to grow as a leader.

Joan also spoke about Generating Excitement among others:

In the work setting, I tend to get excited about topics. It is very hard for me to restrain my excitement, and in that way I think it flows over to other people. They either catch and want to participate, or I find out why they don't share my enthusiasm and see if that will help.

Finally Joan described her perception of nursing as a Higher Calling:

My desire for closeness with God and that desire flowing over into wishing benefit for the people whom I serve. If I think that the highest calling in life is to be so close to God that I can pray to him, share my every living moment with him, then I also want that for my nursing. I think that is an ideal of being whole, then I want that for other nurses too. I don't proselytize; I just hope for them that they can share the same ideal.

I think that we nurses give selflessly of ourselves and often don't think about taking care of our own needs. Out of the positive characteristics, which is the prime example for a nurse, I would say, it is that of commitment. We are very resourceful; we take what is at hand, and we fashion what is needed, always making sure that the needs of the patient are cared for above all else.

Sue, a 56-year-old, doctorally prepared nurse practitioner in women's health working in a private practice, noted that she served patients by:

providing good care and assessing and diagnosing and managing problems as they come up with and also serving as a sounding board for them when they have health problems or issues. I also serve my profession by serving on professional boards and organizations. I would find service in a lot of different ways but mostly in trying to help better the lives that I interact with.

One of Sue's most significant nursing servant leadership characteristics was Listening:

> In myself and other nurse leaders I think there are a lot of things we do to communicate that we are listening to people. I think one of the things that we do is to rephrase what someone says in our own words to make sure they know we are trying to understand what they are telling us. We do a lot of head nodding and head shaking to confirm that we are in tuned to what they are saying. We give verbal feedback sometimes, by saying "I understand what you mean" or "I can see why that would have been a difficulty for you." Sometimes we also use touch to show that we are listening, so we might put our arm around somebody who is having a difficult time or (if) they are failing a course or they have a bad diagnosis or marital problems. We also have colleagues that are having a difficult time, so we may encourage them to come see us so they have a sounding board. We may make suggestions on how they can confront a problem. For me all of those would indicate that I was an active listener.

Sue spoke about the concept of Crossing Over and trying to put herself in the place of patients who are suffering:

> For example, when I used to work labor and delivery, sometimes someone would come in with a fetal demise, totally unexpected death of her baby. Here she carried the baby for 9 months, and she comes into labor and delivery, and we can't find the heart beat. At that point in my career, the early parts, I had never had any children, so that I couldn't speak from personal experience, but I had had losses in my life, like death of grandparents, or illnesses in the family, that I think I could draw upon that made me more empathetic towards what they were going through. I know you can never assure somebody that everything is going to be alright, but I think you can tell them you are there to offer support.

Sue spoke of the desire to always Do the Best for her patients as the rational for her continuing to graduate nursing education:

> My desire is probably one of the biggest reasons why I've always kept my hands in clinical and why I pursued advanced nursing degrees, because I felt like at the undergraduate level, I

had some tools to help with healing a whole lot. But every time I went back for more education then the level of kind of healing things I could do got greater and greater. I was able to do diagnosis, I was able to manage, prescribe. By expanding my education, I also expanded the skills that I had in terms of healing. There were lots of experiences along the way that patients and colleagues taught me how to be better at helping serve other people. One of my patients was dying of breast cancer, and she used to come to my office every single week, and we would talk about what she was going through: she had a daughter in nursing school, and she wasn't going to live to see her daughter graduate. She knew her husband was suffering because his first wife had died of breast cancer, and here she was the second wife dying of breast cancer. A lot of the things that she suggested to me on how I could help other people really helped me a lot. I could translate those in caring for other patients, not just with breast cancer but other challenges. She taught me that the quality of life means a lot. She had some options to make decisions about really invasive treatments. She had to decide when to stop seeking those treatments. That was hard for me as a nurse. You want to give everybody everything because you hold out hope that there is going to be a miracle cure. She taught me a lot about giving permission to say enough.

Sue described the importance of Making Connections in her care of patients and families:

If I can get consensus by being very positive, that is my preferred method of working with other people. There have been times when I sort of had to use my position or some kind of authority to move an agenda forward. But that certainly isn't my preferred style. I do believe in team health care with the patient and family at the center of everything. I think positive input is the better way to persuade people than authoritative style. When I have the option, I would much rather seek consensus than use authority to persuade people.

I also do think it takes a village, and the way other people will get things done may be very different from the way I look at things as a nurse. If we really want to make a difference, we are probably going to have to work and play well together and not just be in our own discipline.

Sue gave an example of going Beyond the Ordinary and providing a nurturing environment in her practice:

There are a lot of ways I try to provide a nurturing environment. One is to make myself accessible to other people so they know they can reach me. The other thing is encouragement; for example, in my clinical practice I work with a young woman who was working as a nursing assistant but she really did not have any long-term goals for herself. We use to meet and talk and chat after we were done seeing patients. She decided she wanted to pursue a career in nursing, and now she is enrolled in a community college. It has been a struggle for her. She has had to work really hard to do okay. One of the ways I think I provided a nurturing environment is that I invited her to come to formal and informal studies sessions. If she is having trouble mastering content, she can come and talk with myself. She has talked to my daughter and my husband, and we have provided some tutoring. As a result of the tutoring she got an 89 on her last exam. It is those little sorts of successes in life that make it all worthwhile. I think by being a woman's health nurse practitioner, I think women are wired differently than men, and we give different kinds of support to each other than men do is by virtue of our genetics and the way we are raised. I think that by being a women's health nurse practitioner I am able to interact with a whole bunch of women and provide support they may not be able to get at home.

Sue concluded:

Somehow you have to have some kind either religious or philosophical or spiritual grounding that makes you want to help others and also that allows you to let others help you. There has…to be some sort of fundamental route that motivates you to interact with the human condition so that we can improve the lives of not only other people but ourselves.…We will grow and be better people as a result of these kinds of interactions.

Matthew, a 51-year-old nurse anesthetist working in a university-affiliated medical center, described the meaning of service in his role:

Service in terms of anything is just doing things for other people to try to make the world a better place or to give back to others. It is the same with nursing: the amount of shifts that I work; nights, weekends, and holidays are the schedules that I have done. Even if you are sick you go into work because you don't want to let them down, your patients and your coworkers. There is a calling; that is doing more for others than for yourself. I believe in that; that is why I have been doing this since 1982.

For Matt, Listening was a critical leadership characteristic:

Obviously, you have to listen to your patients. To students when I teach, it is pretty obvious if they understand or don't understand a concept by looking at their faces. They get uncomfortable, they roll their eyes. You have to be attentive to clues from patients and people you are teaching to see if they are following what you are trying to tell them and if are they interested. It is important when you lecture or teach a patient or work with a patient to know that they understand what you are saying. If they are not understanding what you are saying you try to figure out a different way of communicating with them.

Matt spoke of the need to Cross Over and understand a patient or family's concerns:

In my job, in anesthesia, you have to deal with a lot of issues — the family and the patient. Between the pain, the loss, sacrifice, and various things going on in a family's life or the patient's life, I think you have to understand where they are coming from….However, you can't get so caught up in what is going on with them that you can't focus on your job. Certainly I'm use to calling in pastoral care or grief counselors or those kinds of things. I see it (patient and family problems) and understand the importance of it, but there comes a time, and I don't think you as a provider should get so caught up in how badly the patient's family feels and what is going on that you can't function.

Matt continued:

In anesthesia I have a very specific focus and the same with ICU nurses, you have a very specific focus, and you can not get caught up too much in the psychosocial, spiritual, and all that when you are having to do a technical job. If you don't make a quick decision or follow through or are not technically proficient, the patient might get worse or die. The point is that is the easiest part of my job, is I know what to do and I know how to do it, and no matter how confusing the situation is I am able to do my job. I distance myself in that way just by intellect. I think there comes a time when being so emotionally wrapped in a situation you are not going to be able to function. I've been able to do that for many years of my career because I have dealt in (stressful) environments…where you don't have the luxury of empathizing too much because you really have a job to do….The good news is it doesn't just have to be you. Bring in a grief counselor, someone to talk with the family while I'm in the OR giving anesthesia for someone who might die. It is a lot easier having someone out there totally distant from what we are trying to do, talking to the family.

Matthew described the nurse anesthetist as a patient Advocate:

I believe we are patient advocates. No matter what a surgeon or med student or somebody that is not doing a really good job wants to do, I have the authority and responsibility in my role to say, "You are not doing any good for the patient right now," or "I question what you are doing." Someone has to be an advocate, and they know what is best. If people aren't talking to the family, the study we are doing now on occupational trauma, at my facility we deal with trauma, we are *it* in the state. There are still things we can do better for the patient and family if the patient is not able to defend themselves or can't any longer and they are going to a nursing home. Then you still have the family to deal with. They have a lot of concerns and issues that have to be addressed. You can always do better. Someone has to serve the family and patient's interest because that is why we are here. We are a serving profession. You sacrifice some of yourself to do what you are going to do. Mentally most people can make the adjustment and decide that you are serving a higher purpose. In some lives it makes a great difference. They change their direction in life; they totally turn around. I've had a few patients that I took care of that are 15, 16, getting ready to graduate high school, bad judgment, bad accident, etc., and they actually come back and see you later and say that they went to nursing school or medical school. It was like a wake up call. Some never learn. You can't save them all. I give anesthesia. I do that kind of technical skill and some cognitive, but the point is it is what I do. I distance myself case to case. They will all get the same care. I don't care who you are and what you did, you are still going to get the same level of attention from me. As long as I continue to do that, I should keep my job. If you start to make a difference in who you are taking care of and you decide one person gets one level of care and another gets another, you need to move on. You shouldn't be doing the job you are doing. When I start thinking that way and let it dictate my practice, I think it is time for me to move on. Until then I feel like I am serving the profession, the patient, and the hospital.

THE PARISH NURSE AS SERVANT LEADER

Parish nursing, or congregational nursing as it is sometimes referred to, was first labeled as such by a Lutheran minister, Reverend Dr. Granger Westberg, around the mid-1980s. In his book, *The Parish Nurse: Providing a Minister of Health for Your Congregation*, Westberg advocated a team approach to health care that would include a pastoral care representative as well as those from medicine and nursing: "This triumvirate of doctor, nurse, and pastor symbolized for me a type of patient care I had always dreamed about" (1990, p. 15). Ultimately Westberg "rediscovered church-based nursing and called it *parish nursing*" (Carson & Koenig, 2002, p. xvi).

Parish nursing was recognized as a specialty area of nursing in 1997 by the American Nurses Association (ANA) Congress of Nursing Practice. The *Scope and Standards of Parish Nursing Practice* was acknowledged by the ANA in February of 1998 (p. iii). Parish nurses serve in a variety of faith communities carrying out the roles of health advocate, health educator, health counselor, health referral agent, and liaison with healthcare organizations. Their "pastoral goal, as representative of his or her faith community, is to care for the spiritual needs of the ill members of the congregation" (O'Brien, 2003, pp. 20–21).

Parish nurses "as ministers of health in congregations, seek to assist people to integrate their faith and their physical/emotional health, and in doing so, to 'live life abundantly' (John 10:10)" (Smith, 2003, p. 11). Essentially, "parish nursing programs are a religious response to help bring wholeness and healing to the faith community" (Stewart, 2000, p. 116).

The servant leadership characteristics of listening, giving, ministering, and nurturing are central to the caring ministry of the nurse serving in a faith community.

Annemarie is a 65-year-old doctorally prepared part-time parish nurse who has ministered to parishioners in their homes, in hospitals, and in nursing homes. Annemarie described the servant leader role of the parish nurse as especially centering on the nursing servant leadership theme of Doing Ministry. The parish nurse's activities also highlighted the servant leadership characteristic of Listening.

> The parishioners that I care for, that I minister to, are mostly older and with a lot of health problems physically; some are cognitively impaired as well. But they all love to have the parish nurse come, as a representative of the church, to minister to them. I help them with any health problems or questions. Sometimes I pray with them, or read the Bible if they want, or sometimes just listen. Really listening is a very big thing in parish nursing. Older folks love to reminisce about the past. Talking about the good things that happened in the past sort of validates their lives and helps them accept where they are now in the journey of life. I think listening is probably the most important part of the parish nursing servant leadership ministry.

THE NURSE EDUCATOR AS SERVANT LEADER

Professional nurse educators serve in a variety of settings that prepare contemporary registered nurses for ministry in today's healthcare system. Nurse educators currently teach in diploma nursing programs, of which there are now less than 100 in the country; associate degree nursing programs; and baccalaureate, master's, and doctoral programs in nursing. The role of the nurse educator is primarily that of teacher, advisor, and mentor, vis-à-vis his or her students. An academic position may also require a faculty member to assume the roles of researcher, public speaker, and author, however, if he or she wishes to be promoted or achieve tenure at the institution.

Some nurse educators, especially those teaching in specialty areas such as nurse practitioner programs, are required to keep current with clinical skills and credentialing, as appropriate to their academic assignments. Four factors are identified as important for the nurse educator to succeed when guiding students in the clinical setting. These include: "(1) agreement among staff, leadership, and educator expectations; (2) acquisition of successful educator characteristics; (3) ability to deal with challenges; and (4) creation and completion of a plan for continually updating skills and assuming various responsibilities" (Mateo & Fahje, 1998, p. 169). Mateo and Fahje observe that "successful educators possess leadership, management, and communication skills, as well as political savvy and clinical expertise" (p. 169). One study of nurse educators in the clinical role revealed that while nurse educators did focus on supervision of students when in the clinical areas, they might have worked harder to "forge links with professional staff" (Griscti, Jacono, & Jacono, 2005, p. 84).

Another important task of the nurse educator relates to the role of advisor and counselor to students preparing for graduation from a nursing program. Currently students, completing an accredited nursing program of study, have a vast array of possibilities for healthcare service open to them. The guidance, advice, and suggestions of potential post-graduation job possibilities can be very helpful in directing a student to a satisfactory and growth-producing professional nursing role. As Kirkpatrick and Koldjeski point out "In a rapidly changing healthcare environment, nurses approaching career planning need a stable core of principles and a flexible set of guidelines from which to consider existing and emerging opportunities" (1997, p. 17).

Some educators serve in healthcare settings, such as hospitals and clinics, as well as in academic institutions. In the hospital-based role, the nurse educator may often function as a consultant to staff as well as a patient educator. Consultation "is one component of the nurse educator's role (which)...is rapidly expanding as the healthcare system changes" (Forsyth, Rhudy, & Johnson, 2002, p. 197). With the aging of our society, resulting in more seriously ill patients being hospitalized and thus the increasing complexity of treatment regimens, the nurse educator in the hospital or medical center may become a critically important mentor and guide for nursing staff at all levels of patient care. It is the nurse educator who can research and teach new and innovative methods of nursing intervention that promote the implementation of evidence-based practice and excellent patient-centered care.

For the nurse educator, either in academia or the healthcare setting, the servant leadership characteristics of listening, advocating, and making a difference bring an important dimension of caring to the community being served.

Teresa, a 38-year-old doctorally prepared nurse teaching adult health nursing in a university, shared her perception of service and leadership:

> Personally I think that service is the utmost important part of leadership. I work in a Christian school, and considering that we are suppose to be Christ-like and Christ came to serve, that

is how we too are supposed to lead through service. And I believe that it is in that service, service means to me that instead of doing for myself, I directly am doing for another person. I'm helping them to grow and to change and to see what it is in themselves that is going to make the student a good nurse or a good leader. And I do that through serving them the best way I can. Right now how I'm doing that is through education and providing information and opportunities for the students to learn and grow.

Teresa highlighted Listening as central to servant leadership in nursing. Her comments also reflect the concept of seeking to unravel the Mystery Behind the Visit:

First of all I personally believe that listening is probably the most important thing we do for each other. I think that it is in listening that we learn what is needed to be done and how we can best help. How do I utilize listening in my everyday work is as students come in to talk with me I try to explore what it is that they really need. So if they say something to me, I don't just take it as face value. I want to hear more what it is that is either deeply motivating them or troubling them. I believe that is done in dialogue.

I had a student come in who was not doing so well academically. I also knew, because I have had a relationship with her now for over half a semester, that she doesn't have the very best background family. In the course of our conversation, talking about academics, she had said previously to me that she had been the primary care provider for her brothers and sister. This is a traditional student. She is at the point where she might need to take custody of one of her brother and sisters. In listening to her and hearing what she was saying, I was able to say to her, "You know, let's back up just a little bit here. We need to find out what is really going on. Is this the best time for you to be in school? Do we need to back up and pull you out of some classes? Do we need to continue on so you can get finished and then be this person who is going to be the guardian for the children? What are your needs in this situation?" And I think it was through listening to her that I could respond better. At least she felt listened to and knew what decisions she needed to make. It was up to her and her different options. It had a good outcome.

Teresa's comments about caring reflected the nursing servant leadership concept of Crossing Over:

> Caring to me is kind of getting inside their skin. To know it is actually to put myself, that I can hear and listen so well, that I can actually be able to relate with it. I had another student that kind of came in with a crisis situation where she has her boyfriend who was just let out of prison and he use to beat her. I could step back and say are "You afraid for your safety." When I found out the information, I was able to hear and empathize with her. I could say "Do you need more time before you take your next test? Because it seems to me right now you are not in the right state of mind to be able to do this. Do we need to step back here now and take some time so you can care for yourself and get back in a safe situation and then take the test a day or two later?"

Teresa also gave an example of being an Advocate for her students:

> We were at this student nurses convention and I had one of my students...and I could tell by looking at her that she was getting more and more stressed. Because of that she didn't come for the last speaker. And the last speaker happen to be the best speaker we had, talking about the importance of presence and was just very motivational, and he had written a book about the topic he was talking about. Since she missed this particular speaker, and I knew she was feeling very stressed, I went and got her a copy of the book. And when the conference was over, I called her out and said "I got this for you because I feel like you would have loved to be here for the speaker, and this is really going to speak to you." So when I got back yesterday, she had e-mailed me and said how much that had touched her.

Teresa explained the importance of Staying Focused as a nurse educator:

> I call it reflective practice, and I think that is very important. I think I continually do that. Even this past weekend, I have been going over everything that happened at the state convention. What is it that went well? I had a group of students that didn't engage, and I had a group that engaged very well. What can I do next time to help those that didn't engage to engage more? If they put something into this, they are going to get

something out of it. But if they don't put anything into this, then they are not going to (get anything out). It is the whole idea of reflecting back on things that have happened, things that have worked and haven't worked, and if they haven't worked now what can I do at the present and even after that in the future that is going to make this work?

The advocacy concept of Protecting and Defending was displayed in other experiences Teresa had with students:

Service to students, in my mind, also means care: taking good care because I am holding them in trust. I think when these students come into my office and share things with me in their personal life that I need to hold that in confidence or that I have this piece of information that might explain why this particular student is really down right now. I do have that piece because I have been entrusted with it. Now it is, what do I do with that information? Sometimes I just need to hold it. Hold it is trust. The other day I had a student come in that had been sexually assaulted. I had this piece of information now in trust and I'm holding, it but because it is such an important thing I need to take it somewhere else along with the student. I think that is what that piece is. It is a piece when they come in and you know something that they have trusted you with, some part of themselves that may not have told me, but in my profession I have learned that I hold in trust and care for, and maybe because of it I am going to treat them a little differently. Not special, but differently, because I have more of the information than the rest of the class does. In the beginning of class when we have prayer, I always say "Can we please hold one another in prayer because we do not know everything that everyone is dealing with right now." I think that is a piece of that too.

Teresa admitted to sometimes going Beyond the Ordinary educational practice in her care for students:

Caring is the willingness to put more into than just the 8-hour day. It is the student that calls me up and says can you come over to your office and go through this with me one more time. And I come over and do that. They are taking their final exams, and because I want them to do well I have many times said they can come in and look at their test and study. I had a group of students say "None of those times work for us. Is there anyway you can come over at 9 tonight and just open the lab for a couple of hours and let us study?" To me it is a sign of commitment that I am willing to go that extra mile for them so that again they will learn and they will grow to the potential that I believe they can if they have that time.

Teresa concluded by sharing some thoughts on nursing servant leadership:

> I think nursing servant leadership is what it is all about. I think that leadership is service, something that we are called to do and responsible for. It is that whole story of the more that you have been given then the more it is going to be called for you. I believe that I have been given many gifts, and because of that now it is my responsibility to use those wisely in service and leadership.

Tom, a 47-year-old baccalaureate-prepared nurse educator in a hospital setting, spoke of service in leadership:

> A nursing leader is someone who can delegate and also do the job himself, (someone who) isn't afraid to do the job, isn't afraid to do any job. There is no job too menial. And constantly thinking of the patient as a person, as a whole person, not just as a case or a diagnosis. As a leader being a good role model to others.

Tom also described the importance of Listening:

> Obviously not all our patients can talk, but the ones that can, I think it helps the patient that you do listen to them. Sometimes they are so anxious, they just need to get something off their chest, and we have to realize that we don't just rush somebody through that just so we can do our job, but that is part of our job: to alleviate their fears and anxieties. This actually has a big impact on them. Not everybody realizes that some people just want to get through that so we can get to do the work, get the job done. A lot of people still do realize that. Patients want to speak and get it off their chest.

Tom included several of the nursing servant leadership concepts in his understanding of his role as a patient educator; these included Making a Difference, Being Grounded, Going Beyond the Ordinary, Becoming an Advocate, and providing a Nurturing Environment:

> If you go back to the reason we went into this in the first place, you realize I do make a difference; I actually help take care of people during the day. Sometimes you don't see it when you

are actually working, sometimes you actually see it when you are out in other life and your kids are talking about what you do. It keeps you going. You are always a nurse....You take ownership of your profession. It's a full-service kind of caring. You have to think of all the different aspects of it. With grounding you own it; you don't just come in, put your time in, and leave. You actually have to put in the type of commitment to achieve the goals that are necessary. You need to do what needs to be done. Sometimes it take extra effort or time.

The other thing that comes to mind is being a patient advocate, especially when it comes to the legal points of concern, the procedures that are being done. Just the care the patient receives and the trust they put in you.

You are not only committed to the care of the patient, but you are committed to your coworkers. Encouraging them to stay the course and encourage people that are new to the profession to continue on, not to drop it and go somewhere else, (being) committed to providing a positive environment. Going beyond the routine that is part of the profession, not just doing what you have to but doing everything you feel needs to be done. Sometimes it takes a lot of extra effort.

Three other nurse educators identified nursing servant leadership themes.

Beyond the Ordinary

For the most part my students have my cell phone number, and they can call me 24/7. They are only supposed to contact me in case of emergency. Of course, that goes along with who defines what an emergency is (for a student). Sometimes they just need me to listen and to care. I have gotten calls at 7:30 a.m., and the phone will ring till 10 or 11 at night. Weekends, Saturdays, Sunday, it doesn't make a difference....For the most part, I answer the phone, answer their questions...I have a student text messaging me now! (45, educator, MSN, medical-surgical)

A Sacred Trust

Viewing nursing as a spiritual calling is very important in working with suffering or dying patients. I see myself as being able to be present to them as Saint Teresa said "to be

Jesus' hands and feet and to look with his compassion on their suffering." My own faith also helps me support them in their suffering and dying because I believe that there is life with the Lord after death and that all suffering has meaning. And I trust that while God does not send suffering, he is with us in the midst of it. (69, educator, PhD, RN, adult health)

Assessing Needs

One of the things that I've had to keep in mind as a head nurse and a supervisor is to be always looking down the road in terms of patient needs, staff needs, hospital needs, and even my own needs. You have to try and anticipate problems and needs in order to keep one step ahead of all of the potential crises that can occur; and believe me they are right there on the horizon ready to zonk you. So, it's a case of always thinking ahead; keeping one step ahead of the "noon-day" devil as they say. (69, PhD, RN, educator, adult health)

THE NURSE RESEARCHER AS SERVANT LEADER

The majority of nurse researchers are found in academic institutions where the conduct of empirical research is considered an integral part of the faculty role. Nurse researchers can also be found in some of the larger healthcare facilities where both the institution's interest and budget are adequate to support the conduct of research. For hospitals seeking the currently prized Magnet status, nursing research is very favorably viewed by the evaluators.* In the ideal nursing research setting an academic institution has its own affiliated hospital or medical center where school of nursing faculty may conduct their studies.

As professional nursing "stretches to enlarge a body of knowledge that is uniquely nursing, the demand for nurses who will participate in research increases" (Ellis & Hartley, 2008, p. 511). Ellis and Hartley point out, of course, that nursing research must be conducted by individuals who are knowledgeable about the research process: "This may be a nurse with a master's degree, but for large studies, for funded research, and in large institutions, the principal researcher is usually a nurse with a doctorate"

---

*Magnet hospital status is an award granted by the American Nurses Credentialing Center (ANCC) to a healthcare facility that meets the ANCC standards for excellent patient-centered care.

(2008, p. 223). Additionally, a nursing research problem and purpose must be selected based on the background knowledge and understanding of the topic on the part of the investigator (Burns & Grove, 2005, p. 82).

One of the most important characteristics of a nurse researcher is the ability to process and organize large amounts of data in order to achieve meaningful conclusions that may be communicated to practicing nurses. Three major thought processes that are important for the nurse researcher to possess are "introspection" or the ability to examine one's own thoughts in depth, "intuition" or "an insight or understanding of a situation or event as a whole that cannot be logically explained," and "reasoning" defined as "the processing and organizing of ideas in order to reach conclusions" (Burns & Grove, 2005, pp. 6–7).

For the nurse conducting qualitative research (the seeking of narrative data reflective of the phenomenon or phenomena under study) six specific attributes are recommended

1. Commitment to transparency — Documentation of a decision trail to justify decisions
2. Commitment to absorption and diligence — Meticulousness and thoroughness in analyzing narrative data
3. Commitment to verification — The process of checking, confirming, and making sure the data and analysis procedures are accurate
4. Commitment to reflexivity — Bracketing or carefully analyzing and documenting…presuppositions, biases, and ongoing emotions
5. Commitment to participant-driven inquiry — The inquiry is driven forward by the participants, not the researcher
6. Commitment to insightful interpretation — Being able and confident in using one's own insight in conducting analysis of narrative data (Polit & Beck, 2008, pp. 551–552).

The servant leadership characteristics of listening, crossing over, assessing, and discerning are especially relevant for the nurse researcher conducting empirical studies, especially among persons who are ill or infirm.

Martha, a 68-year-old doctorally prepared nurse educator and researcher working in the areas of chronic and life-threatening illness, described her research-related activities as encompassing the nursing servant leadership ministry concept a Sacred Trust:

For me the role of the nurse researcher is definitely a servant leadership role. As a nurse researcher, study participants frequently entrust us with very personal and painful accounts of coping with illness, either their own or that of loved ones. These study participants expect us to listen compassionately and caringly to their stories and to handle the data they share with us with the utmost care and confidence. This is a sacred trust. We are blessed to become confidants to the sick and the suffering, and we have an ethical responsibility to protect both the study subjects and the things that they tell us. This is a trust given us by God as nurse researchers.

This chapter has included data reflecting the perceptions and experiences of contemporary nurse servant leaders functioning at a variety of levels: administration, management, clinical supervision (head nursing, charge nursing, and team leading), parish nursing, education, and research. The nursing servant leaders' comments well display the key themes and concepts of nursing servant leadership as identified in the model of servant leadership in nursing presented in Chapter 6. While the term *servant leadership* is, admittedly, relatively new to professional leadership in nursing, the characteristics of the concept have been understood and practiced by nurses since the inception of the discipline. This remains true today and is present in a variety of nursing care environments such as the hospital, clinic, long-term care facility, parish, and community, as described in the following chapter.

REFERENCES

Allen, J., & Fabri, A. M. (2005). An evaluation of a community of aged care nurse practitioner service. *Journal of Clinical Nursing, 14*(10), 1202–1209.

American Nurses Association. (1996). *Scopes and standards of advanced practice registered nursing.* Washington, DC: American Nurses Publishing.

American Nurses Association. (1998). *Scope and standards of parish nursing practice.* Washington, DC: American Nurses Publishing.

Anderson, J. H. (2007). Nursing presence in a community heart failure program. *Nurse Practitioner: The American Journal of Primary Health Care, 32*(10), 14–21.

Andrews, D. R., & Dziegielewski, S. F. (2005). The nurse manager: Job satisfaction, the nursing shortage and retention. *Journal of Nursing Management, 13*(4), 286–295.

Baldwin, K. M., Lyon, B. L., Clark, A. P., Fulton, J., Davidson, S., and Dayhoff, N. (2007). Developing clinical nurse specialist practice competencies. *Clinical Nurse Specialist: A Journal for Advanced Nursing Practice, 21*(6), 297–302.

Barter, M. (2002). Follow the team leader. *Nursing Management, 33*(10), 54–57.

Burns, N., & Grove, S. K. (2005). *The practice of nursing research: Conduct, critique and utilization*. St. Louis, MO: Elsevier Saunders.

Carson, V. B., & Koenig, H. G. (2002). *Parish nursing: Stories of service and care*. Philadelphia: Templeton Foundation Press.

Cherry, B., Marshall-Gray, P., Laurence, A., Green, A., Valadez, A., Scott-Tilley, D., et al. (2007). The geriatric training academy: Innovative education for certified nurse aides and charge nurses. *Journal of Gerontological Nursing, 33*(3), 37–44.

Corrigan, P. W., Lickey, S. E., Campion, J., & Rashid, F. (2000). Mental health team leadership and consumers satisfaction and quality of life. *Psychiatric Services, 51*(6), 781–785.

Cumbey, D. A., & Alexander, J. W. (1998). The relationship of job satisfaction with organizational variables in public health. *Journal of Nursing Administration, 28*(5), 39–46.

Drach-Zahavy, A., & Dragan, E. (2002). From caring to managing and beyond: An examination of the head nurse's role. *Journal of Advanced Nursing, 38*(1), 19–28.

Ellis, J. R., & Hartley, C. L. (2008). *Nursing in today's world: Trends, issues and management* (9th ed.). Philadelphia: Lippincott Williams & Wilkins.

Forsyth, D. M., Rhudy, L., & Johnson, L. M. (2002). The consultation role of a nurse educator. *Journal of Continuing Education in Nursing, 33*(5), 197–202.

Garrison, D. R., Morgan, D. A., & Johnson, J. G. (2007). Management theory. In R. A. Patronis Jones (Ed.), *Nursing leadership and management: Theories, processes and practice* (pp. 13–28). Philadelphia: F.A. Davis.

Glasscock, F. E., & Hales, A. (1998). Bowen's family systems theory: A useful approach for a nurse administrator's practice. *Journal of Nursing Administration, 28*(6), 37–42.

Graham, I. (2003). Leading the development of nursing with a nursing development unit: The perspectives of leadership by the team leader and a professor of nursing. *International Journal of Nursing Practice, 9*(4), 213–222.

Greenleaf, R. K. (1977). *Servant leadership: A journey into the nature of legitimate power and greatness*. New York: Paulist Press.

Griffiths, H. (2006). Advanced nurse practice: Enter the nurse practitioner. *Nursing BC, April*, 12–16.

Grindel, C. (2005). AACN presents the clinical nurse leader and the doctor of nursing practice roles: A benefit or a misfortune. *Medsurg Nursing, 14*(4), 209–210.

Griscti, O., Jacono, B., & Jacono, J. (2005). The nurse educator's clinical role. *Journal of Advanced Nursing, 50*(1), 84–92.

Hartranft, S. R., & Garcia, T. (2007). Realizing the anticipated effects of the clinical nurse leader. *Journal of Nursing Administration, 37*(6), 261–263.

Henderson, S. (2004). The role of the clinical nurse specialist in medical-surgical nursing. *Medsurg Nursing, 13*(1), 38–41.

Kania-Lachance, D. M., Best, P. J., McDonah, M. R., & Ghosh, A. K. (2006). Evidence-based practice and the nurse practitioner. *Nurse Practitioner: American Journal of Primary Health Care, 31*(10), 46–54.

Kerfoot, K. (2006). Reliability between nurse managers: The key to the high-reliability organization. *Nursing Economics, 24*(5), 274–275.

Kirkpatrick, M. K., & Koldjeski, D. (1997). Career planning: The nurse educator as facilitator and career counselor. *Nurse Educator, 22*(3), 17–20.

Laschinger, H. K., & Finegan, J. (2005). Using empowerment to build trust and respect in the workplace. *Nursing Economics, 23*(1), 6–13.

Mateo, M., & Fahje, C. J. (1998). The nurse educator role in the clinical setting. *Journal for Nurses in Staff Development, 14*(4), 169–175.

Newhouse, R. P., & Mills, M. E. (2002). Enhancing professional environment in the organized delivery system: Lessons in building trust for the nurse administrator. *Nursing Administration Quarterly, 26*(3), 67–75.

Nilsson, K., & Larsson, U. (2005). Conceptions of gender: A study of female and male head nurses' statements. *Journal of Nursing Management, 13*(2), 179–186.

O'Brien, M. E. (2003). *Parish nursing: Healthcare ministry within the church.* Sudbury, MA: Jones and Bartlett.

O'Keefe, M. (2007). Regulating nursing. In R. A. Patronis Jones (Ed.), *Nursing leadership and management: Theories, processes and practice* (pp. 69–93). Philadelphia: F.A. Davis.

Pinkerton, S. (2003). Supporting the nurse manager to improve staff nurse retention. *Nursing Economics, 21*(1), 45–46.

Polit, D. F., & Beck, C. T. (2008). *Nursing research: Generating and assessing evidence for nursing practice.* Philadelphia: Lippincott Williams & Wilkins.

Redekopp, M. A. (1997). Clinical nurse specialist role confusion: The need for identity. *Clinical Nurse Specialist: Journal for Advanced Nursing Practice, 11*(2), 87–91.

Rhoads, J., Ferguson, L. A., & Langford, C. A. (2006). Measuring nurse practitioner productivity. *Dermatology Nursing, 18*(1), 32–34, 37–38.

Rogers, L. G. (2005). Why trust matters: The nurse manager-staff nurse relationship. *Journal of Nursing Administration, 35*(10), 421–423.

Seavor, C. (2007). Building teams for productivity and efficiency. In R. A. Patronis Jones (Ed.), *Nursing leadership and management: Theories, processes and practice* (pp. 183–200). Philadelphia: F.A. Davis.

Sherman, R. O. (2005). Don't forget our charge nurses. *Nursing Economics, 23*(3), 125–130, 143.

Smith, P. K. (2003). An important role of the parish nurse: Integrator of faith and health. *Stat Bulletin of the Wisconsin Nurses Association, 72*(9), 11.

Smith, D. S., & Dabbs, M. T. (2007). Transforming the care delivery model in preparation for the clinical nurse leader. *Journal of Nursing Administration 37*(4), 157–160.

Stewart, L. E. (2000). Parish nursing: Renewing a long tradition of caring. *Gastroenterology Nursing, 23*(3), 116–120.

Suominen, T., Savikko, N., Puukka, P., Doran, D. I., & Leino-Kilpi, H. (2005). Work empowerment as experienced by head nurses. *Journal of Nursing Management, 13*(2), 147–153.

Tachibana, C., & Nelson-Peterson, D. L. (2007). Implementing the clinical nurse leader role using the Virginia Mason production system. *Journal of Nursing Administration, 37*(11), 477–479.

Valiga, T. M., and Grossman, S. (2007). Leadership and followership. In R. A. Patronis Jones (Ed.) *Nursing leadership and management: Theories, processes and practice* (pp. 3-12). Philadelphia: F.A. Davis.

Westberg, G. E. (1990). *The parish nurse: Providing a minister of health for your congregation.* Minneapolis, MN: Augsburg Press.

Wiggens, M. S. (2006). The partnership care delivery model. *Journal of Nursing Administration, 36*(7–8), 341–345.

Wilson, J., & Bunnell, T. (2007). A review of the merits of the nurse practitioner role. *Nursing Standard, 21*(18), 35–40.

7 Servant Leadership in the Healthcare Setting

Are you able to drink the cup that I am about to drink?
                                                    —Matthew 20:22

I can give an example of the nursing call to serve in the hospital setting. They admitted an older patient, a man in his later 60s, 2 hours before I was supposed to go off shift. He had colon cancer and had a mass very low in the GI tract and was having surgery the next day. And he had to have enemas 'til clear, and there was obviously a tumor obstruction....Even though I am a pediatric nurse, I volunteered to do the procedure. I tried to be very gentle. You know when you meet an obstruction you need to go very gently, to see how you can maneuver the catheter.

His wife thanked me for being so kind and gentle because her husband was in a lot of pain. I made sure he was medicated, made sure I really took my time when I did the enemas. He went to surgery and afterward to the intensive care, but he didn't make it.

Sometime later I got this beautiful note from his wife, and she said to me in the letter "I just want to thank you so much because those were the last conscious hours of my husband's life. The next morning he went to surgery and had general anesthesia, and went to the intensive care unit and never woke up. And I take so much comfort in knowing that in the last hours of his life in which he was conscious that you helped make him comfortable; you took your time, and treated him with such compassion. You did those repeated enemas in such a way, so carefully, that you weren't creating more pain, more discomfort."

To me all that (care and compassion) was influenced because of my feeling that I am there to serve patients. That is why I am a nurse....I feel that I am blessed to be able to do that.

                                        —Teresa, nurse educator in pediatrics

291

When, many centuries ago, the mother of two of the Lord's disciples asked if her sons, James and John, could be assigned places of honor in his kingdom, Jesus replied: "You do not know what you are asking. Are you able to drink the cup that I am about to drink?" (Matthew 20:22). The Lord's response was meant to illustrate the fact that "in order to share in his kingdom, the disciples must share his cup of suffering" (Harrington, 1991, p. 84). Jesus was "challenging James and John to take very seriously what it means to follow him to glory" (Van Linden, 1991, p. 60). The two brothers immediately asserted: "We are able" (Matthew 20:22).

Of course the disciples James and John had not yet witnessed the Lord's passion and death; I sometimes wonder if the brothers would have been so quick to respond affirmatively to Jesus' challenge if they had observed his suffering. I also wonder if we living Christians can respond so positively when we truly consider the "cup" of suffering and sorrow from which our Lord was asked to drink.

We as nurses, serving in the healthcare setting, are asked to drink of a cup of suffering in witnessing daily the painful illnesses and infirmities of our patients. We are asked to take on the sorrow and the suffering of those for whom we care when, as servant leaders, we seek to live out such attributes as Listening with the Heart, Giving of Ourselves, Ministering, Advocating, Serving, and Nurturing. We are asked not only to drink of the cup but to indeed become a chalice from which others may imbibe strength and courage.

THE NURSE'S CHALICE OF SERVANT LEADERSHIP

I had never really thought of my life as a chalice until I read the small book *Poverty of Spirit* by the famous German theologian Johannes Baptist Metz. In describing the self-acceptance and self-awareness of one's humanity as a basic Christian principle, Metz observed that we demonstrate our desire to follow God's will by embracing the "chalice of our existence" (1998, p. 5). Metz also suggested that the "process of becoming a human being unfolds as a process of service" (p. 4). We nurses can reflect our desire to follow the Lord's mandate to care for the sick by embracing the "chalice of our servant leadership."

The word *chalice* suggests a number of understandings. For Christians the term evokes an image of the cup used by Jesus to consecrate the blessed wine at the last supper. The chalice, in ecclesiastical usage, describes the sacred vessel "used to contain the wine consecrated in the Eucharist" (Livingstone, 1990, p. 100). The concept of the holy cup or chalice of Christ is also referred to in many historical legends as the

Holy Grail. In general understanding, however, a chalice is a goblet or cup to hold liquid for drinking.

I think perhaps I like Johannes Metz's conceptualization of our lives, and thus our nursing servanthood, as a chalice, because it reminds me of the "earthen vessels" scripture: the biblical analogy that teaches that we are all only "clay jars," yet we contain within us the light of Christ. The metaphor of one's life, viewed as a chalice, works very well for us as professional nurses. Look at the example of a hospital staff nurse, a clinic nurse, a hospice nurse, or a nurse in a variety of other caregiving venues. He or she generally begins a work shift full of enthusiasm and energy; ready to take on the challenges of the day. The nurse's "chalice" of servant leadership gifts is full: full of scholarly knowledge, full of technical skill, full of caring and compassion, and full of commitment to duty and a desire to serve, to the best of one's ability, the ill and the infirm.

As the workday progresses, however, the contents of a nurse's "chalice" of caring are continually poured out for those in need. At the conclusion of a shift, a nurse may feel exhausted and empty, a recognition that the contents of his or her chalice of service have been significantly, or even completely, depleted. This temporary emptiness of a nurse's caregiving chalice is, nevertheless, a blessed gift. For it is only in such emptiness that the Lord can fill us with his own healing compassion and love. It is only when we have an open and uncluttered space in our spirit that the Lord can reveal his presence and reenergize us with the blessing of servant leadership.

NURSING SERVANT LEADERSHIP IN THE HOSPITAL

It might be suggested that the contemporary healthcare venue most in need of servant leadership is the modern American hospital. With its complex technology, incredible array of medical and social services, high-powered administrative structure and demanding financial constraints, the modern hospital may seem, at times, like a vast and confusing wilderness to both patients and caregiving staff. Being able to negotiate a steady course though this often bewildering system can be greatly and gently facilitated by the presence of a cadre of servant leaders within the institution.

One of the most stressful and demoralizing conditions of a hospitalization that many patients fear, and which some indeed face, is the loss of dignity brought about by the painful or embarrassing sequelae of an illness or injury. In a letter entitled "Dignity Entrusted," oncology nurse Sandy Focht related the story of one of her patients who bemoaned the loss of dignity associated with his course of chemotherapy treatment; in these situations, however, Focht explained "A patient's dignity is not lost; it is just entrusted to someone who cares" (1998, p. 26). The concept of "promoting patient dignity in the healthcare setting" was the aim of a 2007 nursing journal article, in which the authors sought to "heighten awareness of patient dignity, encourage readers to reflect on the concept and apply it to practice" (Matiti, Cotrel-Gibbons, & Teasdale, 2007, p. 46). The authors add that "Self-awareness of knowledge, skills, and attitude is a prerequisite for supporting patient dignity" (Matiti et al., 2007, p. 46). Interestingly "maintaining respect and dignity" was also suggested as important dimension of nursing support for the families of those who are seriously ill (Haugh & Salyer, 2007, p. 319).

While a number of servant leadership characteristics are relevant in providing nursing support for a hospitalized patient's dignity, those that might be highlighted, related to the above nursing suggestions, are protection of a patient's dignity (supported by Listening to his or her concerns and Advocating for the patient's situation) and Assessment — Assessment of one's own abilities and skills, as suggested by Matiti et al., and Assessment of the needs of the other, as in the patient's need to preserve some semblance of dignity despite the side effects of a disease or therapeutic regimen.

Another potentially challenging condition of hospitalization for a patient or family is that of the anxiety/depression phenomenon, often associated with a fearful or life-threatening diagnosis. If the anxiety and depression are in fact situational, related to the hospitalization, rather than a chronic problem, a spiritual caring intervention may be helpful. In a discussion of the spiritual needs of hospitalized patients, it was reported that symptoms of depression may "parallel spiritual distress" and that caring spiritual intervention may provide patients with "inner strength, peace, comfort, wholeness, and enhanced coping patterns" (Davidhizar, Bechtel, & Cosey, 2000, p. 24c). Some specific spiritual interventions reported by nurses as helpful in comforting anxious or depressed hospital patients include "holding a patient's hand, Listening, laughing, prayer, and being present with the patient" (Grant, 2004, p. 39). A few less frequently used interventions identified were "massages, therapeutic touch, music therapy, guided imagery, and meditation" (Grant, 2004, p. 39).

The nursing servant leadership characteristics most supportive for the anxious or depressed hospital patient are Listening with the Heart and Becoming an Advocate. Nurse servant leaders' recognition of the emotional needs of a hospitalized patient will lead to their caring and Listening with an open and receptive heart. This attitude and behavior by a nurse may, in turn, be exactly what is needed to gently encourage the anxious or depressed individual to embrace a posture of hope and trust, rather than one of fear and sorrow.

As well as patients and families, a nurse servant leader, functioning in an administrative or management role, must be concerned about the care and needs of staff members for whom he or she is responsible. In this era of sophisticated and complex therapeutic hospital procedures, nursing staff members are challenged as never before to provide excellent patient-centered care. The financial constraints of modern healthcare systems also can pose difficulties for nursing staff, many of whom are overburdened not only with heavy patient assignments but also may become buried under an ever-growing mountain of paperwork.

The hospital administrator, manager, head nurse, charge nurse, or team leader can engender both commitment and support from staff through embracing a philosophy and spirit of servant leadership. A nursing servant leader whose staff members witness a leadership style that places their needs and concerns above those of the leader, will be both appreciated and respected. The nursing servant leader in the hospital setting will strengthen and enhance the organizational functioning of the overall facility, as well as the department of nursing service.

In an article entitled "Shared Governance and 'Servant Leadership' are Drawing Nurses to New Hospital," it was reported that the hospital's chief nursing officer (CNO) had adopted the model of servant leadership as a strategy for both recruiting and retaining nursing staff (Weber, 2004, p. 2). At the time the article was written the chief nurse reported that the hospital had only "six full-time openings among a staff of 110 registered nurses" (p. 2). The CNO, Terry Ritchey, commented: "My job is to serve those who report to me and are under my care. I tell people 'I'm here to remove barriers and frustrations. I'm the caregiver for the caregivers'" (p. 3).

Regina, a 35-year-old master's-prepared nurse practitioner, currently working as charge nurse in a hospital critical care unit, described a philosophy and practice of nursing leadership totally consistent with the philosophy and practice of servant leadership in the hospital setting:

> Yesterday while working in the ICU, there was a nurse who had a very, very busy assignment, and I was in charge. After the shift, she was so stressed she started to cry. I was able to talk to her and let her know the situation was going to be handled. I got the director involved and was able to resolve the situation. But I showed compassion to that nurse. I could have said, "Yes, I'm in charge, but that is her patient population." I knew that it was our patient, my patient as well. So I had compassion. I cared for the patient, the nurse, and the entire ICU team. Every day as a charge nurse when having 14 patients,

and being in charge, I have my 2 patients I'm responsible for, but I also have the entire ICU which consists of 14 patients, plus the physicians, plus the techs, plus the nurses, plus the housekeepers—the entire team. I use compassion. I use my listening skills to help me be an effective nurse leader.

Regina described the nursing servant leadership characteristic of Giving of Yourself:

Giving is indeed one of the greatest strengths of a servant. Each day I give of myself to my patients. Just the fact that sometimes I pray for my patient without them knowing and those that do know that I'm praying for them I bring my heart, the blessing of God, with me every day. I give of myself to take care of my patients as a positive energy that I bring to the environment. Positive energy brings healing. That instant I know that Christ is with me and thru him I know to heal. He told us to go out and heal the sick, so I know that as nurses we are healers. So for anyone to say nurses will never be wounded, and we don't have any emotions, it is absurd and bizarre; it is unethical. Nursing is a duty from God. God gave us the compassion that we need, the empathy, the healing for our patients.

Regina also spoke about the importance of the nursing servant leadership characteristic of Assessing Needs, both her own and those of hospital patients and staff:

Assessment, as a charge nurse, I have to assess myself, assess my environment, and every patient who is critical: Are they crashing? Are they stable? I have to be very vigilant at all times. I have to be aware of the needs of others such as staff, also. Nursing brings it out in you. Assess if a family gets upset, to be aware of that, if you want to fix the situation.

Regina described advocacy in terms of motivating others and also highlighted the nursing servant leadership concepts of Generating Excitement and Embracing a Higher Purpose:

One of the leadership characteristics of a hospital nurse, I believe is to be a servant, especially as an advanced practice nurse, to advocate for other people, to encourage them and motivate them to do positive things: motivating staff nurses to go back to school for higher education or advance roles; motivating the housekeeper to do a better job, perhaps to move up and be a registered nurse; motivating the registered nurse to become an advanced practice nurse. Each day we motivate our patients, the staff, and ourselves to move forward. Each day I communicate my excitement about being an adult nurse practitioner. I tell people you *have* to do it. You need to move forward. I encourage them. It is a higher purpose. It is a conceptualization in a higher purpose in nursing — not just the education part, the religious part. I'm a Christian. I believe in Jesus, and he has called me to be a nurse for a purpose. This is what I was meant to be: to be a nurse, to be a servant. So when people are hurt and sick, when it comes to nursing, I can put it out to Christ. I am not going to change their religion, I am not going to force my religion on them. But I can care for them in a Christian way...It is a higher purpose.

Linda, a 27-year-old baccalaureate-prepared charge nurse working on a medical-surgical unit of a large city hospital, spoke very positively about the meaning of service in the practice of a nursing leader:

To be a good leader means to put yourself in the service of others, to offer yourself to others in whatever they need — whether it be with patient load or for questions for advice or mentorship. I think that service is the heart of being a good leader in nursing. I don't think it is just a dimension or part of leadership, I think it is the basis of understanding how to be a good leader. Because that is what you demonstrate to others, and they too will pick up that understanding of what it means to be a leader and what it means to never forget your vocation and profession as a nurse.

Linda also shared her understanding of Listening as a nursing leader:

When I think of listening in my role as a leader, I think of not just listening with your ears but listening with all your senses. I think listening, in the sense of being a leader, or as a role model, means not just listening to what the person is verbally telling you but also listening to the person as a whole, the nonverbals, given the holistic approach to listening, which is knowing that that person may not be telling you something for whatever reason. You know that the way your body language or gestures mean something completely different. Allow yourself to listen to what the person is truly saying. Listening not just with your ears but also looking at the person and trying to listen to what their heart is telling you.

Linda spoke of listening as allowing a nurse to Cross Over, to understand the needs of a new staff member:

> I think understanding in my role as a nursing leader means that I am trying to put myself in the other person's shoes without any limitations. Maybe as I have experienced it in my nursing leader role it would be putting myself in the other person's shoes with no limitations in regards to feeling for that person or how they would feel if I was in that position without thinking about my status or my experience or my title. As an experienced nurse, a lot of time experienced nurses tend to forget how it is as a new graduate nurse. When you first get out there and you first start taking your first load of patients, the anxiousness and the feeling of hopelessness (occurs) at time when you can't help a patient out for whatever reason.

Linda emphasized, as did a number of nursing leaders, the importance of assessing one's own need to occasionally Take Time Out, especially when working in a high-powered hospital setting:

> Especially in the hospital setting, we always need to take time out and breathe and really just relax and understand what has been the important topic of the day. What have you learned? If you just continue to go, go, go without taking a minute to really think and process through what you have learned, because everyday is a new learning experience, then you are not really being a good nursing leader. I think you need to regroup, in the sense of just really absorbing and processing what your day has been like or what your experience has been like—thinking it through and understanding it.

Linda added an additional nursing servant leadership characteristic that she labeled "intuition":

> I think a kind of leadership in my mind, I understand as intuition. I can tell you that sometimes, as a nurse, you can walk in the room and see a patient. You don't have to look at vital signs or anything, just look at the patient in the eyes and know that something is wrong. You know automatically just by entering the room that something is not right. There have been so many times when I have not followed my intuition and walked away or not checked something and something has gone bad. I think you don't learn that until you become

a nursing leader, and that is one of the characteristics of your leadership: using your intuition, listening to your intuition, to yourself, being about to foresee when something is going to happen, being able to be a step ahead of your actions. It is very hard for other people to understand, but I think that intuition is a huge part of being a good nursing leader. That is one of the characteristics I didn't have as a new nurse.

Similar to Linda, Naomi, a 49-year-old master's-prepared supervisor in the critical care area, described the importance of both intuition and Crossing Over and trying to put yourself in the place of your patient or their family members:

> (Nursing) is really about being intuitive and spiritual....When you see nursing as a calling, you go to this higher level, which is the vocation level, which has a spiritual dimension to the profession. It elevates it even more. I think if I didn't see (nursing) this way I think I would probably be more the professional where you do things by the book....I think I might do things a little differently. I think that whenever there is another human being involved, you see yourself as in a (vocation), you really understand, "My God, I can make it better." And the reason that I think I see it that way is because if it were me, one of my favorite mottos is, and I ask this of the nurses I work with all the time: "If that woman was your grandmother, was your mother, was your sister, if that person was someone near and dear to you, how would you treat them?" (The patient) is somebody's mother or grandmother, and they (the family) are holding you to take care of her like she was your mother or grandmother. That is the charge you have as nurses. Take care of these people like they were your own. That is the ministry way of looking at nursing; that is the vocational way of looking at it....There is more of an interpersonal and connecting way of looking at it when you are looking at people from a ministry, a vocational point of view.

Veronica, a 50-year-old associate degree RN and charge nurse in a recovery room, described the nursing servant leadership concept of Giving of Yourself:

> In learning what was expected of me in giving of myself in nursing, that's when I felt the calling and that this is where I should be...all of the pieces just fell into place as far as education for

nursing as opposed to other professions I was considering.... (my nursing school) embraced nursing as a vocation. That is what nursing is about, and you are going to give of yourself, and when it is 3 o'clock or 3:30 you may not be going home....There are so many nurses that I know, for instance I work in oncology, and they are wonderful at it, and this is where they want to be....I think that is a calling....I think (these nurses) see nursing as a vocation. They don't generally talk about those things, but when you see them at the bedside you can tell that they are there to serve and care for patients. It's not just a job.

Janet, a 40-year-old, diploma RN, working as a team leader in a hospital clinic, gave an example of Listening with the Heart even when carrying out a physiological nursing assessment:

When you are doing a nursing assessment, if you are listening for breath sounds and the heart you are using an instrument that facilitates your ability to hear. When you are taking a history and so forth, you are listening not only with your ears but you are also looking at that person for emotional response or change of tone, their attentiveness or their change of attentiveness. It is not just listening verbally, but nonverbal is just as important, if not more so. If you are speaking to someone and you are taking a history and they are describing a situation, say they said to you they fell and you are trying to get some more details about how that happened, you are noticing changes in their demeanor, or you ask a question and you asked in a different way and the answer seems to change, you start to think maybe there is more going on. You start thinking, "Is there abuse, or is this just an accident?" I think you have to use all your listening skills. Your listening is directed by listening with your heart.

And, Monica, a 38-year-old master's-prepared nurse with many years of hospital experience spoke of the importance of Doing Ministry as part of her understanding of her vocation of service in nursing:

Perceiving nursing as a ministry has always influenced my nursing. Totally. Totally. That's why, if somebody needs spiritual care during my shift and I haven't (time), you know it is most important. Of course, first things come first, like getting them pain medication or somebody's prescribed meds or treatment. But as soon as I get time to talk with them or pray with them that is definitely priority....so (seeing nursing as a vocation) informs all of my practice. That is my priority.

Monica gave an example of Ministry in her nursing:

Shortly after I came out of school, one of our patients was taken down for a routine X-ray...but they got air in the tubing...and it gave her a stroke....She had the initial stages of cancer...and her diagnosis and prognosis weren't real good, but she was newly diagnosed, so she may have had a while to spend with us yet. But she came back in a coma. And they started IVs to keep her hydrated and put her (in a room) next to the desk... all this was real new to me...I hadn't handled much life and death....And after the family and doctor's discussed her case, they decided to quote "Let her go"! And I said "What does this mean?" And they said "We'll let her go peacefully"....I prayed with her whenever I worked with her. I thought in case she could hear me I thought this was the best thing I could do for this lady. So, I prayed for God's comfort for her and... peace, knowing she was beloved by him and that he would take care of her through this....I was hoping it (prayer) would be help-ful to her if she was still hearing...And by the end of two or three weeks she blinked and started talking to us. And it was slow speech at first, but within a day or two she was totally back....And she said: "I didn't know much what was going on. But every now and then I could see. I knew it was the girls in white, and I could hear your prayers."

Two hospital nurses, Peggy, a 52-year-old master's-prepared charge nurse in cardiac rehabilitation, and Caroline, a 60-year-old master's-prepared team leader working in mental health described how perceiving nursing as a calling helped in their daily work of Being There to Serve and Staying Focused on their vocations. Peggy reported:

When we went to 12-hour shifts, I think made a difference on wanting to do the quality that is necessary at the beginning of the shift and the end of the shift. Wanting to be a good charge nurse that you don't just go and read a book when everybody else is working. You have to help people (staff nurses) too. And that seeing nursing as a calling makes it easier on your coworkers as you collaborate. When you get into the work-force, the place that you are working reflects your values.

Peggy added:

Sometimes I see nurses getting angry and saying "That is it! I'm not doing this." But by saying "This is a calling. This is where I'm supposed to be. Maybe I'm supposed to learn from this. I can see this as a new release to go forward, to be consistent and to keep going on." I see making relationships out of this going through the hard times with my other staff members. Because I am not the only one experiencing it (a problem). I can see it in other nurses too.

Caroline supported Peggy's view of nursing as a "calling":

Nursing is a very human endeavor. We are all humans and are committed to one another; we all have a responsibility to one another, whatever your religious background...there is a purpose for our lives....I think nursing is the highest calling to serve....I think you are always a nurse. It is like when you are ordained, you are always a minister. I think nurses always remain nurses and have that very special privilege to be able to be connected to other people and to each other. To feel that other people need you and want you and will benefit from your presence....I think what nurses do transcends their own lives. I think it takes a nurse out of himself or herself to be caught up with the concerns of other people.

The concept of the nurse's vocation; the mission of Being There to Serve and to help others was also poignantly described by two hospital nurses: Vickie, a 58-year-old oncology research nurse, and Sheila, a 53-year-old head nurse of a critical care unit. Vickie spoke about how she tried to Make a Difference in her patients' lives:

Virtually all of our (cancer) patients are in some way or another in a psychological, emotional, or spiritual crisis at some point, and they all address it in different ways....And of course, one of the things you run into is like "Why should I get treatment? I trust God." Then I like to explain to them that God does help those who help themselves, not in those words specifically. It is terribly important. This is an area where many people would be hesitant to go to a psychologist or a psychiatrist, but they will talk to their nurse. Sometimes this is kind of a burden, and it is a little difficult. On occasion you seek outside help who is really just beyond what you can do. But most times people just need to talk, get it off their chest. And if you were just there to do a 9-to-5 job you would probably say "I have paper work to do." And I do have a lot...you get writer's cramp by the time you finish....And yes it is all stacked up on my desk, but it is more important to be with the patient. I think it makes a difference. I know it makes a difference. If I were in their place, I would want a nurse there if my loved ones weren't there. God didn't put you here for anything else but to help your fellow human beings.

And, Sheila spoke of how seeing nursing as a calling helped her get through each day:

> Seeing nursing as a vocation, I think, helps you get through the day. There are so many other professions...that can't say what we do (helping people) at the end of the day just because of what we do. They are helping people but in a very different way, and I don't think they would call their jobs vocations...I think it is common for nurses to just type our work as a vocation....If you don't see nursing as a vocation and were caring for sick or hospice nursing or working with the mentally disabled, those areas of nursing, if you didn't look at nursing as a service, you would not continue on. I think when people reach that point that they are not happy serving others, then they need to move on....I don't think it would be a bad idea, now that there is such a nursing short-age, to advertise nursing as a service. I think you might get a certain person who is interested in nursing for that reason. It is a higher service and might encourage people to go into the profession.

Finally, a subtheme of the key nursing servant leadership theme Being There to Serve was nurses going Beyond the Ordinary in their practice of their profession. This was exemplified in two nursing leaders' anecdotes. First, Bonnie, a 36-year-old team leader on a pediatric unit, related her response to a parental request:

> I had a patient who was a new baby having surgery, and the surgery had to be done before 12 weeks. I had taken care of him for a couple of weeks before the surgery and the day of the surgery, the mom said to me: "Can you have the Chap-lain come up before he goes to the OR?"....They wanted him baptized before the surgery, and they asked me to be an

honorary godparent. This is an experience you will never forget. I will always remember that family forever. It definitely helped me to view nursing as a vocation to serve....And there have been experiences when families have asked me to pray with them...and I think that also helps me to view nursing as a vocation.

The second anecdote was a story shared by Diane, a 55-year-old manager of a high-risk perinatology unit in a hospital:

I joined in the meetings at our hospital, the perinatal loss committee...a brand new committee that we had put together based on patients' needs. People who have been through lost pregnancies and got no recognition of the loss....our patients would come back and tell us, I need someone to help me through this grief, I need someone to recognize that I had this loss. I need to talk to people....I evolved as chairman of the committee, and we put together a memorial for these people, and we do it every year for all the women who lost their babies. We asked the hospital to donate some land, a small area in front of the hospital. We planted plants and made a memorial garden for all the babies who were lost at our hospital so women can go there (to grieve). Many times, if it is a very early loss, the women have nothing to show for it, no place to go. No tombstone, no grave, nothing to hold on to. And they have had this tremendous loss. As a result of dealing with this committee, it has made a huge impact on my practice and how I perceive life and death in medicine.

NURSING SERVANT LEADERSHIP IN THE LONG-TERM CARE FACILITY

The modern long-term care facility, commonly referred to as a nursing home, can surely be said to vie with the modern hospital in the need for servant leadership within its administrative and caregiving ranks. Today's long-term care facilities undertake the health support and maintenance of the most vulnerable members of our society, the frail elderly. Some long-term care patients are materially poor, having used up savings and other financial resources prior to the need for institutional living. Other frail elders are experiencing social poverty, having lost many of their supportive family members and friends to death or disease. Often a spouse, sibling, or child will, for some years, take on the role of primary caregiver for a beloved family member only to have his or her own health fail after the death of the one for whom he or she has cared. It is not unusual for a newly admitted nursing home resident to be the surviving spouse or a sibling of a recently deceased family member.

An added stressor in contemporary long-term care is the fact that most elders admitted for residential maintenance are now much sicker than they were some years ago. This has partly to do with the advent of better geriatric health care in the community and continual media warnings that older adults take proactive healthcare behaviors such as exercise, eating a healthy diet, and undertaking frequent screening exams for such conditions as heart disease, hypertension, and breast and colon cancer.

Another reason why today's long-term care residents requiring skilled care are more ill than in the past relates to the advent of "continuing care communities," (CCC), sometimes simply labeled "retirement communities." The continuing care community is a unique kind of retirement community, generally admitting elders 65 or older, who are seeking a secure setting where health care is readily available when and if it is needed. In the CCC an older person may be admitted to one of three levels in the facility: independent living, for those who are active and able to care for themselves; assisted care, for elders who need some help with activities of daily living such as meal preparation, laundry, and medications; and admission to a nursing center for the very frail elder who is usually bedridden and needs complete 24/7 care. It is the latter level of the CCC that equates to today's free standing long-term care nursing home; it is for this group of elders, especially, that the spirit of servant leadership among caregivers is a critical element of patient-centered care.

Some years ago I conducted an in-depth case study of a long-term care facility. Although it was officially labeled a nursing home, the facility had some similarities to the contemporary CCC in providing three levels of care. The nursing home's first floor housed what was called a domiciliary care unit. In that unit each resident had a private room (with bath), which they were allowed to furnish with a number of their own possessions such as a comfortable recliner chair, lamps, plants, pillows, and a TV set. These residents were allowed free access to all of the nursing home's service areas and came together in one main dining room for meals. The home's second, third, and fourth floors housed residents who needed assisted or semiskilled care; on these floors the resident rooms were less personal; some were double-occupancy. The majority of the assisted care residents also attended meals in the main dining room with the exception of the third-floor group who were suffering from mild to moderate cognitive impairment. The fifth or top floor of the nursing home was reserved for those individuals who needed skilled nursing care; the majority were bedridden. The rooms were furnished in the style of a usual hospital room with electric beds, tray tables, and private bath or bedside commode (O'Brien, 1989).

Having recently visited a modern continuing care community, I learned that the needs and concerns of the elders in the CCC's three areas of residence, independent living, assisted care, and the nursing center, were very similar to those I had encountered in my nursing home study. I was told by a CCC staff member that now even elders admitted to the independent care areas were older and more debilitated than in the past; many were forced to use wheelchairs or mobile carts, walkers, or cane's to ambulate. The assisted care group was decidedly fragile physically and, for some, cognitively. Deficits in cognition, as well as physical disabilities, was a primary reason for the initiation of assisted care. The residents of the nursing center were, in the main, bedridden or geri-chair bound, and needed continuous 24/7 care as in the nursing home's skilled care unit.

For the resident of a long-term care facility, whether a more traditional nursing home or a continuing care center, especially those requiring partial or complete care, such nursing servant leadership characteristics as listening, giving, ministering, assessing needs, and nurturing are a blessing and deeply appreciated by the residents. Even elders residing in an independent living area within a long-term care facility (LTF) often feel a deep sense of loss and loneliness because of having to leave a previous home. For many the move has meant giving up a multiplicity of former support systems such as extended family, friends, neighbors, and church members. Although the LTF attempts to provide some of those support structures, the fact of an individual being forced to move to either a nursing home or continuing care community can be threatening. For a number of elders, the move in itself represented the fearful beginning of a "slippery slope" into the advanced aging process, a process which can include both physical and cognitive impairment and ultimately death.

In a nursing study of 95 elderly nursing home residents it was revealed that while "losses in later life can prove overwhelming to older adults," some elders coped very well achieving "a spirit of acceptance and serenity" (Bickerstaff, Grasser, & McCabe, 2003, p. 159). One spiritual nursing intervention that was found to increase nursing home residents' inner peace and well-being was "active listening" or Listening with the Heart (Hicks, 1999, p. 144). While the aging process is generally considered a time of physical decline, an elder's spiritual life may grow and deepen (Gaskamp, Sutter, & Meraviglia, 2006, p. 8).

A nursing servant leader who is able and willing to Listen with the Heart to a resident's fear or unhappiness can promote a feeling of understanding and acceptance on the part of the institution; this can greatly enhance a spirit of welcome for a newly admitted individual. Another nurse–patient interaction that may bring peace and happiness to many elders consists of allowing time for the patients' reminiscence or the sharing of previous joyful or successful life experiences. A listening nursing servant leader gifted with a spirit of caring as well as an understanding of the importance of reminiscence to his or her residents, can become a treasured "friend" among caregivers in the LTF. Even listening to just a few words describing the accomplishments of a resident's previous life can support an elder's positive self-image and spirit of hope, when positively received by a servant leader. While admitting that caring for physical needs is a primary activity in nursing homes, nurse practitioner Theris Touhy asserts that nurturing hope in LTF residents is critical to the individuals' spiritual well-being" (2001, p. 45).

Also, in the LTF, where so much of a resident's former autonomy and control have been lost, the servant leadership characteristic of advocacy is a blessed gift. So often elders resist admission to an LTF because they fear that everyone will be constantly telling them what to do. They are also fearful that there will be no one to protect and defend their rights and wishes. As one elderly single woman, anticipating and fearing LTF admission, commented:

> I've always lived alone and been able to control my life. Now I'll have people telling me when to get up, when to get dressed, when to eat, where to go, when to go to bed. I'm not in charge of my own life anymore.

The potential LTF resident's fear relates to being forced to do things the way he or she might not want to do them; that is, be coerced to behave in a certain way. LTF servant leaders, as advocates, can help residents understand why a certain schedule of activities might work for their good; to help them realize that their lives would be safer, happier, and more peaceful in such a structured setting, rather than living alone with no one to support or care for them.

Finally, as in the hospital setting, nursing servant leaders assigned to roles of administration and management need to be deeply aware of and sensitive to the needs and concerns of the staff members in their charge. Providing skilled nursing care in an LTF is not easy, especially for those residents who are more debilitated physically and cognitively. The philosophy and spirit of servant leadership, if modeled by nursing administrators, can, however, filter down to influence the behaviors of staff members toward those under their care.

One of the most important characteristics of the servant leader manager in LTFs, as well as listening, ministering, and advocating, is nurturing the environment. Nursing home and continuing care community administrators and managers need to be able to devise creative ways of making geriatric nursing in an LTF exciting, challenging, and fulfilling, especially for younger nursing staff in the facility. This may be done through such activities as the institution of in-service conferences highlighting new trends in gerontological nursing, periodically sending individual nurses to attend major geriatric nursing conferences around the country, and occasionally rewarding dedicated staff with some hours off for geriatric journal reading.

The above creative strategies not only support and enhance the provision of excellent geriatric patient-centered care in the facility but will represent to staff the administration's commitment to the growth of their nursing personnel serving in a long-term care environment. The LTF's gerontological nurses will feel that they are valued and respected by the top management of the facility if the institution is willing and ready to invest in their continuing education. This attention to the growth of the LTF nursing staff promotes a positive professional self-concept among the facility's gerontological nurses and hopefully assists in both recruitment and retention of skilled and caring geriatric staff, which will, in turn, nurture the overall environment of the facility.

Kathryn, a 58-year-old associate degree nurse who worked with elders, spoke of how viewing nursing as having a Higher Purpose supported her geriatric nursing:

> I treat patients as if they were part of my family, specially the geriatric folks. People deserve to be treated with dignity and respect and care. Believing that nursing is a vocation impacts that. I just treat everyone with the understanding that they are spiritual beings and we are all children of God. I have a theory that if I hurt you, I hurt me, and then when we help one another, we are helping each other. I would want someone to give me the best possible care.

Kathryn added:

I think people coming into nursing today, they don't understand how demanding it is. It takes a lot. It can be very drain-
ing, but it is also what we are there to do. And we do the best
we can for these sick folks....There are days when I have to
remind myself to leave (personal problems) at home. In order
to take care of the patients, I don't have time for personal
issues. That is due to my spiritual beliefs.

Kathryn admitted to the difficulty of contemporary nursing but
reasserted her concept of perceiving nursing as a Caring Vocation, the
subtheme of Embracing a Higher Purpose:

I just want to help people who are sick and suffering. And
every time I tried to stay away from nursing and try something else because I am so frustrated with the bureaucracy and
the craziness from the administration, I had to get back to it
because I cannot tolerate any other job or career that doesn't
involve caring and helping people.

Debbie, a 25-year-old geriatric nurse currently completing a master's degree as a geriatric nurse practitioner, spoke poignantly about the
meaning of nursing for her:

Nursing is something that I feel is not just an occupation. It is
something that I feel I would do even if I were never trained; I
think I would portray the characteristics of a nurse. I would be
a nurse without any monetary compensation if I could afford
to do so. Although I am sometimes frustrated at work with
the circumstances, I am never frustrated with the patients. I'm
always there for the patients. I'm always there for the patients
100%. The reason that I love my job is because I love caring for
the patients. I love taking care of their needs, and my service
to them above all else is the reason that I am a nurse.

Debbie described the importance of Listening to her patients:

When you are listening with your heart, you are listening to
what is *not* said, listening for a concern which might be different than an initially stated interest. Many times I have realized
that what the patient says is not what the patient really wants
to talk about. This past weekend I had an extremely anxious
patient who was in the hospital for headaches. They weren't

sure why she was having the headaches. She would call me constantly complaining of pain and asking for very frequent medication, more than I was able to provide for her. The more I sat and talked to her, the more I realized that pain was only part of her problem. She was scared, she did not know what was wrong with her, and she was worried that the doctors would not figure out what was wrong. She told me several times that she felt like she was losing her mind. The more I talked to her the less anxious she seemed to become and the less she called for pain medicine. I believe this is an example of listening to what the patient really needs. She really didn't need pain medicine. What she needed was someone to talk to and someone to listen to her and someone to reassure her that everything was going to be okay.

Deb spoke about the concept of Crossing Over or identifying with even the older patients:

I believe that to be a good nurse, you truly have to identify with the patient. For example, one weekend I had a patient who was walking with a walker and expected to go home the next day. The following weekend and subsequent weekends thereafter, she was still there in the hospital. I spoke with her about how she felt because she was still in the hospital, and she expressed her disappointment because she had so much to do because her daughter was getting married. We talked about the new developments that had kept her there in the hospital. More than just listening I empathized with her. I understood that she was excited to go home, and I really put myself in her position so I could try to understand her disappointment.

Debbie asserted the importance of Advocacy, especially patient Advocacy, as a characteristic of the nursing leader; this included the nursing servant leadership concept of Making a Difference:

As nurses, our job is to serve others, to protect and defend others and make a difference in their lives. I believe that in day-to-day patient care, nurses do make difference in lives of patients. It may just be a smile or remembering certain facts about a patient and asking the patient about it again that makes them feel like they are worthwhile and that they are more than just somebody in a bed to you, that they have characteristics and qualities that you relate to on a personal level. I try to do this with my patients. I try to remember things about them or their families. Show them that they mean something to me and that I cherish the relationship that we have more than just a nurse-patient relationship but also as two human being relating to each other.

Deb added:

I have been committed to the same institution for several years. I am committed to the patients there. Everyday that I go in I try my best to work with the patients. I try to leave all the stress and emotional influences that are going on in my outside life and truly focus on my patients when I'm at work. Nursing is more than a job. To me it's not just 7 to 7 and leaving. Leadership and service includes really just doing what the patients need and staying as long as you need to stay to get done with what will help the patients.

NURSING SERVANT LEADERSHIP IN THE COMMUNITY

Individuals in today's society work longer than in years past; many older adults do not retire or even plan to retire until well into their 70s. Some of this has to do with financial need; others choose to work longer because they enjoy continuing to feel like active and productive members of the community. Still other elders, while not needing to work for financial recompense, undertake full-time volunteer activities, which not only support their physical and mental health but provide satisfaction and the joy of accomplishment now that participation in the work of a former life career is over.

Elders remaining longer in the community leads also to a greater need for health care in the community, be it related to community health nursing, community-based nursing, or home health care. For some working or volunteering elders such community health nursing programs as blood pressure screening can be lifesaving. Community-based health workshops providing dietary education and guidance on physical exercise for an older adult can keep elders functioning in their activities much longer. For those more frail elders who choose to remain in their own homes, the visits of a home healthcare nurse are essential in being able to maintain the independence of living in a familiar space; the home care patient is living independently, either with or without continual or periodic presence of supportive family members.

Nursing in the community setting, with myriad new and sometimes complex healthcare initiatives, can be as challenging as hospital or long-term care nursing, if not more so. Thus, again, the philosophy and practice of servant leadership among nursing caregivers is both a necessity and a blessing to the community of need. It is important, however, when discussing nursing in the community, to distinguish between the terms *community-based nursing, community health nursing,* and *home healthcare nursing.*

Community-Based Nursing

Community-based nursing is defined as "nursing care directed toward specific individuals and families within a community. It is designed to meet needs of people as they move between and among healthcare settings. The emphasis is on a 'flowing' kind of care that does not necessarily occur in one setting" (Hunt, 2005, p. 15). Community-based nursing "refers to the wide variety of settings other than institutions in which nursing is practiced. It includes public health, home health, ambulatory care, occupational health, and school nursing" (Ellis & Hartley, 2008, p. 96). In these settings "the patient/client is in charge....The nurse serves as an educator, a guide, a resource person, and an advocate, but health action is taken by the client and the family" (Ellis & Hartley, 2008, p. 96).

Maria, a 66-year-old master's-prepared nurse working as team leader currently working in mental health, spoke of her past experience in community nursing:

> I have never earned a lot of money, but I have always worked in areas that I felt were important to patients. I worked in intensive care for many years. I worked supervising new graduates; I was a head nurse several times....I worked in emergency rooms....Later, I worked in the community in lots of places that didn't have much money but lots of need, like AIDS patients and homeless patients. So I would have to say my sense of trying to help people who need help and aren't getting much help, was my overriding concern in community nursing.

And, Linda, a 27-year-old master's-prepared hospital charge nurse, described a future role that she envisioned in community nursing:

> I think that as I am more experienced and have transcended or developed into the nursing leader role, I have thought more so

about my community. As part of my master's program, I have decided that I actually want to work for my (ethnic) community. I want to work for the people that are in need. I've pretty much decided that the population that I want to work with are the low-income, noninsured — probably the immigrant populations, which is what our community has a high influx of now. I want to give to the people in need. That is the community I want to work with. I think it is an example of how community is built into the aspect of the role of nursing leader.

Another example of a nurse working in a community-oriented role is that of Barbara, a 45-year-old nurse, trained in the law, who deals with medical-legal issues, in her practice. Barbara described the meaning of service in her profession:

> With respect to service, I think of it as a commitment that I am willing to give the community, the people of the community in my professional role. What I am able to do is to bring some of the background that I was blessed to be able to give: getting a good education in nursing and being able to come back and get my law degree. I see it as a combination and a responsibility to use that set of skills and background and knowledge to go out into the community and help somehow add to and benefit those around me. I do it with a great passion for health policy and health care where I bring the clinical and legal and policy perspectives to try to advance things that will overall lead to a healthier community both physically and holistically.

Barbara explained how she was able to Cross Over and advocate for patients in the community:

> In my role just prior to this, I worked with various healthcare clients to help them understand what they needed from policy. Working with my Medicaid providers, I think I became more passionate, and it showed in my advocacy for the client. I tried to really understand what the poor needed and how difficult it was for them to navigate through the healthcare system. I tried to put myself in their shoes so that I could then advocate and use my words to help other people understand the responsibility that the state has to that population and how difficult it is for people not to imagine it is just easy because it is for them.

Barbara described how her current community-oriented nursing role supported her conceptualization of nursing as Embracing a Higher Purpose:

I think it was a great length of time it took me in ultimately getting there to make a commitment to what I do now, which is public policy, public service. I left my private-sector role with clients and took a great leap of faith, and it was because I believed I could work just for the community. I think I realized that I was responding to a higher call.

Barbara added:

I am now combining my health background and legal background and a sense of commitment. I watch the delivery of health care and the business aspect of health care evolve. I've seen in the past what has occurred with respect to hospitals. In my community there is a potential closing of one of our health centers, so I use my background and what I know of the last 15 years in an intuitive sense and combine with the great need that it is in the community to be able now to be on the forefront calling for specific measures while others are leaning back and shying away from it. They don't see the real potential and don't understand the impact on the community. When you spend any time, whether it is a short amount of time or long amount of time in a clinical setting where people are dying or hit with an illness—healthy one day, sick the next, it forever changes the way that you vision time and a sense of need. There will never be enough time, there will never be enough money, but you see the reality of it at the bedside, and it allows you to go ahead and move forward or have the strength or courage to move forward.

Community Health Nursing

Community health nursing, which may be carried out with individuals or groups, has a predominant responsibility to the overall population. Community health nursing (sometimes called public health nursing) "is defined by its role in promoting the public's health" (Hunt, 2005, p. 15). Hunt adds "community health nursing is a subset of community-based nursing (it has)...a definitive philosophy of practice and requires specific knowledge and skill" (p. 15). The "defining characteristic of community health nursing is its focus on the health of population groups" (Clark, 2003,

p. 174). Some tenets of community health nursing include "population-based assessment," "primary prevention given priority," "obligations to reach out to all who might benefit from an intervention," "dominant concern for the greater good of all," and "stewardship of available resources" (Clark, 2003, p. 174).

A classic historical example of community or public health nursing is that of the care of poor immigrants initiated by Lillian Wald at the Henry Street Settlement House in New York City (Lillian Wald's work is described in Chapter 2).

Ada, a 58-year-old nursing educator with a background in public health, pointed out the importance of Being There to Serve the underserved:

> I think one of my jobs that I loved the most was public health. I think at that time I made maybe a subconscious decision that I wanted to be involved in the greater good, not just individual illnesses, through the broader perspective of public health. I loved public health, and I loved working with clinics and working with the underserved and running a variety of clinics in the state health department. That was very fulfilling.

Home Health Care Nursing

Home health care nursing is "the delivery of quality nursing care to patients in their home environment; it is provided on an intermittent or part-time basis…a fundamental purpose of care is to foster patient self-management…the patient's caregiver or family and home environment (which included community resources) are viewed as critical elements of a plan of care" (Rice, 2006, pp. 12–13). Some characteristics of home health nursing include the following: "Home health nurses provide care to patients across the life span, from the prenatal through the postdeath periods. Home health nursing stresses the holistic management of personal health practices for the treatment of diseases or disability. Practice embraces primary, secondary, and tertiary prevention; assistance to families with coordination of community resources and health insurance benefits; and delivery of healthcare services in a patient's home" (American Nurses Association, 2008, p. 3).

Because many individuals with life-threatening illnesses continue to choose to remain at home as long as possible, visits from a home health care nurse can provide helpful advice and support as a disease progresses toward the end-of-life stage. The home health care nurse's consultation and encouragement can facilitate a patient's compliance with a prescribed treatment regimen and assist with the management of such problems as anorexia, pain, and depression. In the majority of cases family members become the "core" of end-of-life care and thus "the home health clinician can play an important role in easing the burdens often experienced by the caregiver" (Ruder, 2008, p. 131).

Nurse servant leaders in the community, whether ministering in a community-based nursing, community health nursing, or home health nursing setting, need to employ all of the characteristics of servant leadership in their caregiving or staff-supporting activities. Community nursing servant leaders must continually seek to find creative ways of organizing and carrying out excellent patient-centered care in the community.

Community nurse servant leaders are also called upon, in their various caregiving activities, to operationalize the concepts of listening with the heart, giving of themselves in providing compassionate care, assessing patient and family needs, discerning appropriate decisions, and nurturing the community environment. The nursing servant leader working in public health nursing, community-based health care, or home healthcare nursing becomes a teacher, a mentor, an advocate, a friend, and a caregiver to many of his or her patients. Each of these roles has attached to it unique and specific responsibilities that only a nurse with the heart of a servant leader can truly embrace.

Becky, a 43-year-old baccalaureate prepared home health care nurse, specializing In maternal–child health care, described her role as a servant leader:

> As a nursing leader I think my service that I provide with a specialty in maternal child is that caring and that understanding for the population that I take care of. It is not just the nursing duties but applying all the nursing skills that I have and experience that I have to individualize each person—and the ability to reach that person where ever they are and what they need help with.

Becky added:

> As a nurse dealing with other people, listening, I think listening, to them is the most valuable activity. Sometimes you have to look at (nonverbal) cues from other people to see what exactly they need. Usually there is a concern that comes out originally, and then when you are talking to them further and getting to build a rapport with them, they usually give you different signals on what they can help you with. Often when

dealing with the whole family an issue for one person might not be the issue for the other person, so it is sometimes implied and sometimes very vague. But it always should be addressed, and that is my role as the nurse.

Becky continued with a description of patient Advocacy:

As a home health care nurse often I go into their environment, and I am able to realize exactly how people live, and I personalize their life much easier. With women I usually have an easier time to empathize because I am a woman, and also with my culture, being Hispanic, I take those all into account. The example I can think of is a woman that had just come into the country and was given WIC tickets, tickets to take to the supermarket to get free food, but she spoke only Spanish, and they were all in English. I identified with her in that, helping her to understand that in this country, we are treated as Americans. But, I saw her in another way: that she was a woman that needed food but didn't know how to go get it. So that is where my nursing leadership came in, and I helped her and guided her to get her nutritional food stamps or whatever she needed. I put myself in her shoes and imagined being illiterate and from a different country and needing that additional support and not being able to ask for it.

Assessment of Needs of her home health care clients was a significant part of Becky's role:

In my experience in nursing a lot of the interventions that I have done is healing women, especially the ones that have had stillborn babies: just that gentle touch, that guidance that they can make it through this, that this is going to be a very hard part in their life. It might be a small back rub or just touching their hand, but it helps them through this. It also might go right towards the family members too. They need the same thing as that woman who is actually experiencing the miscarriage of the stillborn. They need guidance on how they can help themselves and help the patient.

Becky also spoke of the importance of Discerning a Decision:

I think Discerning to me is ethically based and also religiously based: what's right and wrong. I often see myself as coming back to when there is a tough decision to be made; if it about a patient or about me personally, I always have to go back to my bases, my religious background, and think what is right or wrong—and what do I want out of the whole picture versus just that moment. I think you have to guide your patients, not imposing on them, but just telling them where you are coming from and just reaching an understanding.

As with Linda and Emily, described earlier, Becky identified "intuition" as an important servant leadership characteristic for the home healthcare nurse:

Intuition, I think is very important. I learned that very early on in my career from nurses who had been nursing for a while. They would tell me what was going to happen, and I never realized it. I think I definitely have to use my intuition now when I'm in home health care. I'm on my own. So when the patient has a slight inclination that something could go wrong, that is the patient that I watch a little more carefully. And that is the one that I'm saying "I'm not exactly sure what is happening," but I want the patient to be well aware of what she should do in case of an emergency. Intuition sometimes come in to staff also where you know that there are certain indicators that things are going to go wrong and that you need more staff. And you can't explain at the moment because the census is low, but you know for sure that something will hit because you are in charge and you see how the unit works. And that happens with experience. I think intuition comes with experience and experience with a certain population or a certain unit. It's very hard to pin down why you feel that way about something, but you know that you do—that's intuition.

Becky concluded her remarks by focusing on the joy of serving others and going Beyond the Ordinary as part of the vocation of nursing:

When you serve other people they give you much more than you give them. It just seems like a win-win situation....The kind of commitment you give to the patients is that you provide them the best care. I think as a nurse, continuing your education and being up to date is very important. The next is the commitment that you make to your fellow nurses that you are doing your job so they don't have to follow up behind you and clean up or do extra because of you. A caring activity of nursing is providing the best care. You go above and beyond; you stay to work extra. Going above and beyond in any way when you are working....As a home healthcare nurse explaining to patients exactly what is needed for good maternal care and providing them with a connection with their doctor, telling them how they need to talk to the doctors or anybody else to get the information they might need.

Marilyn, a 55-year-old diploma RN and supervisor of a home health care unit, spoke to the nursing servant leadership characteristic of Listening:

I think you always need to listen. I think if you know people well enough you are always listening to what is not being said. I feel that I am a fairly good judge of people and can tell what is being said and not being said. An example is with a new secretary that I have, who is experiencing financial difficulty, and listening to her ask for a specific day off. I knew that it was more than just a day off or something. One thing lead to another and she actually confided in me. We were able to get her the assistance that she needed.

Marilyn also noted the importance of caring for a nursing leader:

I think caring is the greatest strength of servant leadership. Caring as a nursing leader is trying to make things the right way. Sometimes it doesn't work out that way, but you are always trying. Connect with other people constantly, and taking their concerns and try to help them come up with a solution that is agreeable.

Marilyn identified Advocacy for staff as another important nursing leadership characteristic:

Always be there to protect the staff and hopefully make a difference. Nursing is advocating and protecting. You are serving the needs of others. It is constant. It is constant. I think guiding new nurses so that they can believe that you believe in the institution you work in (is crucial), so they can go home and say they love it there or like it and can focus on what they can do. Nursing leaders can do that because they have contact with a larger population of employees. I can go and listen to what is going on with inpatient care with a whole new prospective because I am not in that "every man for himself" situation. And it really is a unique place to be.

And, Cecilia, a 51-year-old baccalaureate-prepared nurse working in maternal-child nursing, spoke of the nursing servant leadership theme Making Connections in her home health care nursing experiences:

(You make connections caring for new moms); you were their nurse, and they took pictures of you. You were a part of the family, so in that respect it (nursing) made a big impact. I did postpartum, then I did labor and delivery, and then I did home health for mothers and infants. And that was very gratifying, because I got to go into the homes and help them to breastfeed and take care of the their infant. We were really able to make an impact on education, on the environment. We were caring for patients, caring for the families. Sometimes we set out to do one thing, we set out to go (to a home) for one reason, and while we were there we got caught up in other things that were also needs of the family. So it was definitely making a connection and definitely a service to the family.

NURSING SERVANT LEADERSHIP IN THE PARISH

Parish nursing, or faith community nursing, is one of the newer specialty areas of nursing within which an understanding of the concept of servant leadership is inherent. Most contemporary parish nurses, serving as healthcare liaison between a faith community and its ill members, undertake the role on a purely volunteer basis. This is not because the role of the parish nurse is not valued by the congregations in which the nurse serves. The volunteer nature of the role is generally a matter of finances; that is, most churches do not have a budget allocation for healthcare services; yet many pastors, church councils, and congregation members are supportive of initiating a parish nursing program within their churches.

The concept of the church as a family of faith community, concerned about the physical and mental health of its members, is a tradition that harkens back to the era of the early Christian church. A primary role of the first church deacons and deaconesses was to visit the sick in their homes: "the church was viewed by its members as a community wherein all of one's needs might be addressed: physical, emotional, social, and spiritual" (O'Brien, 2003, p. 16). Some ill church members were even brought into the homes of the deacons and deaconesses and cared for in spaces called *diaconias* or Christrooms (O'Brien, 2008, p. 26).

Contemporary parish nurses carry out a number of activities that "encompass the full range of wholistic health care and include providing health screenings, actively listening to parishioners' life stories, making referrals to healthcare providers and support services, advocating for healthcare access and healthy behaviors, and offering spiritual support" (Bokinskie & Kloster, 2008, p. 20). Rev. Deborah Patterson, executive director of the International Parish Nurse Resource Center (IPNRC) in St. Louis, Missouri, identified eight specific advocacy roles for parish nurses:

1. Help obtaining access to care.
2. Serve as health navigator.
3. Serve as a patient advocate in the healthcare system.
4. Work to acquire needed services in a community.
5. Mobilize for the health of neighbors.
6. Raise awareness of legislative issues related to health.
7. Advocate for environmental health concerns
8. Work for others in developing countries (Patterson, 2007, p. 35).

Several nursing studies have explored the impact of parish nursing on the recipients of the nurse's advocacy and intervention. The research *The Gift of Faith in Chronic Illness: An Experiment in Parish Nursing* documented the importance of parish nursing for a group of chronically ill adults marginalized from practice of their faith by illness. In analyzing both quantitative and qualitative study data it was found "that the intervention provided by parish nurses and parish health ministers resulted in positive increases in the variables of spiritual well-being, including the concepts of personal faith, religious practice, and spiritual contentment, as well as in hope and life satisfaction among the project participants" (O'Brien, 2003, p. 283).

In the study *Parish Nursing: Meeting the Spiritual Needs of Elders Near the End of Life*, analysis of both quantitative and qualitative data revealed that "elders spiritual needs were amenable to the interventions of a parish nurse" (O'Brien 2006, p. 33). The study concluded that the findings were "significant for documenting the difference parish nurse ministry can make in promoting and facilitating spiritual well-being in the lives of chronically ill, frail elders" (O'Brien, 2006, p. 33).

A grounded theory research study exploring spiritual interventions carried out among 10 practicing parish nurses revealed a core process category labeled "Bringing God Near," which included the phases: "trusting God, forming relationships with the patient/family, opening to God, activating/nurturing faith, and recognizing spiritual renewal or growth" (Van Dover & Pfeiffer, 2007, p. 213).

For a parish nurse servant advocate, as noted earlier, the philosophy, spirit, and behavioral characteristics of servant leadership are embedded within the conceptualization and role activities identified for parish nursing. Parish nurses listen, give, minister, discern, and make a difference in the lives of the members of the faith they serve.

Annemarie, 65, a doctorally prepared parish nurse working part-time, identified all three subthemes of the nursing servant leadership theme: Doing Ministry, Making Connections, being the Wounded Healer, and seeing her parish nursing as a Sacred Trust from God:

> Doing parish nursing is a wonderful ministry. Right now I'm still working so I can only do it part-time, but it's become a real joy in my life. Our parishioners, especially the older folks which is most of who I see, need so much and are so grateful for everything you do. They are alone, many of them, and felt unconnected to the church and to other parishioners if they can't get out to services any more. So the parish nurse makes that connection between the church and the person who is homebound. It not exactly home care nursing, but it has some of the elements of it. Often times too, I can use my own experiences, times when I've been sick and alone, to help me understand what they are going through. It's like they say using your own "wounds" to understand someone else's; that idea of the "wounded healer." I can be that sometimes, I think. Parish nursing is a very special kind of nursing. It's called *nursing*, but it's ministry too, and so there is a sacredness to it. There is sacredness to all nursing, but it just seems a little more present in parish nursing. I guess that's because we do specifically try to attend to patients' spiritual needs as well as their physical problems.

NURSING INTUITION IN THE HEALTHCARE SETTING

Although the concept of intuition was not addressed by enough study participants to warrant identification as a key theme of nursing servant leadership, it was mentioned specifically by four members of the group as being linked to servant leadership concepts of Listening with the Heart, Crossing Over, and Staying Focused. Although most practicing nurses admit to the importance of intuition in their clinical interactions, the literature notes that "in today's evidence-based research climate" intuition may be "denigrated because it is difficult to investigate and quantify" (Truman, 2003, p. 42). Intuition is, however perceived as a "useful tool that needs to be recognized in nursing" (Truman, 2003, p. 43). Although admittedly a "complex concept," intuition is described as "a valuable source of knowing" that nurses need "to embrace" (Smith, 2007, p. 17).

In a study to explore 262 nurses' understanding and use of intuition, it was concluded that intuition "is the result of a complex interaction of attributes, including experience, expertise, and knowledge, along with personality, environment, acceptance of intuition as a valid behavior, and the presence of absence of a nurse/client relationship" (McCutcheon & Pincombe, 2001, p. 345). And, in research to examine surgical and intensive care nurse's expertise, the nurse's use of and understanding of intuition was also considered with the finding that "both intuitive and analytical elements" need to be recognized in assessing clinical competence (King & Clark, 2002, p. 322). Research on novice nurses' use of intuition revealed that novice nurses were more likely to use intuition to guide decisions "if they are older, have had more hospitalizations, and experience more social support" (Ruth-Sahd & Hendy, 2005, p. 450). Intuition was considered an important enough nursing concept that nurse researchers developed a tool to measure intuition as used by nursing students (Smith & Thurkettle, 2004, p. 614).

Three nursing leaders, Linda, Emily, and Becky, cited earlier in this chapter, shared comments related to the relevance of intuition associated with their role as servant leaders. A fourth nursing leader, Mary Theresa, a doctorally prepared nurse educator currently teaching in a university setting, not only described her perception of the importance of intuition in nursing but also related a powerful case example of an experience of using intuition in her past clinical practice:

> Listening with your Heart is very important to help a nursing leader cross over to try and understand what a person, a patient, is going through. But sometime they don't always want to tell you what's going on with them. Sometimes, male patients especially, don't want to seem like they're complaining, or anybody for that matter. And I think that's when you have to kind of intuit what's going on or what might be going on. You have to stay focused. Intuition is a big, big thing in nursing practice, and any nurse with any amount of experience will tell you that. You can almost always trust a nurse's intuition.

Mary Theresa added:

> You have to use intuition with children also. They especially won't tell you if they are hurting or don't feel good because

they want to go home or they don't want another needle. And sometimes it's not that they're holding back; they just don't know when something is wrong with them physically.

I remember one situation, a long time ago, when I was working in a kidney transplant unit. We had a beautiful, bright little 10-year-old who had just had a transplant. She was a sweetheart and never complained. One evening I went in to check on her at bedtime, for PM care, and she just didn't look right. Her output (urine) was okay. I checked all her vitals, and they were not significant. I asked her how she felt, and she just kept saying "Okay." But I called the transplant team anyway and said, "Will you look at this child? Something's not right. I just feel it even though I can't document it with numbers." The resident came, and her transplant surgeon, who was still in the house, and by the time they arrived her BP was dropping and she was perspiring. They rushed her to surgery and discovered she was bleeding. I never forgot that instance of using intuition to call for help when I just knew a patient didn't look right.

This chapter has explored the concept of nursing servant leadership in a variety of nursing environments including the hospital, the clinic, the long-term care facility, the community, and the parish. Contemporary nurses working in these settings shared insightful and poignant stories that reflect many nursing servant leadership characteristics as identified by the overall nursing leader population interviewed in the study Called to Serve. It is anticipated that the concept of servant leadership in nursing, which is just beginning to be appreciated by current healthcare facilities, will eventually be adopted as the model of leadership for nursing departments across the country. Nursing leaders who undertake to embrace the model of servant leadership describe the value of this model not only for enhancing patient and staff satisfaction but also for providing much joy and professional satisfaction for its practitioners.

REFERENCES

American Nurses Association. (2008). *Home health nursing: Scope and standards of practice*. Silver Spring, MD: Author.

Bickerstaff, K. A., Grasser, C. M., & McCabe, B. (2003). How elderly nursing home residents transcend losses of later life. *Holistic Nursing Practice: The Science of Health and Healing, 17*(3), 159–165.

Bokinskie, J. C., & Kloster, P. K. (2008). Effective parish nursing: Building success and overcoming barriers. *Journal of Christian Nursing, 25*(1), 20–25.

Clark, M. J. (2003). *Community health nursing: Caring for populations.* Upper Saddle River, NJ: Prentice Hall.

Davidhizar, R., Bechtel, G. A., & Cosey, E. J. (2000). The spiritual needs of hospitalized patients. *American Journal of Nursing, 100*(7), 24c–24d.

Ellis, J. R., & Hartley, C. L. (2008). *Nursing in today's world: Trends, issues and management* (9th ed.). Philadelphia: Lippincott Williams & Wilkins.

Focht, S. (1998). Dignity entrusted (Letter to the editor). *America, 179*(2), 26.

Gascamp, C., Sutter, R., & Meraviglia, M. (2006). Promoting spirituality in the older adult. *Journal of Gerontological Nursing, 32*(11), 8–13.

Grant, D. (2004). Spiritual interventions: How, when and why nurses use them. *Holistic Nursing Practice: The Science of Health and Healing, 18*(1), 36–41.

Harrington, D. J. (1991). *The gospel according to Matthew.* Collegeville, MN: Liturgical Press.

Haugh, K. H., & Salyer, J. (2007). Needs of patients and families during the wait for a donor heart. *Heart & Lung: The Journal of Acute and Critical Care, 36*(5), 319–329.

Hicks, T. J. (1999). Spirituality and the elderly: Nursing implications with nursing home residents. *Geriatric Nursing, 20*(3), 144–146.

Hunt, R. (2005). *Introduction to community-based nursing* (3rd ed.). Philadelphia: Lippincott Williams & Wilkins.

King, L., & Clark, J. M. (2002). Intuition and the development of expertise in surgical ward and intensive care nurses. *Journal of Advanced Nursing, 37*(4), 322–329.

Livingstone, E. A. (1990). *The concise Oxford dictionary of the Christian Church.* NY: Oxford University Press.

Matiti, M., Cotrel-Gibbons, E., & Teasdale, K. (2007). Promoting patient dignity in healthcare settings. *Nursing Standard, 21*(45), 46–52.

McCutcheon, H. J., & Pincombe, J. (2001). Intuition: An important tool in the practice of nursing. *Journal of Advanced Nursing, 35*(3), 342–348.

Metz, J. B. (1998). *Poverty of spirit.* Mahwah, NJ: Paulist Press.

O'Brien, M. E. (1989). *Anatomy of a nursing home: A new view of resident life.* Owings Mills, MD: National Health Publishing.

O'Brien, M. E. (2003). *Parish nursing: Healthcare ministry within the church.* Sudbury, MA: Jones and Bartlett.

O'Brien, M. E. (2006). Parish nursing: Meeting spiritual needs of elders near the end of life. *Journal of Christian Nursing, 23*(1), 28–33.

O'Brien, M. E. (2008). *Spirituality in nursing: Standing on Holy Ground* (3rd ed.). Sudbury, MA: Jones and Bartlett.

Patterson, D. (2007). Eight advocacy roles for parish nurses. *Journal of Christian Nursing, 24*(1), 33–35.

Rice, R. (2006). *Home care nursing practice: Concepts and application* (4th ed.). St. Louis, MO: Mosby Elsevier.

Ruder, S. (2008). The challenges of family member caregiving: How the home health and hospice clinician can help at the end of life. *Home Healthcare Nurse: The Journal for the Homecare and Hospice Professional, 26*(2), 131–136.

Ruth-Sahd, L. A., & Hendy, H. M. (2005). Predictors of novice nurses' use of intuition to guide patient care decisions. *Journal of Nursing Education, 44*(10), 450–458.

Smith, A. J. (2007). Embracing intuition in nursing practice. *Alabama Nurse, 34*(3), 16–17.

Smith, A. J., & Thurkettle, M. A. (2004). Use of intuition by nursing students: Instrument development and testing. *Journal of Advanced Nursing, 47*(6), 614–622.

Touhy, T. A. (2001). Nurturing hope and spirituality in the nursing home. *Holistic Nursing Practice: The Science of Health and Healing, 15*(4), 45–56.

Truman, P. (2003). Intuition and practice. *Nursing Standard, 18*(7), 42–43.

Van Dover, L., & Pfeiffer, J. B. (2007). Spiritual care in Christian parish nursing. *Journal of Advanced Nursing, 57*(2), 213–221.

Van Linden, P. (1991). *The gospel according to Mark.* Collegeville, MN: Liturgical Press.

Weber, D. (2004). Shared governance and 'servant leadership' are drawing nurses to new hospital. *Patient Care Staffing Report, 4*(7), 2–4.

8   The Spirituality of Servant Leadership in Nursing

You are my servant whom I have chosen.

—Isaiah 43:10

If I did not have that spiritual deep grounding, that persistence of faith that tends to support you in your nursing career, I am afraid I would be relying on other alternatives to make me happy. I really believe that spirituality is very healing not only for the patient but also for the nurse who is a servant leader. It is a reflection of who you are as a person....You have to have some kind of belief in yourself and in a higher being in a meaningful, purposeful way of what it is to be not only yourself but a nurse too. You have to have the spiritual aspect in your nursing life in order to survive.

—Agnes, supervisor, medical outpatient clinic

I think having a spiritual commitment to your profession, to your calling, is an aspect of being a good nurse, an aspect of the role of a nurse servant leader. You are going beyond the usual expectations. Nursing is obviously not just a job; you do what you do at work or the institution but also away from there. If somebody was to know you away from the hospital they would know that you show the same characteristics away from your normal nursing environment. That is what the role of a nursing servant leader is. You are showing leadership because that is your way of life, helping others. Caring for other is your vocation as a leader. Viewing nursing as a calling adds a definite spiritual dimension to the profession. (Linda, charge nurse, medical-surgical unit).

Although the philosophy of servant leadership, as originally described by Robert Greenleaf in 1977, did not have an overtly religious undergirding, the concept can, by its very nature, be considered spiritual in the broadest sense of the word. Greenleaf asserted that "the servant-leader is servant first…(servant leadership) begins with the natural feeling that one wants to serve, to serve first" (1977, p. 27). By describing a servant leader as an individual whose first interest is that of serving others, Greenleaf distinguished the servant leader from the person for whom leadership is first, one who seeks a leadership role "perhaps because of the need to assuage an unusual power drive or to acquire material possessions" (1977, p. 27).

The philosophy of servant leadership, as understood by Greenleaf, describes not a self-serving leader but a self-giving leader, one who puts the needs and concerns of those he or she serves before personal interests. This can lead to an interpretation of servant leadership that is deeply humanitarian for some and deeply religious and for others. A nonreligious understanding of servant leadership presents a humanistic philosophy of caring that places the good of others in the human family, especially others for whose leadership one is responsible, as a central concern of the leader; the leader sees servant leadership as moral and good for the functioning of an organization and for all of its members.

A religious understanding of the concept reflects a model of servanthood as presented in spiritual teachings such as those of the Judeo-Christian tradition. In both Old and New Testament writings, as discussed in Chapter 3, the concepts of service and servanthood are taught as the ideal attributes for one who wishes to live a holy and religiously attuned life. In the Torah or Old Testament passages the concept of service is particularly related to service of the God of Israel: "The Lord, your God, shall you fear; him you shall serve, and by his name alone you shall swear" (Deuteronomy 6:13). New Testament passages reflect Jesus as a role model of the servant leader in mandates such as: "Whoever wishes to become great among you must be your servant, and whoever wishes to be first among you must be slave of all. For the Son of Man came not to be served but to serve, and to give his life as a ransom for many" (Mark 10:42–45).

Thus there can be found both a spiritual and a religious significance to the philosophy of servant leadership as identified and described by Greenleaf as well as by others who have followed his lead in exploring the concept.

THE SPIRITUAL GROUNDING OF SERVANT LEADERSHIP IN NURSING

The philosophy of servant leadership, especially as described by Greenleaf, supports the firmly held belief of many spiritual and religious people that it is in fact "better to give than to receive." For those of the Christian community, the concept is reflected in the well-loved prayer attributed to St. Francis of Assisi: "Lord make me an instrument of your peace." In the prayer, Francis is believed to have prayed that in being instruments of peace, we should seek "not so much to be understood as to understand," "not so much to be loved as to love." This advice is based on the philosophy that it is "in giving that we receive."

Thus, the prayer of Saint Francis is very much in concert with the concept of servant leadership that teaches that those who embrace its spirit and spirituality receive satisfaction and success through giving first to others before attending to their own needs. And, Francis' concept of each person being a peacemaker is also related to the servant leadership theme of one being a healer in society. As Greenleaf, a devout Quaker, observed, "Servant-leaders are healers in the sense of *making whole* by helping others to a larger and nobler vision and purpose than they would be likely to obtain for themselves" (1977, p. 240). This spirituality is reflected in Ken Blanchard and Phil Hodges' book *Lead Like Jesus: Lessons from the Greatest Leadership Role Model of All Time*, in which the authors observe: "Self-serving leaders think they should lead and others should follow. Servant leaders, on the other hand, seek to respect the wishes of those who have entrusted them with a season of influence and responsibility" (2005, p. 47).

The majority of nurses are, by the very essence of their calling and their profession of caring for the sick, natural servant leaders. They choose to undertake the vocation of nursing, with all of its challenges and difficulties, because they are men and women who embrace the spirituality of giving to others; they recognize, in the words of Francis of Assisi, that it is truly in giving that one receives. Nurses are servant leaders in body, mind, and spirit.

Frequently nurses are stretched almost to the limit of their physical abilities in working long hours, with heavy patient loads or overwhelming staffing responsibilities; they may go home physically exhausted, especially after the 12-hour nursing shifts initiated in some contemporary hospitals. Nurses must constantly pursue continuing education, keeping their minds alert and becoming educated to new medical knowledge and new technologies upon which a patient's life may depend. And nurses give constantly of their spirits, listening with a caring and empathetic heart, to the worries and concerns of their staff, their patients, and their patients' families. Nursing servant leaders often expend a great deal of energy agonizing over the problems and concerns of those they lead; this is the vocation of nursing. This is the vocation of servant leadership. This is the spirituality of servant leadership in nursing.

THE MINISTRY OF SERVANT LEADERSHIP IN NURSING

Following acceptance and understanding of the spirituality of servant leadership in nursing, one might also consider the nurse servant leader to be a minister in caring for the sick. The outcome of a qualitative study of spiritual care activities among 66 professional nurses, which I conducted several years ago, was the labeling of the nurse as "anonymous minister." Data elicited in the study interviews identified three dominant themes that revealed nursing to be a ministry, albeit an anonymous ministry, that is, ministry not generally charted, reported, or written about. The nursing ministry themes included a Sacred Calling, Nonverbalized Theology, and Nursing Liturgy (O'Brien, 2008). The theme of a Sacred Calling was demonstrated in nurses' comments such as: "When I was 16 I felt a calling to be a nurse; it's like a sacred calling" (p. 101). *Nonverbalized Theology* was a term used by a doctorally prepared nurse study participant: "I can be there (with patients) to be a person of the love of God....You want to alleviate suffering, convey hope, bring love...but there is no theology being verbalized. It's a nonverbalized theology" (p. 109). And, the theme of Nursing Liturgy was applied to anecdotes containing stories of nurses praying with or for their patients. One poignant example was the experience of Cathy who related an incident of several nurses and a young physician holding and praying with a dying anencephalic infant: "We prayed and we sang hymns and we just held her and loved her until she died. It was her special ritual to go to God" (p. 118).

In a 1994 article in the *Journal of Advanced Nursing*, Joanne Widerquist and Ruth Davidhizar asserted with their article's title "The Ministry of Nursing," that nursing could indeed be considered a ministry. The authors point out that "Historically, the nursing profession has roots in the Christian concept of ministry. A caring ministry called for persons to serve their neighbors who were in need physically or spiritually...Many of the caring qualities of today's nurses are pastoral in nature, and contribute richly to healing. Examining nursing as ministry provides an opportunity to consider the nature of nursing as it moves into the 21st century" (p. 647). The relatively new concept of parish nursing (O'Brien, 2003a) is described as ministry and as a "growing practice within the churches to restore a ministry of health and healing" (Stoll, 1997, p. 18). The parish nurse is clearly considered "a registered professional nurse who, as a member of the ministerial team, provides holistic nursing services to the members of the congregation (Schank, Weis, & Matheus, 1996, p. 11).

The term *ministry* is also included as central to the definition of nursing offered by Judy Shelly and Arlene Miller in their 2006 book, *Called to Care: A Christian Worldview of Nursing:* "Christian nursing is a ministry of compassionate care for the whole person, in response to God's grace toward a sinful world, which aims to foster optimum health *(shalom)* and bring comfort in suffering and death to anyone in need" (p. 244).

Thus, any nurse leader, especially those embracing the philosophy and practice of servant leadership, might be considered ministers. The ministry of the nursing leaders who participated in the study Called to Serve, is clearly reflected in the 9 identified nursing servant leadership themes and 16 subthemes:

1. Listening with the Heart: The Sounds of Silence, the Mystery Behind the Visit
2. Giving of Yourself: Crossing Over, Compassionate Care
3. Doing Ministry: Making Connections, the Wounded Healer, a Sacred Trust
4. Assessing Needs: Being Grounded, Taking Time Out
5. Becoming an Advocate: To Protect and Defend
6. Discerning Decisions: Staying Focused
7. Making a Difference: Doing Your Best, Generating Excitement, a Nurturing Environment
8. Being There to Serve: Beyond the Ordinary
9. Embracing a Higher Purpose: A Caring Vocation

These behavioral themes express the unique and caring ways in which nursing servant leaders minister to those for whom they are responsible, whether patients, family members, or healthcare staff.

NURSING SERVANT LEADERSHIP IN THE VISUAL ARTS AND POETRY

In discussing his conceptualization of hermeneutic phenomenological research, the method upon which the servant leadership in nursing study described in this book was based, Max van Manen (1990) suggests that the investigator may look at artistic sources related to the phenomenon under study in order to "glean thematic descriptions" (p. 96). Included among these artistic sources are visual art forms (such as sketches and prints, paintings, stained glass, and sculpture) and poetry. It was noted by van Manen that "for the artist as well as the phenomenologist, the source of all work is the experiential lifeworld of all human beings. Just as the poet or the novelist attempts to grasp the essence of some experience in literary form, so the phenomenologist attempts to grasp the essence of some experience in a phenomenological description" (pp. 96–97). "A genuine artistic expression," van Manen adds "is not just representational or imitational of some event in the world. Rather, it transcends the experiential world in an act of reflective existence" (p. 97). Visual art and poetry allow one to express spiritual feelings intensely. Artistic representations of life experiences may be employed to elucidate the investigator's understanding of the phenomenon under study; in this case that of servant leadership in nursing.

Sketches and Prints

In my office there are two artistic depictions of nurses, both of which continually remind me that nursing is a spiritual vocation of servant leadership as well as a profession. One piece is a framed black-and-white ink sketch that displays "a 1950s-era nurse elegant in white uniform and cap, with a dark cape billowing out over her slender shoulders. The nurse is pictured with open arms, standing under a life-sized crucifix. The motto on the poster, an advertisement for membership in the National Council of Catholic Nurses, reads: 'Nursing…a pathway to sanctity.' The imagery of the sketch and its message remind the observer that the nurse's calling is truly a holy vocation of offering oneself in the service of others. The sketch also supports the fact that the nurse's calling can indeed become a 'pathway to sanctity'" (O'Brien, 2003b, pp. 22–23). The nursing servant leadership theme reflected in this sketch is Giving of Yourself.

The other bit of nursing artwork, kept over my office desk, is a colorful poster containing the print of a photogravure of John Morton-Sale's "The Red Cross of Comfort" originally painted in 1939. In the picture a young soldier is sitting in a reclining chair with a blanket over his knees and a wide bandage covering his forehead and eyes. A nurse is pictured standing behind the soldier gently touching the edges of his bandage as if testing it for comfort. The nurse, whose facial features express tender care and compassion, is dressed in a long blue gown overlaid with a full white apron bearing the Red Cross symbol across her chest. This picture reminds one, also, of the spiritual vocation of nursing service especially as witnessed by the loving concern of Red Cross and military nurses, many of whom have risked their lives to provide care to those injured in combat. A nursing servant leadership subtheme reflected in this print is that of Compassionate Care.

Paintings

In her elegant book, *Nursing, The Finest Art: An Illustrated History* (1996), M. Patricia Donahue has compiled a splendid collection of pictures of magnificent paintings that reflect the spirituality of nursing leadership. Three examples reflect the themes of nursing servant leadership. The late 18th-century work "Christ Healing the Sick in the Temple" by Benjamin West (p. 72) pictures Jesus surrounded by the ill and the infirm whom he seeks to heal in the name of his Father. The painting reminds one of whence came the Christian tradition of caring for the sick and reflects the nursing servant leadership theme Embracing a Higher Purpose. Georges de La Tour's "St. Sebastian Nursed by St. Irene," c. 1638 (p. 89) depicts St. Irene removing an arrow from the leg of St. Sebastian and reflects the hands-on care associated with the nursing vocation of service to those in need. This image contains within it the nursing servant leadership theme of Doing Ministry. Pablo Picasso's 1897 painting entitled "Science and Charity" pictures a bedridden women being attended on one side by a physician taking her pulse and on the other side by a nursing Daughter of Charity caringly offering a cup of water (p. 68). This work displays the teamwork of a nurse and a physician sharing the care of their patient. It reflects the nursing servant leadership theme of a Nurturing Environment.

Stained Glass

The Florence Nightingale window, installed in the Washington National Cathedral in Washington, DC, in 1983, contains six vibrant stained glass panels representing various dimensions of Nightingale's life and ministry:

1. St. Thomas Hospital, London
2. Hospital nursing
3. Nightingale's childhood
4. Nightingale's book *Notes on Nursing*
5. The Crimean mission
6. Nursing education

The individual panels picture Nightingale's spirituality in caring for the sick, in teaching, and in writing, nursing roles in which her servant leadership was born and flourished. In all of her leadership roles Nightingale reflected the nursing servant leadership subtheme of a Caring Vocation.

The Saint Christopher window, installed in St. Christopher's Chapel of the Mary Breckinridge Hospital, Hyden, Kentucky, depicts in lovely stained glass colors of red, gold, blue, and green, the saint carrying the Christ child over a stream. The window was installed in a wing of the original Hyden Hospital at the request of its founder and the founder of Frontier Nursing Service, Mary Breckinridge. As Breckinridge initially wrote in her autobiography *Wide Neighborhoods: A Story of the Frontier Nursing Service,* "In the new wing for Hyden Hospital, whenever it is constructed, we shall build St. Christopher's chapel. For this we have a glorious fifteenth-century French stained glass window of St. Christopher and the Christ child, when he carried him over a ford like ours...If the Frontier Nursing Service had a patron saint it could not be other than St. Christopher, on whose help we counted when we carried children on the pommels of our saddles through treacherous fords" (1981, p. 362). The St. Christopher window was originally located in the New York home of Mary Breckinridge's cousin who commissioned stained glass experts to dissemble the window and ship it to Hyden, Kentucky, for the hospital chapel.

The St. Christopher window provides a poignant reminder of the spiritual essence of the servant leadership of Breckinridge and her followers in the Frontier Nursing Service who carried so many ill and injured children to safety and health. Breckinridge listened and responded to the desperate need for health care for the children and families in rural Leslie County, Kentucky. She heard their cries for care with the nursing servant leadership ability of Listening with the Heart.*

Sculpture

One of the most powerful reminders of servant leadership in trauma nursing is the beautiful memorial sculpture of British Nurse Edith Cavell, located in St. Martin-in-the-Fields, near Trafalgar Square, London. The white marble statue, set against a 40-foot-high gray granite cross, contains the last recorded words of Edith Cavell prior to her execution for assisting English soldiers to escape from German-occupied Belgium. Her oft cited comment was "Patriotism is not enough. I must have no hatred or bitterness for anyone." Also inscribed on the cross are the place, date, and time of Edith's execution by a German firing squad: Brussels, Dawn,

---

*The servant leadership of Mary Breckinridge is discussed in detail in Chapter 2, "The Spiritual Heritage of Servant Leadership in Nursing."

October 12, 1915. On the back of the monument is the inscription: "faithful unto death", and on each of the four sides are the words: humanity, sacrifice, devotion, and fortitude. The Cavell monument reminds all nurses of Edith Cavell's self-sacrificing servant leadership in protecting and defending to the death the wounded soldiers for whom she cared. Her life poignantly and powerfully reflected the nursing servant leadership theme of Being There to Serve.[†]

The lovely statue "The Spirit of Nursing," located in section 21 (sometimes called the "Nurses Section") of Arlington Military Cemetery, in Arlington, Virginia, was created as a memorial to honor nurses who served in World War I. The 10-foot-high marble monument was sculpted by Frances L. Rich and unveiled in 1938. Below the statue of a nurse wearing a flowing uniform of the era, is a plaque with the words: "This monument was erected in 1938 and rededicated in 1971 to commemorate devoted service to country and humanity by Army, Navy, and Air Force Nurses." The statue is a reminder of the spirituality of servant leadership not only of all those military nurses buried at Arlington Cemetery, but also of current military men and women serving in this country and abroad. These men and women truly embody in their caring ministry the nursing servant leadership subtheme of To Protect and Defend.

Another magnificent monument to the spirituality of servant leadership in military nursing is Glenna Goodacre's bronze Vietnam Women's Memorial, dedicated on November 11, 1993. The memorial statue portrays a group of three military women, one of whom, a nurse, is tenderly holding a young wounded soldier across her lap; the image evokes a memory of another woman, so many centuries ago, holding the broken body of her crucified son. The other two women are supporting their military colleague, one by appearing to be watching for enemy intrusion or allied support from the sky; the other quietly sitting by the nurse's side holding the fallen soldier's helmet.

The Vietnam Women's Memorial "culminated 10 years of effort begun by Minnesota RN Diane Carlson Evans who served in Vietnam" and who "strongly desired to see a monument to women veterans" (About the Vietnam Women's Memorial Project, 1995, p. 1). The monument is a testament to those military nurses who, themselves touched by the pain and suffering of war and conflict, reflect the empathetic spirituality of nursing servant leadership subtheme of Crossing Over.

[†]The servant leadership of Edith Cavell is also described in Chapter 2, "The Spiritual Heritage of Servant Leadership in Nursing."

Poetry

In considering poetry that reflects the spirituality of servant leadership in professional nursing, Henry Wadsworth Longfellow's classic work "Santa Filomena" immediately comes to mind. In this work Longfellow immortalized Nightingale as "the Lady with the Lamp." The poem celebrates Nightingale's ministry to wounded soldiers in the Crimea with such poignant passages as: "Lo! In that house of misery,/ a lady with a lamp I see/Pass through the glimmering gloom/ and flit from room to room./ And slow, as in a dream of bliss,/ the speechless sufferer turns to kiss/ his shadow as it falls,/ upon the darkening walls./ ...A lady with a lamp shall stand,/ in the great history of the land,/ a noble type of good,/heroic womanhood" (1857, p. 23).

Nightingale's nursing ministry in the Crimea significantly affected not only the care but the very survival of many of Britain's wounded soldiers thus demonstrating the important nursing servant leadership theme of Making a Difference.

An anonymously authored epic poem, reflecting the spirituality of the nursing vocation, is "Mary's Nurse," published as a centerfold in the December 1929 issue of the *American Journal of Nursing*. In the poem a nurse caring for a young mother-to-be is meditating on how it might have been for Jesus' mother-to-be in the stable at Bethlehem. In her musings the nurse imagines that Joseph, seeing that Mary's time was close, may have sought out a neighbor woman, a nurse, and begged her help. This local nurse was envisioned as thinking to herself how "glorious...twoud be" to help bring the awaited messiah into the world, but she reflects "I can only bring some comfort now, to poor young girl in wretched cattle stall" (p. 1445). If Joseph had tried to express his thanks, Mary's nurse is thought, by her imaginer, to have responded with the words reflecting her vocation: "It is not hard...to nurse the sick for those whose lives are given so. To tend the maimed, the ill. That is a joyous life, a life complete" (p. 1445). This epic poem well exemplifies the nursing servant leadership theme of Assessing Needs.

A 1954 nursing journal issue published a poem reflective of a nurse's caring and commitment and of a nurse's spiritual vocation of service. "A Nurse's Night Prayer" evokes the memory of Jesus' teaching in Matthew 25:35-36, "For I was sick and you cared for me." In the poem a nurse mused that she was seeing the Lord himself in a poor ill patient and offered the thought: "I looked at my patient there in his bed,/ but I felt I was seeing the thorn-crowned head,/ and the lashed body, all ripped and torn,/ of my Jesus on the Cross, so forlorn" (Maher, p. 30). This poem reflects the author's spiritual embrace of her vocation and demonstrates the nursing servant leadership theme of Being Grounded in one's commitment to serve.

A poem included in another 1954 nursing journal is the classic work "To Be a Nurse," which begins with the line: "To be a nurse is to walk with God/ Along the path which the Master trod" and ends with the words "The Great Physician, Christ, is working through you" (Hain, p. 57). This poem exemplifies the author's sense of a nurse's spirituality. It reflects the servant leadership theme of a Sacred Trust.

More contemporary poetry, reflecting the spirituality of nursing, may be found in works such as "Standing on Holy Ground": "The Nurse reverently touches and is touched by the patient's heart,/ the dwelling place of the living God./ This is spirituality in nursing,/ This is the ground of the practice of nursing, /This is holy ground" (O'Brien, 2003a, p. iv). In this poetic meditation, the nurse is reminded of the treasured place in which he or she stands as a nurse, the importance of the holy and caring environment in which nursing must be carried out. The work is reflective of the servant leadership theme of Staying Focused so critical to patient healing.

In the poem "Veronica: A Nurse's Meditation" are found the lines: "I wash the gentle, weathered face with a clean soft towel and I think of Veronica./ I am rewarded with the Blessed image of the human Son of God" (O'Brien, 2003b, p. 98). The nurse is reminded of the sacredness of the calling to serve the sick; that in caring for any ill or injured person, he or she is also caring for the Lord. The nurse who wipes the face of a homeless man, also wipes the face of Jesus, as Veronica did so many centuries ago. The nursing servant leadership theme demonstrated in this meditation is that of Becoming an Advocate.[‡]

In the poem "The Lord of the Nursing Home" are the lines: "You are there, O Lord of the nursing home,/ in the kindness and compassion of a geriatric nurse/ who caringly keeps watch at the bedside of a dying patient" (O'Brien, 2003a, p. 196). The importance of the nurse spending caring time with a patient is acknowledged. The fact is highlighted that the nurse represents the presence of the Lord in her commitment of time and energy, which are never lost. Taking time to be present to a suffering patient may be as meaningful a caring activity for the nurse as to the ill person. The work demonstrates the nursing servant leadership theme of Beyond the Ordinary routine care.

[‡]A more detailed account of Veronica's ministry is contained in Chapter 2, "The Spiritual Heritage of Servant Leadership in Nursing."

And in the meditation "The Nurse with an Alabaster Jar" we find: "To rend a nurse's alabaster jar;/ to pour out the costly ointment/ of caring/ of concern/ of tenderness./ Is that not what Jesus meant by his loving invitation:/ 'Come, follow me'"? (O'Brien, 2006, p. 6). Nurses are reminded that the extravagant giving of their caring, their concern, and their tenderness is a blessing not a waste; they should never be afraid of "breaking open" the alabaster jar of their hearts. "The Nurse with An Alabaster Jar" reflects the nursing servant leadership theme of making Discerning Decisions.

A PARABLE OF SERVANT LEADERSHIP IN NURSING

It was Christmas Eve at the small Midwest hospital and everyone — well, at least all of the nursing staff — anticipated a quiet evening. No elective surgeries had been admitted for the past few days, and all of the patients who were able to be discharged had been sent home for the holiday. The only patients left were a few seriously debilitated elders, like Catherine McNearny, scattered throughout a medical-surgical unit.

Catherine or "The delightful Miss M," as the nurses liked to call her, was 85 years old and a real joy to care for. Her hospitalization had begun almost 3 months earlier when she fell on her way to church one rainy fall morning. Catherine had made the pilgrimage to morning Mass at St. Cecilia's every day for almost 20 years, ever since retirement from her position as a local elementary school teacher. But on that fateful day, the wet, slippery leaves Catherine had always feared won out, and she ended up lying on the pavement with a badly fractured hip.

Catherine McNearny was a single lady but was interested and involved in everything and everyone around her. This was no sour spinster but a woman who loved and was loved, especially by the 3rd graders she had nurtured and taught for over 40 years.

After the initial surgery to repair her fractured hip, Catherine was the soul of patience and good humor. She never complained and always had a smile and a thank-you for even the smallest gesture of caring from the nursing staff. Her one dearest hope, however, was to return to her small house as soon as possible so she could welcome the neighbor children again for milk and cookies, as she had been doing for so many years.

Sadly, however, a rapid discharge was not to be. Catherine developed a nasty infection at her operative site, as well as a serious case of pneumonia and a variety of other age-related complications. She had no real family left but several faithful neighbors and a close friend did come to visit. As the holidays neared, however, her acquaintances became caught up in their family responsibilities and the visits dropped off. And to make matters worse, her dear friend, also a retired teacher, suffered a stroke and had to be admitted to a nursing home. And so, on this Christmas Eve, at St. Joseph's Hospital, in an almost deserted unit, Catherine McNearny was alone.

There were a number of brightly colored Christmas cards that the nurses had affixed to the wall above Miss M's bed and a small Christmas tree, delivered by the Gray Ladies hospital volunteer corps. But Catherine knew there would be no joyful midnight Mass for her at St. Cecilia's this year, a ritual she had treasured since childhood.

Anne O'Donnell, RN, MSN, AFNP, a 28-year-old nurse practitioner, was serving as the house supervisor at St. Joe's that Christmas Eve. As Anne made her nursing rounds, and there really wasn't much to "round" considering the dearth of patients in the house, she rejoiced at the thought of her own Christmas Eve plans. In just a few hours Anne would be "off duty" and on the road to her family home in a neighboring town. If there was not too much traffic she should be home in plenty of time to join her parents, three sisters, and two brothers for their parish midnight Mass. One of the best parts of Christmas Eve was looking forward to a great family party, hosted by her parents, after the service. Anne hadn't seen some of her siblings in months. She couldn't wait!

As Anne headed down the hall to the supervisor's office, she happened to notice that Miss M's call light was on. As she stepped into the room, Anne could see that Catherine was in pain even though she smiled brightly and thanked the nurse for responding to her light. After getting her patient some water and medication, Anne decided to visit for a while as she still had a little time before her shift ended.

The two began to reminisce about Christmases past and Catherine asked Anne how she would spend the rest of her Christmas Eve. Something in Catherine's slightly wistful tone made Anne hold back from sharing her joyful anticipation of the midnight service followed by a family party, Christmas cookies, and presents. Instead Anne asked Catherine if there was anything special she could do for her that Christmas Eve. Catherine replied kindly that she was fine; that one of her neighbors had brought in a small TV set so she could participate in a televised midnight Mass from her hospital room, and she was looking forward to that.

Without missing a beat, Anne admitted to Catherine that her family parish was in a neighboring town and added that she was not sure if she would be able to get there in time for Mass. She asked Catherine if she would like some company for the televised midnight service in her room. That way, Anne explained, together they could form a small hospital parish community, and it would be almost like being in church. And afterwards, Anne suggested, they could share a cup of Christmas punch, courtesy of the hospital kitchen.

Catherine's eyes filled with tears as she joyfully accepted. She would not be alone for Christmas Eve after all!

Nursing supervisor and nurse servant leader Anne O'Donnell would not have the joy of being with her beloved family that Christmas Eve. She would attend her own parish Mass in the morning. There is no doubt, however, that the reward she received, in giving up her own plans in order to befriend a lonely elder on that blessed night of the Lord's birth, brought gifts of happiness and fulfillment that her nurse's heart would treasure forever.

REFERENCES

About the Vietnam Women's Memorial project. (1995). *Nebraska Nurse, 28*(2), 1.

Blanchard, K., & Hodges, P. (2005). *Lead like Jesus: Lessons from the greatest leadership role model of all time.* Nashville, TN: Thomas Nelson.

Breckinridge, M. (1981). *Wide neighborhoods: A story of the Frontier Nursing Service.* Lexington, KY: University of Kentucky Press.

Donahue, M. P. (1996). *Nursing, the finest art: An illustrated history.* St. Louis, MO: Mosby.

Greenleaf, R. K. (1977). *Servant leadership: A journey into the nature of legitimate power & greatness.* Mahwah, NJ: Paulist Press.

Hain, R. (1954). Capping exercises. *The Catholic Nurse, 3*(1), 53–57.

Longfellow, H. W. (1857). Santa Filomena. *Atlantic Monthly, 1*(1), 23.

Maher, A. (1954). A nurse's night prayer. *The Catholic Nurse, 2*(4), 30–31.

Mary's nurse. (1929). *American Journal of Nursing, XXIX*(12), 1444–1445.

O'Brien, M. E. (2003a). *Parish nursing: Healthcare ministry within the church.* Sudbury, MA: Jones and Bartlett.

O'Brien, M. E. (2003b). *Prayer in nursing: The spirituality of compassionate caregiving.* Sudbury, MA: Jones and Bartlett.

O'Brien, M. E. (2004). *A nurse's handbook of spiritual care: Standing on holy ground.* Sudbury, MA: Jones and Bartlett.

O'Brien, M. E. (2006). *The nurse with an alabaster jar: A biblical approach to nursing.* Madison, WI: NCF Press.

O'Brien, M. E. (2008). *Spirituality in nursing: Standing on holy ground* (3rd ed.). Sudbury, MA: Jones and Bartlett.

Schank, M. J., Weis, D., & Matheus, R. (1996). Parish nursing: Ministry of healing; Parish nurses provide holistic nursing services to members of church congregations. *Geriatric Nursing, 17*(1), 11–13.

Shelly, J. A., & Miller, A. B. (2006). *Called to care: A Christian worldview for nursing.* Downer's Grove, IL: InterVarsity Press.

Stoll, R. I. (1997). Parish nurse ministry growing. *Pennsylvania Nurse, 52*(8), 18.

Van Manen, M. (1990). *Researching lived experience: Human science for an action sensitive pedagogy.* New York: State University of New York Press.

Widerquist, J., & Davidhizar, R. (1994). The ministry of nursing. *Journal of Advanced Nursing, 19*(4), 647–652.

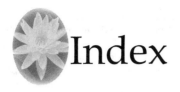

Index

DATE DUE
